CW00429578

# PRIMARY CARE
## —— FOR ——
# PHYSICIAN ASSOCIATES

Sofia Hiramatsu

*Physician Associate in General Practice*
*Matrix Education Founder and OSCE Course Tutor*

Muhammed Akunjee

Nazmul Akunjee

*MRCGP CSA Course GP Facilitators*
*GP Appraisers and GP Trainers*

Orders please contact: Sofia Hiramatsu

Email address: info@matrixeducation.co.uk

Website: www.matrixeducation.co.uk

*A British Library Cataloguing in Publication Data*
A catalogue record for this title is available from The British Library

ISBN 978-1-913713-36-2

First published by Compass-Publishing UK 2021

Copyright © 2021 Sofia Hiramatsu – Matrix Education

All rights reserved. This work is copyright. Permission is given for copies to be made of pages provided they are used exclusively within the institution for which this work has been purchased. For reproduction for any other purpose, permission must first be obtained in writing from The Matrix Education department.

Cover design © Lauria Idrisee

Typeset by The Book Refinery Ltd, www.thebookrefinery.com

Printed in the UK by CMP - Dorset

# Contents

## 8. EAR, NOSE AND THROAT — 277

## 9. OPHTHALMOLOGY — 319

## 10. FEMALE HEALTH — 335

## 11. MUSCULOSKELETAL       405

## 12. DERMATOLOGY       463

# Introduction

General practice (GP) throws up a mix of patients presenting with a whole range of confounding and complex symptoms. Once qualified as a physician associate (PA), if you choose to work in GP, you will be expected to deal with a variety of these patients.

The PA curriculum is wide ranging and covers the plethora of medical specialities that GP PAs need to have knowledge of. This book was written with the GP PA in mind. It includes over 120 common symptoms that patients present with and that may also come up in your national exams.

For each symptom, a comprehensive consultation framework has been included to guide you through the best approach for dealing with the presented complaint. This book has been specifically written to save you hours of time researching and it will hopefully become your companion to ease you through your exams and into your future as a fully fledged PA in primary care.

This book includes guidance such as what questions to ask, eliciting relevant past medical history, social history, etc. The framework then guides you on which examinations would be relevant and what investigations should be requested. Each topic will also advise you about the possible differential diagnoses and evidence -based ways of managing these.

We hope that you find this book to be a useful aid to help you excel in your exams and for you to continue to use well into your qualified PA years!

# About the Authors

## Ms Sofia Hiramatsu

Sofia Hiramatsu is a qualified PA and has been working in general practice since early 2018. She has worked as a PA lead for the Welbourne primary care network in Haringey, and undertaken locum and salaried work in primary care, from walk-in and urgent-care centres to a number of GP surgeries across London. She qualified in 2015 from Coventry University, with a BSc in Human Biosciences, followed by a PA Postgraduate Diploma from the University of Birmingham. Her special interests include dermatology, minor surgery and medical education. She has completed training in minor surgery, which is approved by the Royal College of General Practitioners (RCGP) and NHS England. In addition, she is the founder of Matrix Education, the first company providing products and services tailored to students and qualified PAs in the UK. This includes the development of the Matrix app that follows the PA curriculum, and the introduction of objective structured clinical examination (OSCE) courses in preparation for the PA nationals taught by registered PAs. In 2020, the company developed Matrix Appraisals, an online portfolio and appraisal toolkit made specifically for PAs.

## Dr Muhammed Akunjee

Muhammed Akunjee has been a GP principal in London since 2007. He has worked as the mental health lead for Haringey Clinical Commissioning Group (CCG) and spent five years as a CCG board member as well as a clinical director. He has undertaken consultancy work for primary-care procurement projects, both in the UK and the Middle East. He qualified from Guy's, King's and St Thomas's Medical School in 2002 and completed his Membership of the Royal College of General Practitioners (MRCGP) in 2006, gaining a distinction. Whilst at medical school, Dr Muhammed was awarded a number of prestigious awards, including the War Memorial Clinician Exhibition, a distinction in the Practice of Medicine (POM), the KCL Lightfoot Award, a British Medical and Dental Student bursary, the Rayne Institute Research Prize, and the Leukaemia Research Bursary. During his GP registrar year, he was also awarded first prize for the Roche / RCGP Registrar award which was for a paper on miscommunication between secondary and primary care. He is a GP appraiser for NHS England as well as a British Medical Association (BMA) book-award appraiser.

He completed a Postgraduate Certificate in Medical Education at the University of Dundee and a Certificate in Diabetes at Warwick University. He has also completed a

Postgraduate Certificate in Business Administration at Liverpool University. He has attended the London Deanery's Introduction to Teaching in Primary Care course, and has taught and examined clinical skills at Imperial College, London. He is an avid medical book writer and has had a number of articles published in peer-reviewed journals.

# Dr Nazmul Akunjee

Nazmul Akunjee completed his GP vocational training in 2011 and is currently a GP principal in a large North London practice. He has published a number of articles related to examination skills in peer-reviewed journals and has been appointed as a GP appraiser by NHS England (London). He is currently the clinical director of the GP Haringey Federation (federated4health) as well as the GP IT lead for Haringey CCG. He is now a GP trainer for Health Education North Central and East London. Nazmul Akunjee passed and excelled at his Clinical Skills Assessment (CSA) exam in February 2011, passing all 13 stations at the first attempt. Since then, he has been involved in one-to-one private CSA coaching as well as group tuition with GP registrars. He completed the London Deanery's Introduction to Teaching in Primary Care course in June 2011, and has taught and examined medical students at University College London Medical School.

# BMA Book Awards

Nazmul Akunjee and Muhammed Akunjee are both authors of *The Easy Guide to OSCEs* series published by Radcliffe. In 2008, their book *The Easy Guide to OSCEs for Final Year Medical Students* was commended in the BMA book awards. Their second publication, *The Easy Guide to OSCEs for Specialties,* was highly commended in the BMA book awards the following year in 2009. The work *Clinical Skills Explained* was highly commended at the BMA book awards in 2013.

# 1

# Challenging Consultations

## Complaints

The number of complaints is rising in the consumer-driven society that we live in. Patients' demands are increasing, and they are expecting higher standards of care than ever before. When their expectation is not met by the service provided, a complaint is likely to be generated. People incorrectly assume that most complaints are around neglect, poor care or clinical negligence. However, research shows that most complaints centre around poor communication between patient and clinician, or attitude.

The key to responding to a complaint is to allow the patient to vocalise and vent their concerns, and then to respond to them according to local policies and protocols. Most situations can be diffused by apologising and explaining to the patient what steps you will take to ensure that similar mistakes will not happen again.

» Cues – Pick up on any cues that the patient is getting angry, such as changes in body posture (moving to standing from being seated), raising their voice, clenching their fists or becoming fidgety.
*'I can see that you are unhappy; please do tell me about it so I can help you.'*

» Avoid – Do not be defensive or deny responsibility. It is important not to blame anyone without establishing all the facts. Do not be evasive when the patient asks you any questions, as this may appear as if you are trying to cover their problem.

### Establishing Events

» Establish reason – Try to establish why the patient wants to complain. Ask what happened and what went wrong.
*'Tell me exactly what happened.'*

» Listen – Allow the patient time and space to express their story. Be empathetic.
*'Thank you for telling me.'*

» Acknowledge – Recognise why the patient is unhappy and acknowledge their response. Show appreciation to the patient for raising the complaint.
*'I am grateful that you have brought this to my attention.'*

» Apologise – Apologise even if you feel the complaint was not warranted; this should be offered as early as possible.

*'I am sorry that happened.'*

## RED FLAGS

If the patient is not responding to your efforts, is getting abusive or threatens violence, then you should explain to them that you are feeling uncomfortable and may terminate the consultation if they continue to behave that way.

Patients may wish to lodge a complaint for a wide number of reasons. It is important to be confident when dealing with a patient who wishes to complain, and to be able to advise them clearly regarding what will happen next. Many clinicians simply advise the patient to go to the practice manager to make a complaint, having spent the last five minutes explaining their complaint to you. This will invariably irk the patient and possibly may make them feel even more frustrated. A better course of action would be to inform the patient about the procedure and tell them that you will record the complaint and escalate it to the practice manager on their behalf.

## Management

✓ Offer reason – Provide an honest explanation summarising the series of events. If a mistake happened, then inform the patient how and why it occurred. If there are some mitigating circumstances surrounding the mishap, then these can be stated without justifying the mistake.

✓ Explanation – Explain to the patient the practice's complaints procedure. Do not simply tell the patient to speak to the practice manager. Offer to ensure that the patient's complaint is seen through, and offer to take personal responsibility if appropriate.

**Complaints procedure – Explain the complaints procedure and protocol to the patient:**

› All complaints should be dated.

› Verbal complaints should be recorded in writing.

› All complaints should be acknowledged in writing within 48 hours of receipt.

› A full investigation will take place within 10 working days.

› A practice meeting may be organised to establish all facts; a patient can attend if they so wish.

› A written response will be given within two weeks.

✓ Prevention – State what immediate measures you have taken to rectify things and minimise the risk of recurrence.

*'We can try to prevent this from happening again by...'*

These actions include significant event analysis, practice protocol, education event/retraining for the clinician, or adding alerts to notes.

✓ Escalation – If the patient is still unhappy, then you should advise them how to escalate the issue. If the local complaints resolution fails, the patient may be directed to the local Clinical Commissioning Group (CCG) complaints officer, NHS England or to the Care Quality Commission (CQC) directly. Alternatively, the patient may refer their complaint to an independent review panel of the NHS Complaints Independent Complaints Advocacy Service (ICAS) or the Patient Ombudsman. Patients may be guided to Patient Advice and Liaison Service (PALS) or ICAS at any time.

✓ Follow-up – Offer the patient a convenient follow-up appointment if relevant. If a complaint is being made, explain when the patient should expect to get a response.

---

## References

Care Quality Commission (2018). *Regulation 16: Receiving and acting on complaints.* https://www.cqc.org.uk/guidance-providers/regulations-enforcement/regulation-16-receiving-acting-complaints

# Breaking Bad News

Breaking bad news is an important skill that physician associates (PAs) must be able to do well, especially for the national objective structured clinical examinations (OSCE). It is a difficult skill to master, particularly if one has not been trained to do it proficiently or one has not been exposed to doing it on a regular basis (oncology or palliative care). With patients having longer life expectancies, they are more likely to suffer from cancers or chronic illnesses than before.

Bad news is any news that may seriously or adversely affect the patient's well-being and their view about their future. Invariably, it is not about telling a patient their death is imminent, but more commonly may be communicating diagnoses of cancer, HIV, dementia, blindness, or that a couple are infertile and cannot have children. If delivered incorrectly, it may increase anxiety in patients, cause them to misunderstand the prognosis, and lead to increased complaints and patient dissatisfaction.

Adopt an open posture that is calm and inviting. Use the speed and tone of your voice to relax the patient and help soothe them. Ensure that you read the patient's notes fully before they enter the room, to see if there is any documentation that may indicate there might be some difficult news to break (abnormal blood tests, scan, smear results or a letter from the hospital). Consider possible differentials based on the results, and determine what the next steps will be necessary.

» Cues – Pick up on any cues that the patient is expecting some news. Try to establish why they have attended today and what they were expecting.

## TIPS

Do not avoid breaking the news. You should try to inform the patient about what the results mean and not hide any information. It is best to be honest and open. Try to use non-medical jargon as much as possible. If you have to resort to medical terms, then explain what they mean in layman's terms.

## SPIKES – Six Step Protocol for Delivering Bad News

Consider using the **SPIKES** protocol to deliver the news to the patient:

» **S**etting up – Check the notes and rehearse how you want to break the news. Ensure privacy and sit close to the patient. Ensure you are not rushed or interrupted (e.g. by calls or bleeps).

» **P**erception – Check what the patient knows so far and what their understanding is.

» **P**atient's **I**nvitation – Find out how much the patient wants to know.

» Giving **K**nowledge – Fire a warning shot. Give medical facts and avoid jargon.

» Address emotions and show **E**mpathy – Respond to their emotions.

» **S**trategy and summary – Explain the different options available.

## Setting the Scene

» Establish the problem – Ask questions to determine what the problem is.
*'Thanks for coming in today. As we have not met before, may I just ask you a few questions before we speak about the test results today?'*

» Summarise – Summarise what information you have to hand from previous consultations and check with the patient if anything has changed in the meantime. If there has been a change, find out more about what has happened.

» Understanding – Ask questions to determine the patient's understanding.
*'What have you already been told about what is going on?'*

» Concerns – Ask questions to determine whether the patient has any concerns.
*'With your symptoms going on for such a long time, have you considered what may be causing it? Do you have any particular concerns you would like to raise with me today?'*

» Information delivery – Ask questions to determine how the patient would like the information to be delivered.
*'How would you like me to give the information about the test results? Would you like to know everything about them? Or just the main points?'*

## Breaking the News

Ensure that when you break the bad news. you do not do it all in one go, but rather perform it in stages and fire a warning shot first, suggesting that some unpleasant news may follow.

➤ Warning shot

› Ask the patient whether they came alone or attended with someone, and whether they want anyone else present during the consultation today.

*'I'm afraid I have some difficult news to tell you. The results are a little more serious than we had hoped.'*

➤ News

› Provide an honest and clear explanation of what the results show.

*'The results show changes in your scan. Although this may be caused by infection or inflammation, sadly, at this stage, we cannot exclude cancer as a possible cause.'*

## Response

» Having broken the news, *pause* and *await* the patient's response:

> › Crying – Say something like, '*I am really sorry that I have to give you this news. I can see that it has really affected you; this is completely normal.*' Offer tissues.

> › Anger – Say something like, '*You seem quite upset at the moment. That is perfectly understandable. However, I want you to know that I am here to help.*'

> › Silence – Say something like, '*I know this was totally unexpected. Do you want me to carry on? I can understand that it is a lot to take in, so please take your time and tell me when you are ready to carry on.*'

Don't forget to ask about their social history:

» Domestic situation – Ask something like, '*Who lives with you at home?*'

» Support network – Ask something like, '*Have you spoken to anyone about this, such as your friends or family?*'

» Occupation – Ask something like, '*Are you currently working or studying?*'

## NATIONAL EXAM TIPS

In general practice, there is often little opportunity to inform patients that they definitely have cancer, as biopsies are rarely taken. Patients who have had biopsies are likely to be already under secondary care and would usually have been pre-warned about the possible malignant nature of their lesion. In primary care, you will more likely have to explain to a patient something like an abnormal smear or a scan that shows something more serious. In such cases, it is important to inform the patient about the possible sinister pathology, but also to convey to them that the alternative benign diagnoses have not been excluded.

## Management

✓ Referral – If you suspect cancer, consider referring the patient to specialist services via the two-week wait (2WW) pathway if you have not already done so. Explain why you need to refer them and what the hospital may do in terms of treatments and investigations.

✓ Investigations – If relevant, consider referring the patient for further investigations to help confirm or exclude differential diagnoses.

✓ Treatment – Consider explaining what some of the possible treatment options will be; e.g. radiotherapy, chemotherapy, surgery or palliative care.

✓    Prognosis – Be honest if you know the seriousness of the condition.

✓    Give reassurance if applicable – For example, say something like, *'Thankfully, you have been diagnosed very early on and the lesion is small. We have excellent treatments that can control the cells and prevent them from causing any permanent harm.'*

## Safety Netting

»    Support – If the patient does not have any family or local friends, consider referring them to a counsellor, bereavement service or patient-support group, as appropriate.

»    Exit – Offer to call in the receptionist or nurse to take the patient to a quiet room where they can sit and have a cup of tea until they are composed enough to go home. If the patient is due to go home alone, ask if they would like to contact a friend or family member to pick them up.

»    Follow-up – Offer the patient an early follow-up to address any new questions or concerns the patient may have following the news. Allow them telephone access or emergency consultations during this difficult early period.

---

### References

Medical Defence Union (2019). *Breaking bad news.* https://www.themdu.com/guidance-and-advice/guides/breaking-bad-news

# Angry Patients

Occasionally, a patient's display of anger may be directed towards health professionals, particularly when their own illnesses and sense of well-being is affected. Patients may get angry for a variety of reasons, such as receiving bad news or having to wait for a long time. However, their anger may also be a sign of mental illness, personality disorder or substance abuse. The key to responding to an angry patient is to remain calm and not to face anger with anger. Most situations can be easily diffused by apologising and giving the patient time to explain their predicament.

> » Safety – Ensure that the consultation is conducted in a safe, open place. If not, make sure that your colleagues know where you are. Try to be seated close to an exit for a quick escape in the event that the patient becomes physically violent.

> » Cues – Pick up any cues that the patient is getting angry, such as changes in body posture (moving to standing from seated), raising their voice, clenching their fists or becoming fidgety.
> *'I can see that you are unhappy; please do tell me about it so I can help you.'*

> » Avoid – Do not be defensive or deny responsibility. It is important not to blame anyone without establishing all the facts. Do not be evasive when the patient asks you any questions, as this may appear as if you are trying to cover up their problem.

## Establishing Events

> » Try to establish why the patient is in the state they are in. Ask what has caused them to become angry and why.
> *'Tell me exactly what happened.'*

> » Allow the patient time and space to express their story. Be empathetic.
> *'Thank you for telling me. I know it must have been difficult to do so.'*

> » Recognise why the patient is angry and acknowledge their response if it is reasonable. Show appreciation to the patient for raising the complaint, especially if it is of a serious nature.
> *'I can see why that made you upset... I can imagine that it must have been quite difficult for you.'*

> » Apologise even if you feel the complaint was not warranted; this should be offered as early as possible.
> *'I am sorry for the experience you have had.'*

## RED FLAGS

If the patient is not responding to your efforts, is getting increasingly more abusive or threatens violence, then you should explain to them that you are feeling uncomfortable and may terminate the consultation if they continue their behaviour.

## Management

✓ Offer reason – Provide an honest explanation summarising the series of events. If a mistake has happened, then inform the patient as to how and why it occurred. If there are some mitigating circumstances surrounding the mishap, then these can be stated without justifying the mistake.

✓ Prevention – State what immediate measures you have taken to rectify things and minimise the distress; e.g. preventing the mistake from happening again. We can try to prevent this from happening again using a significant event analysis (SEA), practice audit, practice protocol, education event / retraining for the clinician, and/or adding alerts to notes.

✓ Complaints – If they are still angry, explain the practice's complaints procedure. Do not simply tell the patient to speak to the practice manager. Offer to ensure that their complaint is seen through and offer to take personal responsibility if appropriate.

*'If you still feel upset about it, I am happy to run through the complaints procedure with you.'*

## Safety Netting

» Offer the patient a convenient follow-up appointment if relevant. If a complaint is being made, explain when the patient will expect to get a response.

# Domestic Violence

Domestic violence refers to abuse or violence that takes place between adults within the home. Although the word 'violence' conjures up thoughts of physicality, the definition of domestic violence also encompasses verbal abuse, intimidation, sexual assault and even rape. Sadly, domestic violence is a common phenomenon that affects one in four women, with two women a week being killed by their current or former partners. However, it is important to acknowledge that over 40% of domestic violence victims are male, and they may not be forthcoming due to shame or embarrassment.

## The Definition of Domestic Violence

> ➤ Domestic violence has been defined by the Department of Health (DoH) to refer to *'Any incident of threatening behaviour, violence or abuse (psychological, physical, sexual, financial or emotional) between adults who are, or have been intimate partners or family members, regardless of gender or sexuality.'*

### *History*

Approach the topic sensitively in a non-threatening, non-judgmental manner. It can be quite difficult to broach the subject initially, so begin by designing your first few questions to put the patient at ease. Avoid focusing only on injuries without addressing the underlying cause.

» Open questions

> › Ask some general questions about the relationship.

> *'You look upset? Is everything alright at home? Is your partner taking care of you? Do you get on well with your partner?'*

> › Confidentiality – Reaffirm and emphasise that everything discussed is confidential.

> › Pick up any cues such as multiple minor injuries, fractures, multiple Accident and Emergency (A&E) or walk-in-centre (WIC) attendances.

> *'I have noticed that you have a number of bruises/cuts/burns; is everything alright?'*

» Leading questions

> › Ask more direct and leading questions to enquire about possible injuries.

> *'How does your partner treat you? Are you having any problems?'*

> *'Do you ever feel frightened by your partner?'*

> *'Do you feel safe at home?'*

> › Ask them about their partner.

> *'Has your partner ever physically hurt or threatened you?'*

*'Has your partner ever broken or destroyed things that were personal to you?'*

*'Has your partner ever prevented you from doing things that you wanted to do, such as leaving the house or going to see friends?'*

*'Does your partner have any criminal convictions?'*

› Listen – Allow the patient time and space to express their story. Be empathetic.

*'Thank you for telling me. I know it must have been difficult to do so.'*

*'It's not your fault... You are not to blame...'*

› Enquire whether the violence has increased in frequency and severity.

› Ask about alcohol – Ask if the abuser is intoxicated at the time of the abuse.

» Use the mnemonic HARK for questions to ask regarding domestic violence

**Have you ever been...**

› **H**umiliated (emotionally and verbally abused, including put-downs)

› **A**fraid of

› **R**aped (made to have non-consensual sex)

› **K**icked (physically assaulted)

**... by your partner?**

» Ask about past history, including obstetrics (*'Have you had any terminations or miscarriages?'*) and mental health (*'Do you have low mood or anxiety?'*).

» Ask about social history

› *'Who lives with you at home?'*

› Support networks – *'Have you spoken to anyone about this, such as your friends or the police?'*

› *'Are you working or studying at the moment?'*

› *'Do you drink any alcohol, and if so, how often?'*

› *'Do you take any recreational drugs?'*

## RED FLAGS

» Self harm – *'Have you ever felt so low that you wanted to end it all? Have you ever tried to take your own life?'*

» Children – Determine if there are any children in the home and establish if they are at risk. *'Has your partner ever threatened or abused your children?'*

» Partner – Ask if their partner ever sexually abused or raped them. *'Has your partner ever forced themselves on you, even when you did not want to have sexual intercourse?'*

## Subtle Clues to Domestic Violence

Domestic violence is still considered a taboo subject, with women experiencing around 35 episodes of domestic violence (on average) before seeking help. Patients delay presentation for a number of reasons, the most common of which include feeling shame or embarrassment, worrying about reprisals from partners, or fearing that their children will be taken away.

Patients may present with subtle signs and symptoms that may be a clue that domestic violence is taking place. It is important to be aware of these symptoms, which include delayed presentation, multiple injuries (to the abdomen, face and hands), fractures, unexplained bruising, burns, injuries at different stages of healing, a history of LOC and miscarriages.

## NATIONAL EXAM TIPS

Domestic violence is extremely common and is not committed solely by men against women. It is important to broach the subject in an empathetic way, as many partners may find it difficult to talk about the subject for fear of retribution. The patient's records may give an indication that they are undergoing domestic violence, such as unexplained falls or injuries in an otherwise fit and well patient. However, when opening the subject, remember that the patient is an adult and cannot be forced into making a disclosure or taking further action. Always ask whether there are children at home, and consider making a referral to the local child protection services if you are concerned that they are at risk of abuse or neglect.

## Management

✓    Illegal – Stress to the patient that domestic violence is illegal, unacceptable and should not be tolerated. Offer to contact the police if the patient consents. Respect their autonomy if they do not wish to do so.

✓    Children's safety – If children are involved, seek advice from your child protection lead. The child may require transfer to a safe location if they are at risk.

✓    Visa applicants – Reassure the patient that the government supports victims of domestic violence in their immigration applications.

### Safety Plan

»    Escape route – Plan an escape route (stairs, doors and windows) in case you need to leave quickly.

»    Escape bag – Pack an emergency bag that contains money, phone, keys and important documents (e.g. passport). This can be left at a friend's house.

»    Numbers – Have a range of emergency numbers (e.g. friends, 999 and a refuge that you can call).

» Neighbour – Advise a neighbour to contact the police if they hear shouting or suspicious noises.

» Safe house – Have a safe house (with a friend, with family or a refuge) that you can reside at in an emergency.

» Services – Contact the National Domestic Violence Helpline; local services such as women's aid groups, refuges, Relate, the local police domestic violence safety unit and the local housing association.

» Follow-up – Offer open same-day emergency appointments, taking into account that the patient may not be able to attend a routine appointment due to circumstances. Add an alert to their notes not to inform the family (confidentiality), highlighting that the patient is at risk of domestic violence.

## Government immigration policy with respect to domestic violence

» Domestic violence victims can apply for indefinite leave to remain in the country in their own right if they have been victims of domestic violence during the first two years of that relationship.

## Principles of approaching domestic violence

» Support, empathise and listen to the patient, appreciating their capacity to act whilst respecting their autonomy. *'Whatever you decide, we are here to support you.'*

» Document any injuries and take photographs if appropriate.

» If there are children involved, then a referral to child protection services may be necessary. Inform child protection services of the referral and the need to breach confidentiality before doing so.

---

### References

Royal College of General Practitioners (2014). *Responding to domestic abuse: Guidance for general practices.* https://safelives.org.uk/sites/default/files/resources/SafeLives%27%20GP%20guidance.pdf

# Child Protection

Child protection is the process and system by which children are identified as being sufferers of, or at risk of, harm as a result of abuse or neglect.

## Types of Child Maltreatment (According to the DoH)

| | |
|---|---|
| Physical abuse | May involve hitting, kicking, poisoning, burning or any method that causes child harm. Also failing to prevent harm befalling a child. |
| Emotional abuse | This is the persistent emotional mistreatment of a child that results in the stunting of the child's emotional development. It may involve swearing, shouting, or making them feel worthless or unloved. |
| Sexual abuse | This is forcing a child to take part in sexual activities that they do not understand the meaning of. This may include penetrative (anal or vaginal) or non-penetrative (kissing, fondling, etc.) acts. |
| Neglect | This is the failure to cater to a child's basic physical and psychological needs, leading to, impairment of the child's development. It may include failure to provide adequate food, clothing or shelter, or failure to ensure appropriate medical treatment. |
| Fabricated illness | NICE also includes induced illness or the fabrication of a child's illness by the carer of the child. |
| Other forms of abuse | The NSPCC recognises other forms of child abuse, including female genital mutilation (FGM), grooming / sexual exploitation, child trafficking, online abuse, cyberbullying and bullying. |

As professionals, we are often at the forefront when dealing with patients and their children, and it is of exceptional importance that we are to pick up the tell-tale signs of abuse or neglect early, to help safeguard and prevent the suffering of children and young people.

## *History*

» Open questions

> Ask questions about the child's / young person's home life.

*'You look upset? Is everything alright at home? Are your parents or carers taking care of you? Do you get on well with your family?'*

> Reaffirm and emphasise that everything discussed is confidential as long as there is no risk to the child or others.

> › If the child is <16 years and attends alone, check if there is anyone with parental responsibility who can attend with them. Do not request this if the alleged abuse is being perpetrated by the person in question.
>
> *'Have you spoken to your parents about it? Is there a reason why you have not?'*

> › Pick up any cues, such as multiple minor injuries, fractures, multiple A&E attendances, poor growth and dentition, change in emotional state or under-aged sexual activity.
>
> *'I noticed that you have been in and out of hospital a few times with bruises/cuts/burns; is everything at home alright?'*

» Associated history

> › Ask how their mood is and whether they are feeling low or down.
> › Ask how their sleep is and whether they have any recurrent nightmares.
> › Ask about their self-esteem.
> › Ask if they are experiencing any anger.
> › Ask if they have self-harmed or had any thoughts of suicide.
> › Ask if they have any pain when passing urine.

» Past history

> › Ask about issues with orthopaedics (If they have broken any bones, and if so, how this happened).
> › Ask how their mental health is.
> › Ask if they have a learning disability.

» Social history

> › Ask how things are at school, and how is their attendance is.
> › Ask if any social worker is involved or if they have any siblings on the child protection register.
> › Ask if they have any support from anyone (friends, police, school teachers, etc.).
> › Ask if they drink any alcohol, smoke or take recreational drugs.

## Risk Factors for Child Abuse

➤ Environmental – A history of child abuse in the family, or poverty/financial stresses.

➤ Parental – Domestic violence, mental health issues (depression, anxiety, etc.), substance/alcohol abuse or learning difficulties.

➤ Child factors – Physical and mental disabilities, or previously living in care

➤ Leading questions – Ask more direct and leading questions to enquire about possible child abuse

› General – *'Do you feel safe at home? How does your carer/parents treat you? Are you having any problems? Do you ever feel frightened by them? Have they ever hurt you in any way?'*

› Physical – *'Have you ever been hurt by your parents? Have you ever been kicked or punched, or burnt by hot water or cigarettes?'*

› Emotional – *'Is there any shouting? What do they say and how often? How did it make you feel?'*

› Neglect – *'Are you eating and drinking okay? Do you feel hungry? How often do you bathe or change clothes? Who takes care of you when you are sick? Do you have all of your immunisations?'*

› Sexual – *'Have you ever had sex? Who with? Where you pressurised? Have you ever been pregnant? Have you had any itching down below? Have you had any discharge?'*

› Grooming – *'Have you ever had sex with someone older than you? Did they put you under any pressure? Have they bought you any expensive gifts? Where any alcohol or drugs involved? Do they ask you to have sex with their friends?'*

› FGM – Sometimes women are 'cut' down below; *'Has this happened to you when you when you were younger? Has anyone else in the family had this done?'*

## Investigations

» Urine – Pregnancy test if applicable.

## Examination

» Vitals – Blood pressure (BP), height, weight and body mass index (BMI).

» Carer – Observe the interaction between the child and their carer or parent. Is there decreased attachment between the two? Does the carer appear coercive or controlling of the child?

» Physical

› Check for signs of bruising, particularly for clusters, and whether they are a similar shape or size. Are they away from the non-bony parts of the body? Are they on the eyes, ears, cheeks or buttocks?

› Look for any bites, scald marks, or circular cigarette marks.

› Look for any injury to the oral cavity, such as the gums or tongue, or a torn frenulum.

» Neglect – Look at their general appearance. Check whether they are wearing appropriate clothes, and if they are well-kempt and clean. Determine how their are.

» Emotional – Asses whether the child looks fearful or withdrawn.

## BASHH guidelines (2011)

The British Association for Sexual Health and HIV (BASHH) guidelines recommend that you should not perform an intimate examination unless there is an urgent health need to do so. An intimate forensic examination should only be performed by a health professional specifically trained in forensics for sexual assault. This is to avoid evidence being lost or contaminated, and avoids repeating a potentially distressing examination.

## Management

✓ Record clearly all allegations and the examination's findings. Use a body map if there are multiple injuries.

✓ Stress to the patient that any form of child abuse is illegal and should not be tolerated. Their safety is paramount.

✓ Explain that you will have to inform other agencies, as the child or other children are at risk of harm. Try to obtain their consent, but do not let this impede you from making a referral if it is not obtained. Agencies will only be informed on a need-to-know basis.

✓ Health visitors can perform home visits for those under five years old to assess the home circumstances discreetly, where an impromptu GP home visit would not be appropriate. Equally, if they have a social worker, they could visit the home and assess the situation.

*More information*

✓ Surgery lead – If you are unsure what do, or need any advice, discuss with the surgery's child protection lead (usually a senior GP partner).

✓ CCG lead – If they are unavailable, you could contact the local CCG's child protection / safeguarding lead or the named GP for safeguarding children.

## Referral

→ First response team – If you suspect child abuse, but the child is not at risk, discuss this with the child protection agency and make a referral to them to investigate further.

*Emergency*

→ Social worker – Contact the on-call social worker or the National Society for the Prevention of Cruelty to Children (NSPCC) to discuss the case.

→ If you think the child is at high risk now or is a victim of rape, contact the police immediately. The child can be kept in a place of safety for 72 hours.

→ Sexual abuse – In the case of rape or sexual abuse, it is best not to examine the patient. You should refer them to a local sexual assault referral centre (SARC), who would do the examination within 72 hours.

## References

National Institute for Health and Care Excellence (2017). *Child abuse and neglect.* https://www.nice.org.uk/guidance/ng76

# Telephone Consultations

Teleconsulting allows patients better access to medical care, and the consultation is shorter on average, allowing for more patients to be assessed. Although such consultations may be a great advantage for patients, as they are more convenient, timely and quicker than face-to-face consultations, the clinician conducting them must be aware of the key skills and communication skills necessary to ensure that they remain safe, and that they provide an efficient and high-quality service for patients. In the absence of examining the patient, safety netting is paramount to a successful telephone consultation.

## Pitfalls of Telephone Consultations

» Communication – You rely entirely on verbal communication as opposed to non-verbal. Patient cues, body language and facial expression are lost.

» Clinician centred – Consultations tend to be more clinician-centred and less-psychosocial lines of questioning are usually employed.

» Shorter – Consultations tend to be shorter, and include less patient education as well as rapport building is undertaken.

» Misinformation – Occasionally, a clinician may miss out key areas of enquiry such as allergies. You may underestimate symptom severity and tend to think patients are healthier than they truly are.

» Signs – It is impossible to perform a physical examination, so valuable clinical signs may be missed when making an assessment.

## Principles

» Communication;

› Ensure that you use your verbal communication skills to gather as much history as possible. Use active-listening skills to obtain information. Try to clarify and repeat back to the patient what they have said to ensure there is no miscommunication. Make sure that you talk slowly and clearly to aid understanding.

› Cues – Listen out for verbal cues, such as changes in tone of voice and pace, and pauses that may indicate fear, anxiety, pain or depression.

› Active listening – Allow the patient to speak without interruption for as long as they require.

› Repetition – Consider advising the caller to repeat back to you any medical advice (treatments, red flags, etc.) you have given, to check their understanding.

» Telephone-callback request – Establish why the telephone=callback request was made to your staff and what the main issue of concern is.

» Read the medical records and candidate brief thoroughly. Check if there is anything there to give a clue as to what the telephone consultation may be about (e.g. an anxious patient).

## History

» Introduce yourself – Clearly state your name and designation.

» Establish caller – Obtain the patient's name and telephone number (in case the line is cut off). Enquire whether they are ringing about themselves or about another person. If it is the latter, ask if they have consent.

» Rapport – Greet the patient and ask them how you can help.

» Focused history

> Establish in chronological order how their symptoms have developed.

> Ask about the onset, when they were last well, what were the triggers, if they've had any similar episodes and if they have had any contact with anyone with similar symptoms.

» Past history – Ask if they have any previous medical conditions.

» Drug history – Ask if they are taking any medications or have any allergies.

» Family history – Ask if there is any history of such conditions in the family.

» Social history – Ask about their relationships, how things are at home, what their occupation is, and whether they smoke or drink alcohol.

## Investigations

» Request the patient attends the surgery to pick up any relevant investigation forms. Consider sending a community phlebotomist to undertake any requested blood tests if the patient is housebound.

## Examination

» Request the patient attends the surgery if you need to examine them, or consider visiting them at home. Consider using available community nursing services to check height, weight, urine and BP.

## RED FLAGS

As appropriate for the presented complaint, with a lower threshold for children.

Be careful when taking a call where a patient is demanding results for a partner or relative. It is paramount that you confirm who you are talking to and gain explicit consent from the patient to discuss the case with any other parties. In the case of children, it is also important to ensure you are speaking with the carer who has the parenting responsibilities.

## Management

✓ Explain the condition using the patient's own description and terms, as relevant. Ensure you break the information into small chunks, and repeat them to ensure clarity and to reduce the chance of miscommunication.

✓ Treat the condition as necessary. Consider lifestyle changes, self-management and medical options.

✓ If the patient requires a referral, consider whether this can be done without having to see or examine the patient.

✓ If at any point you are unhappy with the consultation, request that the patient attends the surgery. If they are unable to do so, consider whether a home visit is appropriate.

✓ Signpost the patient to alternative methods of treatment, such as self-care, buying over-the-counter (OTC) medications from a pharmacy, or attending urgent care centre (UCC) / WIC /A&E, depending on the severity of and appropriateness to their ailments.

## Safety Netting

» Do not forget red flags – Explain the natural course of the disease to the patient. Also clearly explain the red-flag signs and symptoms for which they should seek urgent medical help via another callback, 111 or by attending the surgery/A&E.

» Offer the patient a convenient follow-up appointment if relevant. Consider bringing the patient back to check if things have improved.

» Thank the patient and check if they are happy with the advice.

---

*References*

van Galen, L.S. and Car, J. (2018). Telephone consultations. *The BMJ,* March 2018. doi: https://doi.org/10.1136/bmj.k1047

# 2

# Cardiovascular

## Chest Pain

Chest pain is a common presentation in primary care. It may arise from a variety of pathological causes, ranging from musculoskeletal (MSK) to an acute coronary event. It is important to take a thorough history and conduct an examination to arrive at a diagnosis. Patients with cardiac-sounding chest pain should be risk stratified for their cardiovascular risk factors. Take into consideration the patient's age, gender and lifestyle when considering potential differentials. No cause is identified in around 16% of patients presenting with chest pain in primary care.

### Risk Factors for Ischaemic Heart Disease (IHD)

➤ Diabetes Mellitus (DM)

➤ Smoking

➤ Hypertension (HTN)

➤ High cholesterol

➤ Family history of IHD

➤ Previous stroke / transient ischaemic attack (TIA)

➤ Peripheral vascular disease (PVD)

➤ Gout

### *History*

» Focused questions

› Site/onset – Ask where the pain is, when they first noticed it and how long it lasts for.

› Character – Ask them to describe the character (sharp, dull, a burning feeling or pressure).

› Radiation – Ask if there is movement of the pain to their arms, jaw or back.

› Triggers – Ask if anything makes it worse or better.

> › Severity – Ask what the severity is on a scale of one to ten.

» Associated history – Ask if they have any shortness of breath (SOB), sudden onset or a cough.

» Past history – Ask if they have had any similar symptoms in the past, a myocardial infarction (MI), HTN, cholesterol or DM. Ask if they have had any previous investigations, an electrocardiogram (ECG), an echocardiogram (echo), an angiogram, or any history of pulmonary embolism (PE) or deep vein thrombosis (DVT).

» Drug history – Ask if they have taken nonsteroidal anti-inflammatory drugs (NSAIDs), steroids, bisphosphonates, nitrates, gastro-oesophageal reflux disease (GORD) medication, oral contraceptive pill (OCP) or hormone replacement therapy (HRT) (additional risk of PE).

» Social history – Determine their occupation, whether they smoke, their alcohol intake is, if they take recreational drugs and if they drive.

» Family history – Ask if there is any family history of IHD or PE.

## RED FLAGS

Haemoptysis, SOB or severe crushing pain at rest. Angina pain that has become acutely more severe or increased in frequency. Reduced walking distance.

## Differential Diagnosis

| | |
|---|---|
| Angina | Cardiac pain (radiating to left arm/jaw). Worse on exercising, after a heavy meal or triggered by cold weather. Relieved by glyceryl trinitrate (GTN) and rest. Check for a worsening of symptoms (change in character or decreasing walking distance). On examination (OE): nil may be found. |
| ACS / unstable angina | Central, crushing cardiac pain (those with DM and the elderly may have no chest pain). Pain at rest, associated with nausea, vomiting, sweating and SOB. May or may not be relieved by GTN spray. OE: patient may be short of breath, sweaty and tachycardic. |
| GORD | A burning sensation over the epigastrium, moving up to the neck. Worsened by lying down or bending over. Acid brash and water brash may be present. Can cause painful swallowing or nocturnal asthma. Relieved by antacids, but related to consuming spicy food, alcohol or hot caffeinated drinks. OE: epigastric pain. |

| MSK | Sharp pain at a specific point. No radiation of pain. Reproducible on palpation and from passive movements. History of colds, coughing or excessive physical activity may be elicited. OE: focal chest tenderness that is worse on movement. |
|---|---|
| PE | Sudden SOB with pleuritic chest pain. May also have haemoptysis and tachycardia. Risk factors: DVT, travel, trauma, OCP and malignancy. OE: tachypnea with calf tenderness. |
| Pericarditis | Sharp, stabbing, retrosternal chest pain (which can radiate to the jaw, the back or the left side of the chest). Pain made worse on deep inspiration (pleuritic) and lying flat, on left side, or on inspiration. Relieved by sitting forwards. OE: pericardial friction rub noted. |
| Aortic dissection | Sudden, severe, retrosternal chest pain that is tearing in character. Radiates to the back. OE: unequal pulses and BPs in both arms. |
| Pneumothorax | Sudden onset of pleuritic chest pain with SOB. Can occur with existing lung disease. OE: reduced breath sounds, increased resonance and a percussion note over the affected area. |
| Herpes zoster (shingles) | Sharp, burning pain preceded by a rash (several days earlier). OE: the rash often has grouped vesicles with a red base, and with a unilateral dermatomal distribution, often affecting the lower thoracic region. |
| Psychogenic | Non-specific recurrent chest pain or tightness, with palpitations. Pain may be described as like an electric shock or jolt. History of low mood, feeling sad or down, and experiencing anxiety. OE: poor eye contact and low affect. |
| Pneumonia | Pleuritic chest pain associated with a fever, productive cough and dyspnoea. OE: coarse crackles with a dull percussion note and fever. |
| Pancreatitis | Acute onset of boring epigastric pain, associated with nausea and vomiting. Relieved on sitting up or leaning forwards, but worse on lying flat. Comes in waves. Risk factors: gallstones, excess alcohol, and raised calcium and triglyceride levels. |

## Examination

»   Vitals – BP (both arms – aortic dissection), pulse (irregular atrial fibrillation [AF]), temperature and respiratory rate.

»   Cardiovascular – Listen for heart sounds, check for reproducible chest-wall tenderness (MSK). Palpate legs for DVT, and check ankles for oedema.

» Respiratory – Listen to the chest (reduced air entry and dullness to percussion for pneumothorax; pleural rub for PE; and crackles for pneumonia).

» Abdominal – Check for tenderness (gallstones, gastric ulcer or pancreatitis).

» Skin – Check for rashes (shingles).

## Investigations

» Bloods – Full blood count (FBC), urea and electrolytes (U&E), lipids, fasting glucose, c-reactive protein (CRP), troponin (if they have had chest pain <72 hours), D-dimer (PE), liver function tests (LFTs), amylase (pancreatitis), and erythrocyte sedimentation (ESR) (infection).

» ECG – IHD (ST elevation/depression, new left bundle branch block (LBBB) and T-wave inversion) and PE (AF, right bundle branch block [RBBB] and S1Q3T3).

» Exercise test – No longer part of the criteria to diagnose angina.

» Chest x-ray (CXR) – To exclude chest infection, pneumothorax and heart failure (HF).

» Others (specialist) – Cardiac magnetic resonance imaging (MRI) / computerised tomography (CT) scan (calcium score), thallium scan, myocardial perfusion scintigraphy and angiogram.

## Management

### Conservative

✓ Advise them to stop smoking, and exercise for at least 30 minutes, five times a week. They should try to reduce stress, improve their diet (five portions of fruit or vegetables, and less fat) and reduce their alcohol intake.

✓ For dyspepsia – Advise them to avoid chilli and spicy food; cut down on caffeine and alcohol; stop smoking; and eat small, regular meals and ensure that the last meal of each day is several hours before bedtime.

### Medical

✓ ACS – Offer a GTN spray, give 300mg aspirin stat, and immediately refer them to hospital (with a letter confirming the meds given). Perform an ECG as soon as possible. Offer oxygen if their oxygen saturation is less than 94%. Avoid giving clopidogrel outside hospital.

✓ Angina – Initiate treatment if their history is suggestive of stable angina, and refer them to the chest pain clinic (within two weeks) for confirmation of the diagnosis.

✓ Dyspepsia – Offer alginates (Gaviscon), proton pump inhibitor PPI (omeprazole) or H2 antagonist (ranitidine).

✓ PE – If suspected, start them on low molecular weight heparin (LMWH). Refer them to secondary care.

✓ MSK/pericarditis – Treat with NSAIDs and reassure the patient. Use steroids for pericarditis in resistant cases.

✓ Aortic dissection – Refer them for urgent admission and intervention.

✓ Pancreatitis – Offer analgesia and refer them to hospital for endoscopic retrograde cholangiopancreatography (ERCP). Advise the patient to stop smoking and stop drinking alcohol.

## Referral

→ Refer them if you are unsure of the diagnosis. Admit them if they are hemodynamically unstable (with tachycardia, tachypnoea, BP <90/60, reduced oxygen saturations, altered consciousness or raised temperature).

## Safety Netting

» Advise the patient to seek medical advice if any red-flag symptoms are present, or if angina persists for 10–20 minutes after resting or is not relieved by a GTN spray. Offer a follow-up appointment in two to four weeks if they are stable.

*References*

National Institute for Health and Care Excellence (2016). *Chest pain of recent onset: assessment and diagnosis.* https://www.nice.org.uk/guidance/cg95/documents/short-version-of-draft-guideline

National Clinical Guideline Centre (UK). (2012). *Venous thromboembolic disease: the management of venous thromboembolic diseases and the role of thrombophilia testing.* Royal College of Physicians (UK).

# Angina

IHD refers to a number of conditions, including angina, unstable angina and myocardial infarction (MI). It is a common condition that affects both men and women, with around two million sufferers in the UK. Men are more likely to suffer from angina than women.

Symptoms classically include crushing central chest pain or pressure located behind the lower-left sternal edge, radiating to the left arm or jaw. It is believed the metabolic products of ischaemia trigger pain fibres that pass to the sympathetic ganglia between the C7 and T4 vertebrae, causing pain within the respective peripheral dermatomes. In stable angina, the pain is brought on by exercise, a heavy meal or cold weather, and it goes once one rests. In unstable angina and MI (acute coronary syndrome [ACS]), the pain comes on at rest, is severe, and may be associated with a feeling of nausea, sweating and breathlessness. The pain is typically relieved or partially relieved by the use of sublingual nitrates (GTN spray). A strong family history of heart disease (atherosclerosis) and risk factors are normally present.

## Risk Factors for IHD

- Hypercholesterolaemia
- HTN
- Smoking
- Male gender
- DM
- Obesity
- PVD
- Raised stress levels
- Lack of regular exercise
- Family history of IHD, strokes/TIA or PVD

## Risk Factors for PE

- Previous DVT/PE
- Recent travel
- Trauma or surgery
- Prolonged bed rest
- Immobility
- Combined oral contraceptive pill (COCP)
- Childbirth
- Cancer

## Diagnosis of Angina by History

Patients with the three following features can be diagnosed with typical angina. Atypical angina has two of these features:

- » Constricting discomfort in the front of the chest, neck, shoulders, jaw or arms.
- » Precipitated by physical exertion.
- » Relieved by rest or GTN within five minutes.

## Risk Factors Making Stable Angina More Likely

➤ Stable angina is unlikely if the pain is prolonged, unrelated to activity, brought on by breathing, or associated with dizziness, palpitations, tingling or difficulty swallowing.

## *History*

- » Focused questions
    - › Ask where the pain is, when was it first noticed and what they were doing at the time, and how long it lasts for.
    - › Ask about radiation (the pain moving to the arms, jaw / or back).
    - › Ask about the character (weight or pressure on the chest).
    - › Ask about the severity (pain score).
    - › Ask about the exacerbating and relieving factors, including exercise.

- » Associated history – Ask if they are sweaty, clammy, breathless and vomit during an episode.
- » Atypical features of angina – Ask if they have nausea, gastrointestinal (GI) discomfort, fatigue, burping or restlessness.
- » Past history – Ask if this has happened before, and if they have had a previous MI, HTN, cholesterol, DM, stroke or PVD. Ask about any previous investigations (ECG, echo or angiogram).
- » Drug history – Ask about all medications.
- » Social history – Ask about their occupation, or whether they are a smoker, or drink alcohol.
- » Family history – Ask whether anyone in their family has IHD or raised cholesterol.

## RED FLAGS

Severe crushing pain at rest with SOB, angina pain that has become acutely more severe or increased in frequency, or a reduced walking distance.

## Differentials

➤ ACS

➤ Pericarditis

➤ Aortic dissection

## Examination

» Vitals – BP, pulse and oxygen saturations.

» Cardiovascular – Heart sounds.

## Investigations

» Bloods – FBC, U&E, cholesterol, glucose and troponin (if chest pain has lasted <72 hours).

» ECG – Pathological Q-waves, ST elevation/depression, new LBBB and T=wave inversion/flattening.

» CXR – To exclude chest infection and cardiomegaly (HTN/cardiomyopathy).

» Do not use exercise ECG to diagnose or exclude stable angina for people without known coronary artery disease (CAD).

## Management

*Conservative*

✓ Lifestyle – Advise them to stop smoking, to exercise for 30 minutes five times a week, to reduce stress, to eat a Mediterranean diet, to reduce alcohol consumption and to try to lose weight to attain a BMI<=25.

*Medical*

✓ ACS – Offer a GTN spray, give 300mg aspirin stat, and immediately refer them to hospital. Perform an ECG as soon as possible. Offer oxygen if their oxygen saturation <94%. Avoid giving clopidogrel outside hospital.

✓ Angina – Initiate treatment if their history is suggestive of angina and refer them to the chest pain clinic for confirmation.

› GTN is to be used as required when the pain starts. This can cause flushing, headaches and lightheadedness.

› First-line – Consider a beta-blocker (b-blocker) or a calcium channel blocker (CBB). If the b-blocker (bisoprolol) CBB is not tolerated or contraindicated, consider a CCB (verapamil/diltiazem); however, this is contraindicated in HF and heart block. Use amlodipine in HF.

> If the symptoms are not controlled, try combination therapy.

> Start with a low dose of nitrate and titrate up (isosorbide mononitrate).

> Consider nicorandil if the angina is not controlled by first-line therapy or if contraindications.

> Second prevention – Consider aspirin, an angiotensin-converting enzyme inhibitor (ACEi), a statin and an antihypertensive if the patient has raised BP. Start aspirin at 75mg, but consider the GI bleed risk. Patients with cerebrovascular accident (CVA) / PVD should continue taking clopidogrel instead of aspirin. Start an ACEi if the patient has DM, and commence atorvastatin at 80mg.

## Referral

→ Consider referring the patient to a cardiologist if their symptoms are not controlled with combination therapy, or they have several risk factors or a strong family history. Consider an early referral if they have previously had an MI, coronary artery bypass graft (CABG), AF, angina, aortic stenosis (AS), or if an ECG shows a previous MI.

→ Post-MI, the patient will be referred to a cardiac rehabilitation programme within two to four weeks to help gradually increase physical activity. The programme lasts 12 weeks.

→ Referring a patient with angina to hospital – Refer them if they present with chest pain within 12 hours with an abnormal ECG, or with chest pain within the last 12–72 hours. If they had chest pain >72 hours ago, perform a risk assessment, and take an ECG and troponin level before deciding on the next course of action.

## QOF

» Maintain a register of patients with coronary heart disease (CHD).

» Monitor their BP and cholesterol yearly.

» Ensure the patient is on aspirin (and/or clopidogrel), an ACEi, a b-blocker and a statin.

## Safety Netting

» Perform a review two to four weeks after initiating or changing medication. The patient should seek medical advice if any red-flag symptoms occur, if angina persists for >15 minutes after resting or is not relieved by a second dose of GTN spray.

## Post-MI Advice

➤ Employment – Patients in employment should try to return to work, depending on the type of employment they are in. Sedentary workers can return within one month, light manual workers within two months and heavy manual workers within three months.

➤ Exercise – Advise the patient to exercise lightly but regularly. They should consider a stroll in the park after two weeks.

➤ Sexual intercourse – This can resume four weeks post-MI. If they are able to climb two flights of stairs briskly pain free, then sexual activity should not be a problem.

➤ Travel – They should avoid driving for four weeks and avoid flying for 7–14 days post an uncomplicated MI and for four to six weeks if it was complicated.

➤ Driving – The patient should inform the Driver and Vehicle Licensing Agency (DVLA), and they are not to drive if symptoms occur at rest, at the wheel, or from emotion. It should be recommended that patients inform their insurance company about their diagnosis of angina.

## Further Advice for Travel and Driving

➤ **Flying**

› Unstable angina – The patient must not fly.

› Stable angina – If the patient can climb a flight of stairs or walk 100 metres without pain/SOB, they may fly.

› ACS/MI – The patient must not fly for one to two weeks afterwards (uncomplicated), or four to six weeks afterwards (complicated).

› Angioplasty – The patient must not fly for five to seven days afterwards.

› CABG – The patient must not fly for 10–14 days afterwards.

➤ **Driving (group one – cars and motorcycles)**

› Stable angina – The patient must stop driving if they experience pain at rest, from emotion, or that occurs at wheel.

› ACS/MI – There must be no driving for one month afterwards, or one week afterwards if treated with an angioplasty.

› CABG – There must be no driving for one month afterwards.

➤ **Driving (group two – lorries and buses)**

› The patient must notify the DVLA for the following, and exercise testing is required.

› Stable angina – They may be relicensed if they have suffered no angina for six weeks.

> ACS/MI – There must be no driving for six weeks afterwards.

> Angioplasty – There must be no driving for six weeks afterwards.

> CABG – There must be no driving for three months afterwards.

## References

National Institute for Health and Care Excellence (2010). *Recent-onset chest pain of suspected cardiac origin: assessment and diagnosis.* https://www.nice.org.uk/guidance/CG95

National Institute for Health and Care Excellence (2011). *Stable angina: management.* https://www.nice.org.uk/guidance/CG126

# Hypertension

HTN is a very common condition that affects vast swathes of the population. As it is often asymptomatic, most cases are found incidentally when visiting the GP surgery or having their BP checked at the pharmacy. Around 90% of hypertensives have no identifiable cause (primary HTN). HTN is a major risk factor for developing CHD, kidney disease and strokes. The higher the BP, the greater the risk of cardiovascular disease (CVD). Hence, all newly diagnosed hypertensive patients should be risk stratified using tools such as QRISK2 to assess their 10-year risk of having a cardiovascular event.

## Classification of HTN

*Stage 1*      Clinic BP of >=140/90, and an ambulatory blood pressure monitoring (ABPM) daytime average or HBPM average of 135/85.

*Stage 2*      Clinic BP of >=160/100, and an ABPM daytime average or HBPM average of >=150/95.

*Severe*       Clinic BP of >=180/110.

*Accelerated*  Clinic BP of >=180/110 and a papilloedema, with or without retinal haemorrhage

## Types of HTN

➤  Primary – No identifiable cause (90% of people with HTN)

➤  Secondary – Underlying cause (renovascular disease or pheochromocytoma)

➤  White coat – Unusually raised BP when measured during clinics, but normal when measured at home

## *History*

»  Focused questions

  ›  Ask about any headaches, drowsiness, visual disturbances, nausea or vomiting.

»  Past history – Ask if they have had renal disease, endocrine disease, cardiovascular disease (CVD), systemic lupus erythematosus (SLE), scleroderma or sleep apnoea.

»  Secondary causes of HTN

  ›  Renal – Ask if they have had renal failure, renal artery stenosis, glomerulonephritis, adult polycystic ovaries or a renal tumour.

  ›  Endocrine – Ask if they have had Cushing's syndrome, acromegaly, hyperthyroidism or pheochromocytoma.

  ›  Others – Ask if they have had coarctation of aorta, aortic valve disease or a pregnancy.

» Drug history – Ask if they have taken COCP, steroids, ciclosporin, NSAIDs or venlafaxine.

» Social history – Ask about their occupation, stress level, and whether they, smoke, drink alcohol or take / have taken recreational drugs (particularly cocaine).

» Family history – Ask if there is a family history of any HTN or any occurrences of the secondary causes.

## RED FLAGS

A >=180/110 BP reading with signs of papilloedema or retinal hemorrhage, or a one-off BP with systolic >220 and diastolic >120. Microscopic haematuria, very high BP with a headache, pregnancy (pre-eclampsia), signs of end-stage organ damage, fits or HF.

## Risk Factors for HTN

➤ DM

➤ Stroke

➤ Raised cholesterol

➤ Smoking

➤ Family history of CVD

➤ Ethnicity

➤ Social deprivation

➤ Stress

➤ Age

## Examination

» BP – Take three separate consecutive readings.

» Cardiovascular – Listen for heart sounds and check peripheral pulses.

» Fundoscopy – Assess the fundi for signs of hypertensive retinopathy.

› Grade 1 – Silver wiring or arteriolar narrowing.

› Grade 2 – Arterio-venous (AV) nipping.

› Grade 3 – Flame and blot haemorrhages or cotton-wool exudates.

› Grade 4 – Papilloedema.

## Investigations

» Bloods – FBC, U&Es including estimated glomerular filtration rate (eGFR), lipid profile and haemoglobin A1c (HbA1c).

» Resting ECG – Left ventricular hypertrophy and left atrial enlargement.

» Urine – Haematuria and proteinuria (renal causes), and urinary catecholamines (pheochromocytoma).

## Diagnosing HTN with HBPM

» Record BP two times a day, preferably in the morning and evening. Take two readings at least one minute apart and whilst seated.

## Management

### Conservative

✓ CV risk – Determine the QRISK2 score to assess the patient's 10-year risk of having a stroke or heart attack. Consider statins if QRISK2 >10%.

✓ Lifestyle – Advise the patient to reduce their salt intake (<6g/day), increase fruit and vegetable intake, and reduce coffee intake. Encourage them to use relaxation techniques and stress management. They should aim for an optimum weight BMI <25, and encourage exercise (for 30 minutes, five times a week). Advise them to stop smoking and reduce their alcohol consumption (<14 units a week).

✓ Driving – They should inform the DVLA if they are a group two driver (buses or lorries). They shoud be disqualified if their systolic BP is >180 or, resting diastolic BP is >100. They may be relicensed if it is controlled with treatment, and there are no side effects.

### Medical

✓ Antihypertensives

› If the patient is <55 years old, give an ACEi or angiotensin II receptor blockers (ARB), but not both or if the patient is pregnant. If the patient is >55 years old or of Afro-Caribbean origin, give a CCB.

› A combination of an ACEi or ARnB with CCB. If a CCB is contraindicated, then give a thiazide-like diuretic.

› Combine all three medications. For a diuretic, use indapamide 2.5mg once a day (od).

› If a fourth drug is needed, add one of the following: spironolactone 25mg of potassium <4.5mmol, a higher dose of a thiazide-like diuretic of potassium <4.5mmol, an alpha-blocker (a-blocker) or b-blocker.

**Side-effects of antihypertensive medication**

› ACEi/ARB – Profound BP drop, dry cough (ACEi only), renal impairment, angioedema, rash (urticaria) or raised potassium. Consider an ARB if an ACEi is not tolerated.

> › B-blocker – Bradycardia, bronchospasm or erectile dysfunction. Avoid in cases of asthma, chronic obstructive pulmonary disease (COPD), HF or heart block.

> › CCB – Pedal oedema, dizziness, flushing or constipation. Avoid rate-limiting agents (diltiazem) in cases of HF or heart block.

> › Diuretic – Erectile dysfunction or DM/SLE worsens. Avoid in cases of gout (increases uric acid).

> › A-blocker (e.g. doxazosin) – Urinary incontinence or postural hypotension.

## Target BP (NICE)

» 140/90 – Target clinic BP <140/90 in people under 80, and <150/90 if over 80.

» 130/80 – Patients with a history of renal, DM, CVD or end-stage organ damage.

» 125/75 – In patients with chronic kidney disease (CKD), if there is proteinuria, then a target of <125/75 should be sought.

## QOF

» Maintain a register of patients with BP. Monitor BP yearly. Ensure the patient's BP remains <150/90.

## Safety Netting

» Follow-up – A review can be performed by a practice nurse or healthcare assistant (HCA) if HTN is controlled. For patients on lifestyle measures only, follow up every three to four months. If they have been started on medication, follow up in four weeks. The patient will need follow up U&Es within one to two weeks if they are on an ACEi, or in four to six weeks if they are on a diuretic.

» Patients will require annual reviews (QRISK2, U&Es, urine dipstick for proteinuria or urine ACR).

» Refer patients who are <40 with stage 1 HTN for investigation of secondary HTN.

» Arrange same-day admission if their BP is >= 220/120, or their BP >180/110 with signs of papilloedema and/or retinal haemorrhage.

---

### References

National Institute for Health and Care Excellence (2019). *Hypertension in adults: Diagnosis and management.* https://www.nice.org.uk/guidance/ng136

# Palpitations

The term 'palpitations' describes a patient's abnormal awareness of their own heartbeat. It may be caused by a wide range of clinical conditions, including anaemia, cardiac disease or even anxiety. In most cases, the cause is unknown; however, common cardiac causes account for just under 50% of cases, and these include tachycardia, atrial/ventricular ectopics or atrial flutter (AF). It is important to be able to distinguish between life-threatening causes and the more benign ones. This can sometimes be difficult as the severity of the symptoms rarely correlates with the seriousness of the underlying condition. For example, significant palpitations may be felt despite the patient being in sinus rhythm; conversely, a patient in ventricular tachycardia (VT) may remain asymptomatic.

## Causes of Palpitations

➤ **Cardiac**
  › AF, Wolff-Parkinson-White (WPW) syndrome or ectopic beats
  › Ventricular (VT or VF)
  › Sinus tachycardia

➤ **Metabolic**
  › Hyperthyroidism
  › Hypoglycaemia
  › Hypo/hypercalcaemia
  › Hypo/hyperkalemia

➤ **Drugs**
  › Alcohol
  › Amphetamines
  › Caffeine
  › Nitrates
  › Thyroxine

➤ **Structural abnormality**
  › Left HF
  › Aortic aneurysm
  › Cardiomegaly
  › CHD
  › Pericarditis
  › PE

- ➤ **High cardiac output**
  - › Anaemia
  - › Fever
  - › Pregnancy
  - › Thyrotoxicosis

- ➤ **Psychogenic**
  - › Panic attacks
  - › Anxiety disorders
  - › Depression
  - › Emotional distress

## History

- » Focused questions
  - › Clarify what they mean by palpitations. Ask when they started, how long they last for, what they have been doing at the time and how often they are felt.
  - › Ask about the character of the palpatations.
  - › Ask the patient to tap out the rhythm. Ask if they feel their heart is beating fast, regularly or slowly.
  - › Ask whether anything makes the palpitations better or worse.

- » Associated history – Ask if there is any SOB, chest pain, dizziness or LOC.
- » Past history – Ask if this has happened before, or if they have any other heart problems or anxiety.
- » Drug history – Ask if the patient has taken salbutamol, TCA, thyroxine or CCB.
- » Social history – Ask about their occupation, their diet (including caffeine/energy drinks), and whether they drink alcohol, smoke or take recreational drugs (amphetamines).
- » Family history – Ask if there is a family history of AF, implantable cardioverter-defibrillator ICDs or sudden, unexpected death (<40 years).

## RED FLAGS

- » Cardiac – Chest pain with a past medical history of CVD or structural heart disease.
- » Syncope – LOC (VT, SVT or a family history of sudden death).

## LOC Guidelines

Refer all patients with total LOC for a specialist cardiovascular assessment by the most appropriate local service. Exceptions are a confirmed diagnosis after an assessment of an uncomplicated faint, and people whose presentation is strongly suggestive of epileptic seizures.

## Differential Diagnosis

| | |
|---|---|
| Ectopic beats | Worse at rest. Patients feel a missed, skipped or 'extra' beat. |
| AF | Sporadically irregular pulse, which may be paroxysmal. Can start suddenly. May be due to thyrotoxicosis or pneumonia. |
| SVT | Sudden onset, where the patient feels their heart pounding with a rapid pulse, dyspnoea, chest tightness and dizziness. Confirmed tachycardia. |
| Hyperthyroidism | Heat intolerance, weight loss, diarrhoea, eye symptoms and tremors. OE: goitre, AF on pulse, eye signs or sweaty palms. |
| Panic attacks | Sweating with hyperventilation, plus perioral tingling. Short lived. Associated with stress. A feeling of impending doom. OE: sweaty palms, tachycardia or tachypnoea. |

## Examination

» Vitals – BP, pulse and temperature.

» General – Any signs of anaemia (conjunctiva).

» Cardiovascular – Listen for heart sounds (murmurs), lung bases (HF) and a raised jugular venous pulse (JVP).

» Thyroid – Perform a focused thyroid exam (palpate the thyroid gland, and check for tremors and exophthalmos).

## Investigations

» Bloods – FBC, ferritin, U&Es, thyroid function tests (TFTs) and fasting glucose.

» ECG – 12-lead ECG and 24-hour tape.

» CXR – Cardiomegaly and HF.

» Echo (for valvular disease and cardiomyopathy).

# Management

## *Conservative*

✓ Lifestyle – Advise the patient to cut down on alcohol and caffeine consumption, and they should avoid cheese and chocolate.

✓ Diary – Suggest that the patient considers keeping a symptom diary to elucidate trigger factors.

✓ Admission – Consider admitting the patient if they are acutely unwell or show signs of significant disease.

## *Medical*

✓ SVT – Try to get an ECG where possible and consider admitting the patient. One can try a carotid sinus massage (except if the patient has IHD or TIA, or is elderly) or the Valsalva manoeuvre. If the attack terminates, refer them to cardiology.

✓ Panic attacks – Reassure them, and advise them of the use of relaxation and re-breathing techniques. Advise them that they should avoid any precipitants or stressors. Consider prescribing a b-blocker (propranolol) for symptomatic relief if there are no contraindications (asthma). Try a selective serotonin reuptake inhibitor (SSRI) or psychotherapy cognitive behavioural therapy (CBT).

✓ Hyperthyroidism – Prescribe a b-blocker for symptomatic relief. Reduce the thyroxine dose if it is drug induced. Try carbimazole, radioactive iodine or the surgical removal of thyroid gland. These options are initiated by secondary care.

✓ AF – Find and treat the cause of the AF (hyperthyroidism, pneumonia, HF, etc.).

**Rate or rhythm control in AF:**

› Rate control – Offer this to all patients except those with new onset AF, AF with a reversible cause or AF-induced HF. Drugs include b-blockers, CCB (diltiazem) and digoxin.

› Rhythm control – Consider this for patients whose symptoms continue despite rate control (not in the case of IHD or structural heart disease). Drugs include amiodarone, flecainide and dronedarone.

› Anticoagulation – Use the $CHA_2DS_2$-VASc score tool to assess the patient's stroke risk. Offer anticoagulants (warfarin or non-vitamin K antagonist oral anticoagulants [NOACs]) to all patients with a score of two or more, or consider it in men with a score of one. Factor in the patient's HAS-BLED score to determine their risk of bleeding (three or more is considered a high risk). Consider a NOAC if warfarin is contraindicated or the patient has side effects. NOACs have a shorter half-life, so compliance is important.

*Stroke and bleeding risk stratification with the $CHA_2DS_2$–VASc and HAS-BLED schemas*

| $CHA_2DS_2$- VASc | Score | HAS-BLED | Score |
|---|---|---|---|
| Congestive heart failure / left ventricular (LV) dysfunction | 1 | HTN (i.e. uncontrolled BP) | 1 |
| HTN | 1 | Abnormal renal/liver function | 1 or 2 |
| Aged >75 years | 2 | Stroke | 1 |
| DM | 1 | Bleeding tendency or predisposition | 1 |
| Stroke/TIA/TE | 2 | Labile international normalised ratio (INR) | 1 |
| Vascular disease (prior MI, PAD or aortic plaque) | 1 | Age (e.g. >65 years) | 1 |
| Aged 65–74 years | 1 | Drugs (e.g. concomitant aspirin or NSAIDSs) or alcohol | 1 |
| Sex category (e.g. female gender) | 1 | | |
| Maximum score | 9 | | 9 |

*QOF*

✓ Maintain a register of AF patients and monitor them yearly. Ensure patients with a $CHA_2DS_2$ score of one or more are on an anticoagulation or antiplatelet therapy.

*Admitting a Patient with Palpitations to Hospital*

✓ A patient with palpitations and any of the following should be admitted to hospital:

> Arrhythmia associated with haemodynamic compromise.

> Life-threatening arrhythmia requiring rapid control (e.g. VT or SVT).

> Significant heart disease (cardiomyopathy or congestive cardiac failure [CCF]).

> It is associated with angina, syncope or severe SOB.

## Referral

Refer the patient for any of the following:

→ If their symptoms are consistent with VT/SVT.

→ If it is suggestive of a serious cause (SOB, chest pain or LOC).

→ If there is a family history of cardiac-related sudden death.

→ If they have structural heart disease.

→ For ambulatory monitoring to capture rhythm during a symptomatic episode.

→ Refer them to a specialist if no underlying cause has been established, but the patient experiences recurrent symptoms.

## When to Refer Patients with Palpitations

> **Urgent**

Refer the patient if they have any of the following:

› Palpitations during exercise.

› Palpitations with syncope or near syncope.

› A high risk of structural heart disease.

› A family history of inherited heart disease / sudden arrhythmic death syndrome (SADS) and a high degree of AV block.

> **Routine**

Refer the patient if they have any of the following:

› A history that suggests recurrent tachyarrhythmia.

› Palpitations with associated symptoms.

› An abnormal ECG.

› A normal ECG but with known structural disease.

### References

Cheshire and Merseyside Strategic Clinical Networks (2012). *Pathways for cardiology symptoms in primary care.* https://www.nwcscnsenate.nhs.uk/files/1414/4543/7970/AF_Pathway_Master_FINAL_OCTOBER_2015.pdf?PDFPATHWAY=PDF

National Institute for Health and Care Excellence (2014). *Atrial fibrillation: management.* https://www.nice.org.uk/guidance/cg180

# Hypercholesterolaemia

Hypercholesterolaemia is the presence of raised cholesterol levels in the blood. It is important, as it can increase the risk of heart disease by way of angina, MI or even strokes. Cholesterol is believed to lead to the formation of atherosclerotic plaques within the arteries that become larger over time, narrowing the artery and restricting the blood supply. Occasionally, the atheroma plaques may rupture, triggering a thrombosis (clot) that may partially or completely block the blood flow through an artery, giving rise to pain or cell death (MI or CVA). The most common cause of raised cholesterol is dietary and is due to eating high levels of saturated fats. It may also occur genetically in the form of familial hypercholesterolaemia.

» Target cholesterol – This treatment can lead to a >40% reduction in non-HDL cholesterol in three months.

## History

» The focus should be on gathering information so that an accurate cardiovascular risk assessment can be performed. Analyse the patient's notes closely for risk factors and blood results. Determine if the patient is obese.

› Cardiac – Ask them about chest pain, if it occurs at rest or exertion, and if there is any pain on walking (intermittent claudication).

› Stroke – Ask if they have any weakness or numbness in their legs.

› Erectile dysfunction – Ask if they have any problems maintaining an erection.

» Past history – Ask if thy have had HTN, DM, CVD, CKD or thyroid problems.

» Drug history – Ask if they have taken steroids, b-blockers, thiazides, COCP or antipsychotic treatment.

» Social history – Ask about their occupation (the type of work may cause a sedentary lifestyle), whether they smoke or drink alcohol, what their diet is like and about exercise.

» Family history – Ask if there is any family history of CVD, anyone with premature CVD (<55 years), any IHD, any sudden deaths, any familial high cholesterol, and if so, what that person's age is.

## Familial Hypercholesterolaemia

» This is an autosomal dominant condition that has an incidence of one in 500.

» It causes early CVD with persistently high low-density lipoprotein (LDL) levels.

» Patients can be referred to specialist lipid clinics for screening and treatment. This is diagnosed using the Simon Broom criteria.

## Assessing the Patient's Level of Exercise

» The General Practice Physical Activity Questionnaire (GPPAQ) is a screening tool used to assess an adult's (16–74 years) physical activity levels.

» The questionnaire takes into account the patient's occupation and the level of physical intensity that arises from that. It also scores the patient's degree of exercises across five domains, including physical exercises such as swimming, football, cycling, walking, housework, childcare, gardening or do-it-yourself (DIY).

# Examination

» Vitals – BMI, waist circumference and BP.

» General – Eyes (corneal arcus), face (xanthelasma) and tendons (xanthomata).

» Cardiovascular – Listen to the heart and assess the peripheral pulses.

# Investigations

» Bloods – Lipids, HbA1c, U&Es, LFTs (fatty liver) and TFTs. Consider creatine kinase (CK) if the patient experiences muscle pain whilst on a statin. If it is raised over five times the normal limit, repeat after one week. If it is still raised, refer them to a lipid clinic. If the aspartate aminotransferase (AST) / alanine transaminase (ALT) is raised, perform further investigations to establish the cause (e.g. non-alcoholic fatty liver disease [NAFLD]).

» ECG – If there is a history of chest pain or erectile dysfunction.

# Management

*Conservative*

✓ Diet – Advise them to avoid fatty food (cheese, cream, etc.). They should grill, bake, poach or steam foods instead of roasting or frying them. If frying, they should use olive oil. Encourage them to eat at least five portions of fruit and vegetables daily, and to eat at least two portions of fish, with at least one oily fish, weekly.

✓ Exercise – Advise them to take 30 minutes of moderate exercise five times per week (until they become slightly short of breath). They should do muscle strengthening activities two or more times a week.

✓ Offer smoking-cessation advice.

✓ Advise them to reduce their alcohol intake.

*Medical*

✓ Statins inhibit the action of hmg-CoA reductase within the liver, during the rate-limiting step in cholesterol synthesis. They should be taken in the evening as most of the cholesterol synthesis occurs overnight.

> › Side effects include myalgia, myositis, rhabdomyolysis and liver impairment.

> › Risk factors for myopathy include being elderly, being female, having a low BMI and having DM.

> › Patients cannot drink grapefruit juice as it can increase the concentration of some statins by affecting the p450 enzyme.

> › NICE recommends taking baseline LFTs before starting the statins, and then repeating at three months and then 13 months after initiation. If the AST remains three times the upper limit, then stop the statin.

> › Contraindications – Pregnant, breastfeeding or have liver disease.

✓ Statins – Offer a statin as follows. Titrate up if the patient does not achieve a >= 40% reduction in non-high-density lipoproteins (HDL) cholesterol in three months; increase up to a maximum of 80mg.

✓ Risk assess – Calculate the QRISK2 before recommending atorvastatin 20mg.

> › If the patient is <85 years, initiate atorvastatin with a patient of QRISK2 of 10% or more.

> › If they have type 2 DM and have a QRISK2 of 10% or more, initiate atorvastatin.

✓ No risk assessment – Offer lipid therapy without the need for a formal assessment in the following cases:

> › If the patient is >85 years, give atorvastatin 20mg.

> › Offer atorvastatin 80mg for patients with CVD.

> › Offer atorvastatin 20mg for patients with CKD3. If eGFR <30, speak to the GP or seek renal advice before increasing the statin dose.

> › Offer atorvastatin 20mg if >40 years and have Type 1 DM, or for established nephropathy.

✓ Alternative

> › Offer fibrate or ezetimibe if atorvastatin is not tolerated.

## Referral

→ Refer them to a dietician if there are concerns about if the patient's diet.

→ Refer them to a smoking-cessation clinic if they smoke.

→ Refer them to health trainers.

→ If they are overweight, refer them to an exercise / weight-loss programme.

### References

National Institute for Health and Care Excellence (2014). *Cardiovascular disease: risk assessment and reduction, including lipid modification.* https://www.nice.org.uk/guidance/cg181

National Institute for Health and Care Excellence (2008). *Familial hypercholesterolaemia: identification and management.* https://www.nice.org.uk/guidance/cg71

# Peripheral Arterial Disease

Peripheral arterial disease (PAD), also known as PVD, refers to the narrowing or occlusion of the arterial blood supply to the legs. It is primarily caused by atherosclerosis. Although the majority of patients with PAD are symptomatic, blood flow may become restricted during exercise or activity, giving rise to the classical presentation of intermittent claudication. In severe occlusions, patients may also feel pain at rest. Patients diagnosed with PAD have an increased risk of significant mortality, morbidity from MI and /or a CVA. A key factor in developing PAD is smoking, and it is important to encourage patients to stop.

## Types of PAD

> **Acute limb ischaemia**

A rapidly developing, sudden reduction in blood flow to the lower limb, resulting in new or worsening symptoms and signs, with a threat to limb viability. Often caused by thrombosis. Presents as an acute onset of pain (hours/days) with a colour change, and lost of sensation and power.

Six Ps:

> **P**ainful

> **P**ulseless

> **P**allor (pale)

> **P**aralysis

> **P**araesthesia (numbness)

> **P**erishingly cold

> **Chronic limb ischaemia**

Consider if there is progressive worsening of cramp-like calf pain on walking or at rest (at night), non-healing wounds to the legs, or absent peripheral pulses.

> **Intermittent claudication**

Caused by reduced circulation to the lower limb, which causes calf pain (less commonly, buttock and thigh pain) during walking or exercise. The calf pain is reproducible from a predicted walking distance and relieved by rest. Peripheral pulses are felt at rest, but may be absent on exercise up to the point of pain.

> **Critical limb ischaemia**

Severely impaired circulation causes an acute risk of limb viability. It presents as burning, relentless leg pain at rest, which is worse at night. Patients may leave their leg hanging out of bed or sleep on a chair. Patients may have suffered from prior intermittent claudication, having a red/purple (dependent rubor) colour to the leg when it is not elevated and early pallor on elevation, reduced capillary refill, absent foot pulses, ischaemic ulcers or gangrene.

## *History*

» Focused questions:

› Ask when the pain first started, how long it has been going on for and where exactly the pain is felt (buttocks, thigh, calf or foot).

› Possible location of occlusion:

- Buttock pain – Stenosis of the aorta (bilateral pain) or common iliac (unilateral pain).

- Thigh pain – An occlusion in the femoral or common inguinal artery.

- Calf pain – An occlusion in the popliteal or tibial artery.

- Foot pain – An occlusion in the posterior tibial or dorsalis pedis artery.

› Ask about the character (cramping, burning or a numb feeling).

› Ask about the severity, and aggravating (walking for long periods) and relieving factors.

› Ask how far they can walk before the pain comes on (claudication distance).

› Ask if there is any pain at rest.

› Ask if there are any associated changes to the leg – colour, feeling cold or skin changes.

» Associated history – Ask if there has been any SOB, chest pain, palpitations, ankle swelling, or erectile dysfunction.

» Past history – Ask if this has happened before, or if there is any history of MI, HTN, high cholesterol or DM.

» Drug history – Ask if they have taken any b-blockers

» Social history – Ask about their occupation, ask whether they smoke or drink alcohol, ask about their diet and exercise, ask about their driving (those in group two must inform the DVLA).

» Family history – Ask them if they have a family history of IHD or PAD.

## Risk Factors for PAD

➤ Gender (more prevalent in males than females)

➤ Age (>50 years old)

➤ BP

➤ DM

➤ Smoking

➤ Hypercholesterolaemia

➤ Family history of PAD/IHD/CVA

> ➤ BMI >30

> ➤ Physical inactivity

## RED FLAGS

> »   Critical ischaemia – Pain at rest, pallor, paresthesia in the foot, cold legs or gangrene.

## Differential Diagnosis

| Spinal stenosis | May present with slowly worsening back pain. Worse on exercise, but the patient has to sit down for a few minutes to relieve the pain. Numbness and tingling may also be associated with it. OE: pain is reduced on spinal flexion forward. No weakness. |
|---|---|
| DVT | Swollen calf, recent long-haul travel or operation. |
| Intermittent claudication | Calf, buttock or thigh pain that is worse on exertion and relieved by rest. Predictable claudication distance. Associated with erectile dysfunction. |
| OA – hip | Hip pain radiating to the thigh or buttock. Worse on weight bearing. Can occur at rest (with less intensity) or in certain positions. OE: antalgic gait, reduced ROM at the hip joint, or present distal pulses. |
| Chronic compartment syndrome | Tight, bursting pain in the calf muscle. Common in athletes. Starts after exercise. Relief on elevation of the leg. OE: Ankle-brachial pressure index (ABPI) is normal. |
| Lumbar radiculopathy | A history of back pain. A burning sensation at the back of the leg. Worse on walking, carrying something or standing, but relieved by sitting or leaning forwards. OE: reduced straight leg raise (SLR), altered sensation in the lower leg, and reduced ankle reflexes. |
| Diabetic neuropathy | Neuropathic pain (burning, shooting or electric-shock like), affecting the feet and legs, which is worse at night, but often relieved by walking (unlike intermittent claudication). |

## Examination

> »   Vitals – BP, pulse and BMI.

> »   Cardiovascular – Listen for heart sounds.

> »   Abdomen – Palpate the abdomen for an aortic aneurysm.

» Arterial leg exam.

> Inspection – Inspect the legs for a colour change (white, blue, purple or black), trophic changes (shiny skin, hair loss or ulcers) and other signs (gangrenous or has amputated toes). Inspect the pressure points (heel and malleoli) for ulcers.

> Palpation – Check the temperature of the legs and the capillary refill.

> Pulses – Palpate the posterior tibial artery, dorsalis pedis artery, popliteal artery and femoral artery.

» Buerger's test – get the patient on the couch and establish the angle of elevation of the leg where it becomes pale. An angle >30 degrees suggests severe ischaemia. Sit them up with their legs hanging off the edge of the bed. Time how long it takes for the leg to return to a normal colour. Redness suggests reactive hyperaemia and chronic lower limb ischaemia, (takes two to three minutes to return to a normal colour).

## Investigations

» Bloods – FBC, U&Es (exclude renal artery stenosis), lipids, HbA1c and a thrombophilia screen if they are <50 years.

» ECG – Look for signs of ischaemia.

» ABPI – Perform an ABPI or refer them to a vascular clinic for this to be done.

» Specialist – Conduct doppler (duplex) studies to establish the site of the disease or an MRI / CT angiography.

### Interpreting the ABPI

In DM, the ABPI can be falsely elevated due to vessel wall calcification:

| ABPI | Classification |
|---|---|
| >1.0 | Normal |
| 0.5–0.9 | Claudication |

## Management

### Conservative

✓ Offer smoking-cessation advice.

✓ Diet – Advise them to eat five portions of fruit and vegetables a day, and less red meat and dairy products. They should eat a normal, healthy diet.

✓ If their BMI is >30, refer them to an intense weight-loss programme.

✓ Advise them to reduce their alcohol intake (<14 units/week).

✓ Encourage them to increase their exercise, primarily by walking as far as possible within their pain threshold. They should attempt to extend their maximum walking distance over time. Evidence shows that supervised exercise therapy for two hours/week for three months has more success than unsupervised exercise.

✓ Advise that they should avoid tight shoes and socks that may injure or reduce the blood supply to the foot. They should avoid causing any trauma to or accidents involving the foot.

### Medical

✓ Treat the risk factors – Patients with DM, HTN and hypercholesterolaemia should be optimally controlled.

✓ Antiplatelets – Consider offering clopidogrel 75mg with symptomatic PVD. If contraindicated, try aspirin (75mg–325mg) or dipyridamole.

✓ Statin – Offer a statin to the patient; e.g. atorvastatin 80mg.

## Referral

→ Consider a referral to podiatry for foot hygiene, including cutting nails or treating corns/callouses. Refer the patient to the vascular department for diagnosis and further treatment options; e.g. naftidrofuryl, angioplasty, bypass or amputation.

## Safety Netting

» Advise the patient to seek urgent medical advice if they notice any pain at rest or features of critical ischaemia.

### References

National Institute for Health and Care Excellence (2012). *Peripheral arterial disease: diagnosis and management*. NICE Guidance. https://www.nice.org.uk/guidance/cg147

# Varicose Veins

Varicose veins are engorged and tortuous superficial veins found in the leg, and they are often unpleasant to the eye. They usually present with venous insufficiency due to incompetent valves causing a reflux of blood and increased pressure in the distal veins. They often appear in pregnancy, due to increased blood volume straining the venous system, hormones relaxing the blood vessel walls, and the uterus increasing pressure on the pelvic veins and the inferior vena cava. Although they are unsightly, they usually do not present as a medical emergency. However, they may cause medical symptoms such as pain, skin ulcers, bleeding and superficial infections.

## Risk factors

> Female gender
> Age (young/middle-aged)
> Pregnancy and parity
> Occupation (those with prolonged standing)
> DVT
> Family history of varicose veins
> Thrombophlebitis
> OCP/HRT

## History

» Focused questions:
  › Ask when they first noticed the varicose veins and how long they have had them for.
  › Ask about the location (thigh or lower leg) and whether there is any pain (aching, heaviness or pressure in the leg).
  › Ask what the aggravating (standing for long periods) and relieving (sitting down, elevating leg or compression stockings) factors are.

» Associated history – Ask if there is a history of oedema (swelling in leg or ankles) or skin changes (itching or ulcers).

» Past history – Ask if the patient as been pregnant, or had a pelvic tumour, surgery or treatments for varicose veins.

» Drug history – Ask if they have taken COCP or HRT.

» Social history – Ask about their occupation, and whether they smoke, or drink alcohol.

» Family history – Ask if there is a family history of DVT or varicose veins.

## RED FLAGS

DVT (calf swelling, and recent travel or an operation), or an abdominal swelling or lump.

## Examination

- » Vitals – BMI.

- » Abdominal – Examine the patient for pelvic or abdominal masses.

- » Venous leg exam
  - › Inspection – Inspect the gaiter area (above the medial malleolus), and the long (groin to medial malleolus) and short (popliteal to lateral malleolus) saphenous veins for eczema, ulcers or oedema. Check for a hemosiderin pigmentation or lipodermatosclerosis.
  - › Palpation – Palpate along the long and short saphenous veins for tenderness (phlebitis) or hardness (thrombosis). Check for peripheral oedema.

## Investigations

- » Bloods – Not routinely performed.

- » Doppler studies – Establish the site of the disease.

- » ABPI – This may be performed to exclude PVD prior to offering support stockings.

## Differential Diagnosis

| Varicose veins | Unpleasant tortuous veins in the leg, along with saphenous distribution. Aching and/or heaviness that is worse at the end of the day, worse on standing, and improved with rest and elevation. OE: dilated veins in the long / short saphenous vein distribution, pedal oedema and skin changes. |
|---|---|
| Saphena varix | Enlarged saphenous vein at the sapheno-femoral junction. OE: cough impulse, a lump in the groin and a bluish tinge that disappears on lying down. This may appear with varicose veins. |
| Thrombophlebitis | The superficial inflammation of a vein. This may cause pain, redness or swelling. OE: a tender and hard vein. |

## Management

*Conservative*

✓    Reassure – If they are mild varicose veins, then reassure the patient.

✓    Weight reduction – If their BMI is >30, refer them to an intense weight-loss programme.

✓    Exercise – Encourage the patient to increase their exercise, primarily by walking as far as possible within their pain threshold.

✓    Pain – Advise the patient to place a hot flannel over the vein to reduce pain.

✓    Position – Advise the patient to avoid prolonged, uninterrupted standing. Intersperse periods of standing with walking or sitting. They should elevate the legs where possible, particularly at night or when seated, which may also provide temporary symptomatic relief. They should put pillows under their foot/feet when lying in bed or use a footstool when seated.

✓    Pregnancy – Educate the patient that varicose veins may worsen in pregnancy but improve after. Advise them to consider wearing stockings. Surgical interventions are not routinely recommended in pregnancy.

*Medical*

✓    Support stockings – Offer graduated compression stockings to control the symptoms and reduce the risk of ulceration. Advise the patient to put them first thing on in the morning just before they get out of bed (the veins are collapsed, so the stockings are easier to put on) and to remove them before sleeping at night. Class 1 stockings are used for mild symptoms. However, in the presence of significant ankle oedema or to prevent recurrent ulceration, Class 2 stockings should be provided.

**Types of compression stockings**

There are three different grades, according to the pressure they exert upon the ankle. They work by reducing the venous reflux via increasing venous pressure in the legs. Class 1 stockings can be purchased over the counter (OTC), whilst Class 2 and 3 require a prescription. Avoid using these in cases of PVD (pressure necrosis). Thigh-length stockings are useful for varicose veins in the thigh and in pregnancy. Knee-length stockings are recommended for varicose veins in the lower leg, swollen ankles and ulcers.

> Class 1 – Mild varicose veins with aching legs or mild ankle swelling; e.g. for long flights

> Class 2 – Moderate to severe varicose veins with moderate ankle swelling, after vein surgery and to prevent recurrent ulcerations

> Class 3 – Severe varicose veins or ankle swelling, and active leg ulcers

**Complications**

- Eczema – Pateints with varicose eczema can be offered moisturising emollients and/or topical mild steroids.

- Thrombophlebitis – Consider antibiotics if infected, or NSAIDs. Thrombophlebitis increases the risk of any underlying DVT.

*Surgical*

✓ Operation – Refer the patient to a low-priority panel if relevant, depending on your area's protocol. Consider this in cases of severe varicose veins. The options include stripping and sclerotherapy. Newer techniques include foam therapy and radiofrequency ablation.

**Complications**

> Pain and heaviness

> DVT

> Haemorrhaging from trauma

> Varicose eczema

> Venous ulceration

> Skin pigmentation

> Thrombophlebitis

> Lipodermatosclerosis

> Oedema

> Atrophie blanche

# Referral to Vascular Service

→ Refer people with bleeding varicose veins to a vascular service immediately.

→ Refer patients to a vascular service if they have any of the following:

> Symptomatic primary or symptomatic recurrent varicose veins.

> Lower-limb skin changes (pigmentation or eczema) that are thought to be caused by chronic venous insufficiency.

> Superficial vein thrombosis (hard, painful veins) and suspected venous incompetence.

> A venous leg ulcer (a break in the skin below the knee that has not healed within two weeks).

> A healed venous leg ulcer.

## Safety Netting

» If the varicose veins bleed, recommend that the patient lies down and lifts their leg above their heart, applies pressure and seeks urgent medical advice.

*References*

National Institute for Health and Care Excellence (2013). *Varicose veins: diagnosis and management.* https://www.nice.org.uk/guidance/cg168

# Deep Vein Thrombosis

DVT is when a blood clot (thrombus) develops within the deep veins, commonly in the legs or pelvis, which may completely or partially obstruct blood flow within the veins. It often causes pain and swelling within the large veins running through the calf or the thigh. It affects one in 1,000 people per year. If treated swiftly, a DVT may not have serious consequences. However, if missed, a clot may break away, forming an embolus, and pass into the arteries of the lungs, leading to a PE.

## Risk Factors

➤ **Permanent**
  › Past medical history or family history of PE/DVT
  › Family history of thrombophilia
  › Obesity
  › > 50 years
  › Vasculitis
  › Cancer
  › Male gender

➤ **Temporary**
  › Immobility (post-op/long-haul flight)
  › Trauma
  › Hormone therapy (COCP or HRT)
  › Pregnancy
  › Chemotherapy
  › Hospitalisation

## *History*

» Focused questions
  › Ask when they first noticed pain in their leg and how long they have had it for.
  › Ask about the location (thigh or calf), character (dull or heavy ache), pain severity or exacerbating factors (e.g. bending the knee upwards).
  › Ask when they first noticed the swelling, how long they have had it for and whether it started suddenly (DVT) or gradually (oedema).

» Associated history – Ask if there has been a change in colour or temperature (warm).

» Risk factors – Determine if they have experienced immobility, travel, operations, trauma or pregnancy.

» Past history – Ask if they have had a previous DVT, PE (lungs), cancer or a clotting disorder.

» Drug history – Check if they have taken COCP, HRT or had cancer treatment (chemotherapy).

» Social history – Ask if they smoke and what their occupation is.

» Family history – Ask if there is a family history of DVT/PE or clotting disorders.

## RED FLAGS

» PE – Chest pain that is worse when breathing in, any breathlessness that came on suddenly or any sudden collapse.

## Differential Diagnosis

| Limb ischaemia | Calf pain that is worse on exertion and relieved by rest. Predictable claudication distance. Associated with Erectile dysfunction. |
|---|---|
| Cellulitis | Localised pain and warmth over the lower leg(s). The patient may feel feverish and/or fatigued. OE: fever, tachycardia, redness and pain over the affected area and a warm rash. |
| Ruptured Baker's cyst | History of sudden onset, sharp pain or tightness behind the knee, radiating down to the calf. A feeling of liquid moving down the back of the leg. OE: redness and swelling of the calf. |
| Thrombophlebitis | Superficial inflammation of a vein. May cause pain, redness and swelling. OE: a tender and hard vein. |

## Examination

» Vitals – BP, pulse (persistent tachycardia), BMI (obesity), temperature and respiratory rate (increased in PE).

» Chest – Auscultate the chest (pleural rub – to identify PE).

» Abdomen – Palpate the abdomen for any masses (pelvic or colon cancer).

» Perform a leg exam.

  › Inspection – Inspect the legs for any colour change (redness). Look for superficial veins (non-varicose veins).

> › Palpation – Feel along the large veins (thrombophlebitis) for tenderness as well as the back of the calf. Check for warmth (DVT or cellulitis). Assess for pitting oedema (unilateral).

» Specialist

> › Measure the calf swelling at 10cm below the tibial tuberosity (>3cm discrepancy).

## Investigations

» Bloods – D-dimer (if negative, DVT unlikely), FBC and CRP (cellulitis).

D-dimer tests have a relatively high sensitivity but low specificity. A negative D-dimer can often exclude a DVT; however, a positive D-dimer does not diagnose a DVT, but would identify that further investigations are warranted. Other causes of a raised D-dimer include pregnancy, liver disease, inflammation, malignancy, trauma and recent surgery.

» ECG – PE signs (sinus tachycardia and S1Q3T3).

» CXR – If PE is suspected.

» Ultrasound (USS) – USS of proximal leg vein.

» CTPA – If PE is suspected.

### Two-level Modified Wells' Clinical Score

| Points | Outcome |
|--------|---------|
| >=2 | DVT likely |
| <=1 | DVT unlikely |

## Management

### Conservative

✓ Offer smoking-cessation advice.

✓ If the patient's BMI is >25, recommend that they lose weight .

### Medical

✓ If DVT is likely (Wells' score of >=2), refer them to hospital/A&E to organise a USS of the proximal leg vein within four hours. If it is not possible to perform a USS within four hours, offer a D-dimer test, give a 24-hour dose of anticoagulant and organise a USS within 24 hours.

✓ If DVT is unlikely (Wells' score of <=1), request a D-dimer. If it is positive, refer them to hospital (see previous bullet). If it is negative, consider an alternative diagnosis.

✓ Pregnancy – Do not use Wells' score or D-dimers. Refer them to hospital/A&E for assessment.

✓ Follow-up on DVT – A specialist may start the patient on an anticoagulant (warfarin or rivaroxaban), typically for three months. Do not offer elastic graduated compression stockings after a proximal DVT. Recommend exercise (regular walking) and elevating the leg when sitting.

✓ Unprovoked DVT – Offer a thrombophilia test and exclude undiagnosed cancer.

✓ Travel – Delay travel until at least two weeks after anticoagulant treatment. Do *not* travel within two weeks of diagnosis of DVT.

## Safety Netting

» Advise the patient to seek urgent medical advice if they notice any SOB, haemoptysis or increased leg swelling.

*References*

National Institute for Health and Care Excellence (2020). *Venous thromboembolic diseases: diagnosis, management and thrombophilia testing.* https://www.nice.org.uk/guidance/ng158

National Institute for Health and Care Excellence (2012). *Rivaroxaban for the treatment of deep vein thrombosis and prevention of recurrent deep vein thrombosis and pulmonary embolism.* https://www.nice.org.uk/guidance/ta261

# Heart Failure

HF is when the ability of the heart to maintain adequate circulation of blood is impaired, which is often due to structural damage (muscle/valve) or functional impairment (ventricular filling/ejection). This can cause symptoms such as SOB, fatigue, peripheral oedema and crepitations (basal). Around 50% of patients with HF die within five years of diagnosis, and it is a leading cause of hospital admissions in the over 65s.

## Causes of HF

- Myocardial – Coronary artery disease (most common cause, e.g. MI) and HTN, cardiomyopathy.
  - Valvular heart disease (AS), arrhythmia (e.g. AF), congenital heart disease and pericardial disease (constrictive pericarditis).

- High output states – Severe anaemia, thyrotoxicosis, septicemia, liver failure and AV shunt.
- Volume overload – CKD and nephrotic syndrome.
- Drugs – NSAIDs, b-blockers, CCB, alcohol and cocaine.
- Other – Sleep apnoea, obesity, haemochromatosis and hypothyroidism.

## *History*

- » Focused questions
  - Ask about dyspnoea; whether it comes and goes, or is there all the time; what the triggers are (sitting up/rest); what makes it worse (walking); whether there is orthopnoea (breathlessness worse on lying flat); how they exercise; and how much walking they do.

- » Associated history – Ask if their sleep is affected, if they have paroxysmal nocturnal dyspnoea (PND), how many pillows they use, and whether they have chest pain, a cough, any phlegm (pink), oedema, palpitations or fatigue.
- » Past history – Ask if they have had HTN, raised cholesterol, angina, DM, an MI or AF.
- » Drug history – Ask if they have taken NSAIDs, b-blockers or CCB, and if they have allergies.
- » Social history – Ask if they smoke, drink alcohol or take recreational drugs.
- » Family history – Determine if they have a family history of HF.
- » Conduct a depression screen.

## RED FLAGS

Cardiac chest pain (MI/ACS), sudden onset SOB and pink phlegm (pulmonary oedema).

## Examination

» Vitals – BP (HTN), pulse (irregular or tachycardia), temperature, respiratory rate, oxygen saturation, weight (increased) and JVP (raised).

» Cardiovascular – Check for a displaced apex beat and listen for heart sounds (AS). Palpate the legs for oedema (HF) and DVT (PE).

» Respiratory – Auscultate the chest for bibasal crepitations and pleural effusion.

» Abdomen – Palpate for hepatomegaly and ascites.

## Investigations

» Bloods – FBC (low haemoglobin [Hb] shows anaemia, and a raised white cell count [WCC] shows sepsis), pro b-type natriuretic peptide (proBNP) (CCF), U&Es, LFTs, TFT and HbA1c.

ProBNPs are amino acids that are secreted when the heart muscle is stretched. They are raised in HF, and used as a screening blood test prior to performing an echo.

› Normal levels <400pg/ml

› Raised levels 400–2,000pg/ml

› High levels >2,000pg/ml

» ECG – CCF (LVH), PE (AF, RBBB and S1Q3T3), arrhythmia and a previous MI.

» CXR – Cardiomyopathy, cardiomegaly, pulmonary oedema and pleural effusion.

» Lung function – Peak flow or spirometry (COPD).

» Echo – HF (ejection fraction <40%) and valvular dysfunction.

» Urine – Urinalysis.

» Others – Transoesophageal echocardiogram (TOE) and cardiac MRI.

## Management

### Conservative

✓ Diet – Advise them to restrict their fluid intake if there is evidence of dilutional hyponatremia, or if there are high levels of salt or fluid consumption. Aim for <6g of salt per day.

✓ Smoking – Offer smoking-cessation advice.

✓ Alcohol – Advise them to reduce their alcohol consumption to <=14 units a week.

✓ Offer the annual flu jab and a one-off pneumococcal injection.

✓ Air travel – Caution those with a severe HF; it is a contraindication for air travel.

✓ Driving – The advice to be given depends on their New York Heart Association (NYHA) class and whether they are a group one or two driver.

### Medical

✓ Initiate an ACEi and b-blocker: 'Start low and go slow.'

> Ramipril – Titrate twice weekly until the maximum tolerated dose reached. Consider ARB if the ACEi is not tolerated or is contraindicated (valve disease).

> Bisoprolol.

> Aldosterone antagonist; e.g. spironolactone 25mg od.

**For dose changes (ACEi, ARB or aldosterone antagonist):**

> U&Es one week before and after each dose.

> Check BP before and after each dose change. For a b-blocker, check heart rate (HR).

> Once the target dose has been achieved, monitor them monthly for three months, then six monthly.

✓ Diuretics – These are used to relieve the symptoms of HF; titrate up and down accordingly. For patients with a preserved ejection fraction, offer a low to medium dose of furosemide (<80mg/day).

✓ CCB – Avoid diltiazem and verapamil in cases of HF with a reduced ejection fraction.

✓ If an ACEi or ARB is contraindicated, seek specialist advice.

## Referral

→ Cardiac rehab – Refer patients with stable HF to exercise-based cardiac rehab.

→ Cardiologist – Refer the patient to a specialty for the management of HF if they have poor symptom control.

→ HF nurse – Consider the referral of stable patients in the community to the HF nurse for dose control.

→ For patients with high proBNP who have a poor prognosis, refer them urgently to a specialist within two weeks.

→ For patients with raised levels, refer them within six weeks.

→ Refer patients with suspected HF and a previous MI urgently to have a transthoracic doppler 2D echo and a specialist assessment within two weeks.

→ Consider admitting the patient if there are any red flags, MI, reduced oxygen saturations (<92%), tachycardia (>130bpm) or tachypnoea (>30 breaths per minute).

## Safety Netting

» If there are any red-flag symptoms (worsening SOB, chest pain or pink sputum), advise the patient to seek medical advice.

---

### References

National Institute for Health and Care Excellence (2018). *Chronic heart failure in adults: diagnosis and management.* https://www.nice.org.uk/guidance/ng106

National Institute for Health and Care Excellence (2014). *Acute heart failure: diagnosis and management.* https://www.nice.org.uk/guidance/cg187

# Phlebitis and Thrombophlebitis

Phlebitis is the inflammation of a vein, and it can be caused by any damage to the blood vessel wall, an abnormality with coagulation, or poor venous flow. When a blood clot forms and is associated with this inflammation, this is known as thrombophlebitis.

Virchow's triad gives the three cardinal risk factors for a clot to form:

> ➤ Hypercoagulability
>
> ➤ Blood flow stasis
>
> ➤ An insult to the blood vessel wall (from infection, trauma or inflammation)

## Other Risk Factors

> ➤ Pregnancy
>
> ➤ Obesity
>
> ➤ OCP
>
> ➤ Smoking
>
> ➤ Thrombophilia

## *History*

> » The lower extremities tend to be affected the most in superficial thrombophlebitis; however, this can also be due to an intravenous cannula.
>
> » Sclerotherapy can cause iatrogenic chemical phlebitis.
>
> » Thrombophlebitis from a varicose vein can present as a tender knot. This can be associated with erythema and potential bleeding as the inflammation moves through the vein wall.
>
> » It is important to look out for septic phlebitis. This can occur due to the long-term use of an intravenous cannula. It is also common in intravenous drug users, who may use equipment that is not clean.

## Examination

> » Examine for any tenderness, swelling or erythema along the vein.
>
> » The long saphenous vein is usually where spontaneous thrombophlebitis develops, often with varicose veins.

## Differentials

> ➤ Cellulitis
>
> ➤ DVT

➤ Lymphangitis

➤ Ruptured medial head of the gastrocnemius

## Investigations

» Usually, no investigations are needed.

» If a septic cannula is suspected, it should be removed and sent for culture.

» Venography should be avoided as the contrast medium can worsen the condition.

## Management

*Conservative*

✓ Elastic support of the limb reduces swelling and eases discomfort.

✓ Severe thrombophlebitis does not usually require bed rest unless there is severe pain on movement. The affected extremity should be elevated.

✓ Exercise reduces pain and the possibility of a DVT. Patients with reduced mobility should be on prophylaxis for a DVT.

*Medical*

✓ Consider topical analgesia, with NSAID creams applied to the superficial vein area.

✓ Hirudoid cream (heparinoid) shortens the duration of the symptoms.

✓ Consider an intermediate dose of low molecular weight heparin for at least one month.

✓ Consider a fondaparinux 2.5mg od for at least 30 days.

# 3

# Respiratory

## Asthma

Asthma is a chronic respiratory disease that is characterised by the inflammation of the airways, hypersensitivity, and reversible, reduced outflow (bronchospasm) obstruction. It is a common disorder with around 5 million people in the UK suffering from it. The exact cause of asthma is not known; however, a complex interaction between genes, infections and environmental exposure are believed to play a part. The main symptoms of asthma include breathlessness, chest tightness, wheezing and coughing (worse at night or early morning). An obvious allergen – such as pets, pollen or foodstuffs – may also be elicited from the patient, and family history is often asthma positive. Asthma patients may also have had eczema as a child or allergic rhinitis (hay fever).

### Suspect asthma in a patient with the following:

» A wheeze, a dry cough, SOB or chest tightness.

» Daily, episodic, diurnal (night or early morning) or seasonal variation.

» Triggers that make the symptoms worse (e.g. exercise, an upper respiratory tract infection [URTI] or emotion).

» Past medical history or family history of atopy.

» Check for occupational asthma: symptoms are better on days away from work or better on holidays.

» Do not use symptoms alone without objective tests, nor should an atopic disorder be used alone to diagnose asthma.

### Pathophysiology

Associated chronic inflammation leads to hyper-responsive airways, which constrict easily in response to a wide range of exogenous and endogenous stimuli, leading to recurrent symptoms and variable airflow limitations.

### History

» Focused questions

› Ask when the cough or breathlessness started and how long the symptoms last for.

> › Ask when the cough is worse (look for diurnal variation).

> › Ask if anything makes it better or worse.

> › Determine whether there are changes with the season, being away from work or after using an inhaler.

> › Ask about the impact on symptoms of exercise, stress, pets, cold weather and pollution.

» Associated history – Ask about wheezing, chest pain or a tight chest.

» Past history

> › Ask about atopy (hay fever, eczema or urticaria).

> › Determine if there have been any asthma attacks in the last year, A&E attendances or Intensive Therapy Unit (ITU) admissions.

» Drug history

> › Ask how often they are using their inhalers and what their inhaler technique is.

> › Ask if they have used any oral steroids in the last year.

» Social history

> › Ask if they smoke, and if so, how many a day.

> › Ask if they do any sports, what they do for work and whether any of these exacerbate their symptoms.

» Family history – Ask if there is a family history of atopy (whether anyone in the family suffers from asthma, eczema or hay fever).

## RED FLAGS

Severe SOB, the inability to complete sentences, exhaustion and confusion.

» RCP questions to assess asthma in the last month

> › *'Have you had any difficulty sleeping because of your asthma symptoms (including a cough)?'*

> › *'Have you had your usual asthma symptoms during the day (cough, wheezing or a tight chest)?'*

> › *'Has your asthma interfered with your usual activities, such as housework, school, etc.?'*

## Examination

- » Vitals – BP, pulse, temperature, respiratory rate and oxygen saturation.

- » Respiratory
  - › Inspection – Inspect for respiratory distress, particularly regarding the use of accessory muscles, barrel chest, tachypnoea and the patient's ability to complete sentences.
  - › Auscultation – Auscultate the chest for a prolonged expiratory phase. Check for a wheeze. Look out for a silent chest.

## Differential Diagnosis

| Pneumonia | They will usually bring up phlegm or sputum, and have a fever, sweat or chest pain when coughing. |
| --- | --- |
| PE | This can come on suddenly, causing pleuritic pain, breathlessness, haemoptysis and calf pain. |
| GORD | Causes heartburn that is worse when lying flat, excessive saliva (water brash) and an acid taste in the mouth. |
| CF | Frequent chest infections and problems since birth. |

## Investigations

- » Blood tests are often not necessary. An FBC could show eosinophilia.

- » A CXR may show an overinflated chest. Request a CXR if the diagnosis seems unclear.

- » Peak flow can show reversibility with a beta-agonist or inhaled steroids.
  - › Monitor the peak expiratory flow rate (PEFR) for two to four weeks if there is any diagnostic uncertainty. A diurnal variation of >20% is a positive result.
  - › You can calculate the following:
    - - Diurnal variation % = (highest - lowest PEFR) / highest PEFR x 100

- » Spirometry can also illustrate reversibility
  - › Spirometry should be offered to all symptomatic patients (with symptoms for less than five years). Results can be affected by an inhaled corticosteroid (ICS).
  - › The first second of forced expiratory volume / forced vital capacity (FEV1/FVC) <0.7 suggests an airflow obstruction. Offer reversibility testing/trial.
  - › An FEV1/FVC >0.7 shows no evidence of obstruction. Remember that a normal result when asymptomatic does not exclude asthma.

> ›  In adults, an FEV1 with >=12% improvement and 200ml increase in volume after a beta-agonist/corticosteroid is a positive result. A result of <400ml in FEV1 strongly suggests asthma. In children, an FEV1 with a 12% improvement is a positive result.

## Management

*Asthma control test*

✓  This is a score out of 25: <20 is poor control, 20–24 is well-controlled and 25 is under control.

*Conservative*

✓  Advise the patient to avoid allergens that may trigger any symptoms. For example, for dust mites, remove carpets, curtains and soft toys; cover pillows and mattresses; perform regular hoovering; and avoid being around cats or dogs if they are found to increase symptoms.

✓  Breastfeeding protects the baby against asthma.

✓  Advise them to stop smoking and avoid passive smoking where possible.

✓  Suggest they reduce their weight and recommend exercise programmes.

✓  Ensure the patient has a personalised care plan in place.

*Medical*

✓  Check their inhaler technique and demonstrate it correctly.

✓  Consider the following definitions:

> ›  Low dose ICS – 400mcg or less of budesonide/beclomethasone or equivalent.

> ›  Medium dose ICS – 400–800mcg of budesonide/beclomethasone or equivalent.

> ›  High dose ICS – <800mcg of budesonide/beclomethasone or equivalent.

*NICE Guidelines*

✓  Review their response four to eight weeks after each change in treatment:

> ›  Offer an inhaled short-acting beta-agonist (SABA) as required (e.g. salbutamol).

> ›  If the patients is using salbutamol inhaler, or their asthma symptoms are occuring three or more times a week, and they have nocturnal symptoms, then add a low dose ICS. A higher dose may be required in previous/current smokers. Start the ICS at twice a day and reduce it to once a day if under good control (maintenance therapy).

> ›  Add a leukotriene receptor antagonist (LTRA) (e.g. montelukast).

> › Add a long-acting beta-agonist (LABA) (e.g. salmeterol). Consider stopping the LTRA if there is no response.

> › Consider changing the LABA and ICS to a maintenance dose and a reliever therapy (MART) regime; e.g. Symbicort/Fostair with a low maintenance dose of ICS. Increase the MART regime to a moderate ICS dose if the asthma is poorly controlled. If there are ongoing symptoms, increase the MART regime to a high ICS dose.

> › Refer them to the GP or specialist care.

### British Thoracic Society (BTS) Guidance

✓ This recommends initiating low dose steroids as a first-line treatment and then consider increasing if the patient is using SABA three or more times a week:

> › SABA PRN plus a low dose of ICS.

> › Add LABA and a low dose of ICS (as a combination if possible).

> › If there is no response to the LABA, stop it and increase the ICS to a moderate dose.

> › Add an LTRA, theophylline or long-acting muscarinic antagonist (LAMA).

> › Refer the patient to a GP with special interest (GPwSI) in asthma or specialist care.

---

## References

National Institute for Health and Care Excellence (2017). *Asthma: diagnosis, monitoring and chronic asthma management*. https://www.nice.org.uk/guidance/ng80

Scottish Intercollegiate Guidelines Network (2019). *British guideline on the management of asthma*. https://www.sign.ac.uk/sign-158-british-guideline-on-the-management-of-asthma

National Institute for Health and Care Excellence (n.d.). *NICE Quality and Outcomes Framework indicator*. https://www.nice.org.uk/standards-and-indicators/qofindicators

# Cough

A cough reflex is the body's first line of defence for preventing any foreign bodies from entering the respiratory tract. Coughing is a non-specific symptom that is due to the irritation of the airways, anywhere from the pharynx to the lungs. It may be caused by a number of unrelated conditions, such as infections, gastric reflux, airway obstruction or foreign-body aspiration. However, most acute coughs are self-limiting and clear up within three to four weeks. When taking a history, it is often useful to distinguish between acute (less than three weeks) and chronic (more than eight weeks) causes while also attempting to rule out the more sinister causes, such as lung cancer and/or a PE.

## History

- » Focused questions
    - › Ask when the patient first noticed the cough, how long they have had it for, and whether it is dry or wet (chesty).
    - › Ask about the frequency, aggravating (exercise, stress or pets) or relieving factors (inhalers, season, work or after eating).
- » Associated history – Ask if they have SOB, chest pain, reduced appetite or weight loss.
- » Past history – Ask if they have taken an ACEi, a b-blocker, NSAIDs, or meds that worsen GORD, OCP or HRT (PE).
- » Social history – Ask about their occupation (industry, farming, coal mining or construction), if they have occupational asthma, and whether they drink alcohol, have taken long-haul flights or have pets at home.
- » Family history – Ask if there is a family history of asthma or CF.

## Causes of the Cough Based upon Duration

- ➤ Sudden onset – Inhaled foreign body, acute PE or pneumothorax.
- ➤ Acute (less than three weeks) – URTI, acute bronchitis, croup or pneumonia.
- ➤ Subacute (three to eight weeks) – Persistent bronchitis/pneumonia or pertussis (whooping cough).
- ➤ Chronic (more than eight weeks) – Asthma, COPD, lung cancer, GORD, TB, postnasal drip, ACEi or bronchiectasis.

## RED FLAGS

Confusion, pleuritic chest pain, weight loss, hoarseness of voice and haemoptysis.

## Differential Diagnosis

| | |
|---|---|
| URTI | Acute cough, coryzal symptoms, fever, myalgia, pharyngitis and otorrhoea. OE: red throat, bulging eardrum, pyrexia and cervical nodes (CNs). |
| Postnasal drip | A feeling of liquid running down the back of the throat, sneezing, and nasal congestion or blockage. OE: inflamed turbinates. |
| GORD | A burning sensation over the epigastrium, moving up to the neck. Worsened by lying down or bending over. Acid brash and water brash may be present. Can cause painful swallowing or nocturnal asthma. Relieved by antacids, but related to spicy food, alcohol or hot caffeinated drinks. OE: epigastric pain. |
| PE | Sudden SOB with pleuritic chest pain. May also have haemoptysis and tachycardia. Risk factors: DVT, travel, trauma, OCP and malignancy. OE: tachypnoea with calf tenderness. |
| TB | Night sweats, haemoptysis, lymphadenopathy and weight loss. OE: Cachectic appearance and lymph node (LN) bilaterally in the cervical chain. |
| Pneumonia | Pleuritic chest pain associated with fever, productive cough and dyspnoea. OE: coarse crackles with dull percussion notes and fever. |
| Asthma | Diurnal variation, wheeze and SOB, reversible with salbutamol/steroids. OE: expiratory wheeze and reduced pulmonary function (PF). |
| COPD | Heavy smoker, productive cough, >35 years old and lacks reversibility on spirometry. OE: cyanosis, hyperinflation and wheeze. |
| Lung cancer | Heavy smoker, weight loss, haemoptysis, hoarseness of voice and finger clubbing. OE: cachectic appearance, LN in the neck in the supraclavicular area, and finger clubbing. |
| Pertussis (whooping cough) | Ongoing cough (>14 days) with paroxysms of coughing (inspiration followed in rapid succession by an expiratory hacking cough, mainly at night), coryza, mild fever, vomiting, inspiratory whoop, and cyanosis/apnoea. Can last from two to six weeks. |
| Pneumothorax | Sudden onset of SOB with pleuritic chest pain. OE: hyperresonance, reduced breath sounds, chest-wall movement, tracheal deviation away, tachycardia and low BP (tension pneumothorax). |
| Bronchiectasis | Chronic cough, daily production of mucopurulent sputum (thick and viscous), recurrent infections, wheeze, haemoptysis and fatigue. OE: coarse crackles (early inspiration) and finger clubbing. |

## Admission for Community-Acquired Pneumonia

BTS suggests using CRB-65, which is a four-point score used to gauge the severity of pneumonia, helping clinicians in GP to decide when to admit patients. Each area has a score of 1 point if present; a total score of 0 does not require admission, for 1–2 consider a hospital referral, and >3 requires urgent hospital admission:

» Confusion (disorientation regarding time, place and person)

» Respiratory rate >30 breaths per minute

» BP <90/60

» >65 years

# Examination

» Vitals – BP, pulse, temperature, respiratory rate, oxygen saturations and weight.

» Respiratory

› Hands – Clubbing and peripheral cyanosis.

› Percussion – Check for a percussion note or vocal fremitus (pneumonia).

› Auscultation – Listen to the chest for crepitations, wheezing and reduced air entry.

» LNs – Examine the head and neck for LNs (URTI and TB).

» Cardiovascular – Listen for heart sounds and palpate the legs for oedema (HF) and DVT (PE).

» ENT – Examine the throat (tonsilitis) and ears (otitis media) for associated features of URTI.

# Investigations

» Bloods – FBC, U&E, ESR, CRP, LFTs and proBNP (CCF).

» Sputum – MCS.

» ECG – CCF (LVH) and PE.

» CXR – To exclude chest infection, TB and lung cancer.

» Peak flow – Asthma, reversible with a beta-agonist.

» Spirometry – COPD (lacks reversibility).

» Specialist – Ziehl-Neelsen (ZN) staining (TB), blood glucose (BG), ventilation-perfusion (VQ) scan or CT pulmonary angiography (CTPA), bronchoscopy and CT chest.

## Management

### Asthma *(see Asthma section, page 79)*

#### Conservative

✓    Advise them to avoid allergens and provide education re inhalers.

#### Medical

✓    Salbutamol, inhaled steroids or LTRA. Follow NICE or BTS guidance. Consider oral steroids in acute exacerbation.

### COPD *(see Chronic Obstructive Pulmonary Disease section, page 90)*

#### Conservative

✓    Advise them to stop smoking (most important) and offer pulmonary rehabilitation.

#### Medical

✓    Offer ipratropium bromide, LABAs, LABA plus ICS, or oral steroids. Provide a rescue pack (oral steroids plus antibiotics).

### PE

✓    If this is suspected, refer them to hospital. Start them on LMWH, and if confirmed, start them on warfarin for three months if there are transient risk factors (surgery, trauma or immobility) or six months if they are permanent risk factors.

### Dyspepsia

#### Conservative

✓    Advise them to avoid chilli and spicy food; cut down on caffeine and alcohol; stop smoking; eat small, regular meals; and ensure that the last meal of the day is several hours before bedtime.

#### Medical

✓    Consider alginates (Gaviscon), H2 antagonist (ranitidine) and PPI (omeprazole).

### Postnasal drip

✓    Advise them to avoid triggers/allergens.

✓    Trial oral antihistamines or nasal steroids.

### TB

✓    Refer the patient to a specialist, conduct contract tracing and instigate triple therapy.

### Drug induced

✓ Stop the ACEi and change to ARB. It may take a few months to settle down.

### LRTI

✓ Initiate antibiotics, considering doxycycline, amoxicillin or erythromycin / clarithromycin. Warn the patient about side effects (diarrhoea/nausea).

### URTI

✓ Reassure them and explain why antibiotics are not needed, advise them to use OTC meds (honey, cough medication containing guaifenesin or dextromethorphan, and paracetamol/NSAIDs) and fluids; consider a delayed antibiotic prescription.

### Whooping cough

✓ Advise them to rest, increase their fluid intake, and take paracetamol or NSAIDs. Offer clarithromycin or azithromycin if their cough has lasted longer than 21 days. Consider erythromycin if the patient is pregnant. Advise them that it may take several weeks for the cough to resolve. Advise them to stop going to school/work until two days after the antibiotics have been completed, or 21 days after the onset of symptoms if they are not treated. This is a notifiable disease.

## Cancer Referral Guidelines (NICE, 2018)

→ 2WW – For unexplained haemoptysis in patients >40 years, with a CXR that suggests lung cancer (pleural effusion, pleural mass and suspicious lung lesion).

→ Urgent CXR is required for the following:

> Two or more of these features in a patient >40 years: cough, fatigue, SOB, chest pain, weight loss or appetite loss.

→ Or a persistent or recurrent chest infection, finger clubbing, cervical/ supraclavicular LN, chest signs consistent with lung cancer (pleural effusion, persistent consolidation) or thrombocytosis.

→ Refer the patient to oncology if you are unsure of the diagnosis.

→ Admit the patient to hospital if they have these respiratory features:

> Respiratory rate >30 breaths per minute

> Pulse/HR >130

> BP <90/60

> Oxygen saturations <94%, or <92% in COPD patients

> Central cyanosis

> › PEFR <33% of predicted value

> › Altered consciousness

> › Use of accessory muscles for respiration

## Safety Netting

» If the cough persists for three to four weeks, perform a review. If there are any red-flag symptoms, advise the patient to seek medical advice urgently; e.g. symptoms indicating a cancer referral if required.

---

## References

National Institute for Health and Care Excellence(2019). *Cough (acute): antimicrobial prescribing.* https://www.nice.org.uk/guidance/ng120

National Institute for Health and Care Excellence (2015). *Suspected cancer: recognition and referral.* https://www.nice.org.uk/guidance/ng12

British Thoracic Society (2009). *Guidelines for the management of community acquired pneumonia in adults.*

www.brit-thoracic.org.uk/clinical-information/pneumonia/pneumonia-guidelines

# Chronic Obstructive Pulmonary Disease

COPD is an umbrella term used to describe chronic lung diseases, including emphysema and chronic bronchitis. It describes a progressive airflow obstruction that is not reversible and does not change markedly over several months. It is the fourth leading cause of death worldwide. The main cause of COPD is believed to be due to cigarette smoking (both active and passive); however, inherited disorders such as alpha-1 antitrypsin deficiency and air pollution have also been implicated. It is more common in men and diagnosis is often made by the time they reach around 50 years of age. The classification of COPD into 'blue bloaters' and 'pink puffers' has been discarded in recent times. Symptoms vary depending on the stage of the disease; however, breathlessness, coughing and excessive sputum production, as well as wheezing and recurrent chest infections are often found.

## History

» A diagnosis of COPD should be considered in patients >35 years who have a risk factor (generally, smoking) and who present with one or more of the following symptoms:

› Exertional breathlessness

› A chronic cough

› A wheeze

› Regular sputum production

› Recurrent chest infections

› The absence of asthma features

» Focused questions

› Ask when the symptoms first started and how long they last for.

› Ask whether their coughing is all the time or if it comes and goes, and whether it is dry or wet (chesty).

› Ask about sputum production and its colour (grey, yellow or green).

› Ask if there is any breathlessness at rest or on exertion, or any wheezing, and whether it is getting worse over time.

› Ask how far the patient can walk before they get breathless, how they cope with stairs, and how far they could walk before.

The Medical Research Council (MRC) dyspnoea scale is used to assess the degree of disability caused by breathlessness in cases of COPD, rather than the severity of the underlying pathology.

*The Medical Research Council (MRC) Breathlessness Scale*

| Grade | Degree of breathlessness related to activities |
|-------|------------------------------------------------|
| 1 | Not troubled by breathlessness except on strenuous exercise |
| 2 | Short of breath when hurrying on the level or walking up a slight hill |
| 3 | Walks slower than most people on the level, stops after a mile or so, or stops after 15 minutes of walking at own pace |
| 4 | Stops for breath after walking about 100 yards or after a few minutes on level ground |
| 5 | Too breathless to leave the house, or brethless when dressing. |

» Associated history – Ask about their mood, if they have suffered any weight loss, and how they are sleeping.

» Past history – Ask them about exacerbations in the last year or if they have had any chest infections.

» Drug history – Ask if they have taken inhalers, or oral steroids in the last year.

» Social history – Ask if they smoke or drink alcohol, and ask about their occupation (coal/hard-rock miners and tunnel workers).

» Family history – Ask if there is a family history of COPD or alpha-1 antitrypsin deficiency.

## RED FLAGS

» Cor pulmonale – Ankle swelling and paroxysmal nocturnal dyspnoea.

» COPD – Early onset symptoms in a non-smoker with no family history.

» Chest pain or haemoptysis – Consider an alternative diagnosis.

## Differentials

➤ Asthma

➤ Pneumonia

➤ HF

## Differentiating COPD from Asthma

In principle, asthma is a condition with a reversible airway obstruction caused by exposure to precipitants, whilst COPD and has an irreversible airway obstruction caused by damage to the lung parenchyma. Be aware that COPD and asthma may co-exist.

| Clinical Features | COPD | Asthma |
| --- | --- | --- |
| Smoker or ex-smoker | Nearly all | Possibly |
| Age <35 years | Rare | Often |
| Chronic productive cough | Common | Uncommon |
| Breathlessness | Persistent and progressive | Variable |
| Waking at night with SOB/wheezing | Uncommon | Common |
| Eczema, hay fever and allergies | Uncommon | Common |
| Diurnal variation in symptoms | Uncommon | Common |

## Examination

- » Vitals – BP, pulse, temperature, respiratory rate and oxygen saturations.
- » Respiratory
  - › Inspection – Inspect for signs of respiratory distress, use of accessory muscles, barrel chest, tachypnoea, cyanosis (central/peripheral), hyperinflated chest, pursing of lips on expiration and raised JVP.
  - › Palpation – Check for hyperresonance.
  - › Auscultation – Listen to the chest for crepitations, decreased breath sounds and wheezing.
- » Cardiovascular – Check for pedal oedema.

## Investigations

- » Spirometry – Post bronchodilator spirometry is used to diagnose as well as to assess the severity of the airflow obstruction in COPD.
  - › COPD is clinically diagnosed via spirometry where there is evidence of irreversible airway obstruction. The QOF requires evidence of reversibility testing with an inhaled bronchodilator; <400ml in FEV1 after a trial suggests COPD.

> › An FEV1/FVC ratio <0.7 (70%) and FEV1 <80% is predicted.

> › If FEV1 is >80% of what was predicted, then the diagnosis is made only if the patient is symptomatic (i.e. has SOB or a cough).

> › Clinically significant COPD is not present if FEV1 and the FEV1/FVC ratio return to normal with drug therapy.

» Peak flow – To exclude asthma (COPD – irreversible).

» ECG/echo – If cor pulmonale is suspected.

» Bloods – These are often not indicated; FBC (anaemia and polycythaemia) and BNP (cor pulmonale).

» Sputum culture (MC&S) if sputum is produced.

» CXR – If there is overinflated chest bullae, suspected emphysema or an unclear diagnosis.

## Management

### Conservative

✓ Severity – Score their severity using the MRC dyspnoea scale, BMI, frequency of exacerbations, exercise capacity and the presence of cor pulmonale.

✓ Smoking – Offer smoking-cessation advice or refer them to a smoking-cessation clinic. Stopping smoking is the single most beneficial intervention that can be offered.

✓ Exercise – Advise them to reduce their weight to a BMI <25; you may recommend exercise programmes. If their BMI is <20, then offer them nutritional supplements to increase their caloric intake.

✓ Employment – Advise them to avoid employment that involves health hazards that may worsen COPD.

✓ Chest physio – Offer chest physiotherapy if the patient has excessive sputum secretions. The active cycle of breathing techniques (ACBT) is a series of breathing techniques that has been recognised by NICE to loosen secretions and help improve severe ventilation issues.

✓ Self management – Refer them to self-management programmes and offer a personalised care plan.

### Medical (Based on NICE COPD Guidelines)

✓ Bronchodilator (SABA) – Initiate SABA (e.g. salbutamol) or short-acting muscarinic antagonists (SAMA) (e.g. ipratropium bromide one qds). If the patient remains breathless or has exacerbations, check their FEV1.

✓ LAMA plus LABA – Add LABA (e.g. salmeterol) and LAMA (e.g. tiotropium od) to those with confirmed COPD or who retain SOB despite SABA or SAMA.

✓ LABA plus ICS – Add LABA plus an ICS in a combination inhaler (e.g. symbicort) or a LAMA.

✓ LAMA plus LABA plus ICS – For those who still have SOB or have recurrent exacerbations, offer a LAMA and a LABA plus ICS combination inhaler (combined triple inhaler; e.g. Trelegy Ellipta od).

✓ Spacer – Consider whether the patient has severe osteoarthritis (OA) or has problems using the inhaler.

✓ Nebulisers – Consider this for those with distressing dyspnoea despite the maximum inhaler therapy. Only continue if this relieves symptoms, increases ADLs, raises exercise capacity or improves lung function.

✓ Oral steroids – Advanced COPD may need long-term steroids. Use the lowest dose possible and monitor for osteoporosis.

✓ Offer oral theophylline after a trial of short- and long-acting bronchodilators, or in patients who are unable to use inhaled therapy.

✓ Mucolytic – Consider this in patients with a chronic cough or sputum production (Carbocisteine 375mg, three times a day [tds]) Continue if benefits are gained after four weeks. Exercise caution if the patient has a peptic ulcer (PU).

✓ Exacerbations – Increase bronchodilator inhalers, give oral antibiotics if there is purulent sputum or an infection, and give prednisolone 30mg for 7–14 days.

✓ Rescue pack – Consider giving a rescue pack of antibiotics and steroids they can keep at home.

✓ Prophylactic antibiotics – Often only started by specialists.

✓ Immunisation – Offer the annual influenza vaccination and a one-off pneumococcal vaccination.

✓ Oxygen therapy – Consider offering in end-stage COPD. These patients should first be assessed by a respiratory specialist. They must also stop smoking to reduce the risk of hazards (burns and fire).

✓ Treatment – Recommend a prescription of prednisolone 30mg od (7–14 days) where they have significant SOB. If they are requiring three to four courses a year, consider osteoporosis prophylaxis. Consider antibiotics for purulent sputum or signs of pneumonia. Consider amoxicillin 500mg tds (five days) or doxycycline (200mg od for one day, 100mg od for four days). Alternatives include clarithromycin 500mg (five days) and co-amoxiclav 625mg tds (five days).

### Long-Term Oxygen Therapy and Travel

✓ Patients with a partial pressure of oxygen (pO2) of <9.3kPa at sea level should consult the airline company and receive supplemental oxygen while travelling. Patients with significant hypoxia (<6.7 kPa) or hypercapnia are advised not to fly. Patients with bullous disease should be informed of the potential risk of developing a pneumothorax during a flight. If you are unsure, seek advice from the GP or a specialist.

## QOF

» A register of COPD patients needs to be updated and maintained yearly. Patients should have a yearly FEV1 and be assessed for dyspnoea using the MRC scale. Those with an MRC of three or more should have oxygen saturations. Consider pulmonary rehab for those with an MRC of three or more. This is contraindicated if they are unable to walk, have unstable angina or have a previous MI.

## Referral

→ Refer the patient to a speciality if there are worsening symptoms, severe COPD, a rapid decline in FEV1, bullous lung disease, cor pulmonale, onset is in someone <40 years, frequent exacerbations, there is a family history of alpha-1 antitrypsin deficiency, frequent infections (bronchiectasis) or haemoptysis (exclude cancer).

→ Refer the patient to occupational therapy or social services if they have poor social support or are having difficulty in remaining mobile at home due to stairs.

## Safety Netting

» If the patient is acutely short of breath, has increased frequency of sputum, or is exhausted, confused or drowsy, they should seek medical advice.

*References*

National Institute for Health and Care Excellence (2018). *Chronic obstructive pulmonary disease in over 16s: diagnosis and management.* https://www.nice.org.uk/guidance/ng115

Global Initiative for Chronic Obstructive Lung Disease (2020). *Global strategy for the diagnosis, management and prevention of COPD.* https://goldcopd.org/wp-content/uploads/2019/12/GOLD-2020-FINAL-ver1.2-03Dec19_WMV.pdf

# Smoking Cessation

Smoking tobacco is the single most preventable cause of premature death in the UK. It is thought that almost 0.5 million hospital admissions each year are due to smoking-related diseases, and over 100,000 smokers in the UK die from smoking-related causes yearly. Around 10 million adults smoke, mostly males, but there is a rising prevalence of female smokers. It is the largest preventable cause of cancer, and it is known to be a significant risk factor for CVD. Whilst the majority of smokers profess to wanting to quit (>70%), only a small number actually go on to do so (<2%/year). Quitting smoking at any age brings many benefits, both immediate and long term. Hence, all patients who smoke should opportunistically be offered support and advice regarding smoking-cessation. About 40% of patients with serious mental health illnesses smoke.

Patients who wish to quit smoking often attend their surgery quite excited, wishing to turn over a new leaf. It is important to enquire as to what the trigger or motivational factor is in their decision to stop today; e.g. having a newborn baby or a recent family death. This can be used to reinforce the need to stop, and acts as a reminder when their motivation may wane. All patients who smoke should be offered brief intervention to help them stop smoking, and they should be signposted to the appropriate services.

## Association of Smoking with Disease

» Cancers – Lung (95%), oropharynx, oesophagus, gastric, lip, colon, bladder and stomach.

» CVD – CHD, CVA/TIA, PVD, erectile dysfunction and HF.

» Respiratory – COPD, exacerbation of asthma and chest infections.

» Obstetrics – Intrauterine growth restriction (IUGR), preterm delivery, stillbirth, miscarriage, ectopic pregnancy, pre-eclampsia, SVT, sudden infant death syndrome (SIDS) and cleft lip.

» Other – Dyspepsia, PUs, osteoporosis, thrombosis, infertility or poor surgery outcomes.

## Benefits of Quitting Smoking

Stopping smoking at any stage of life provides both immediate, and long-term health benefits.

» Financial – Cigarettes are heavily taxed and are expensive. By quitting, one will have more disposable income.

» Skin – One month post quitting, one's physical appearance will improve. Wrinkles may fade, and the grey facial colour will be replaced as circulation improves.

» Respiratory – After three months, breathing should improve and coughing/ wheezing should subside. The lung cancer risk falls by 50% 10 years post quitting.

» Cardiac – One year post cessation, the risk of MI is reduced by 50%.

## History

» Focused questions

> Ask how many they smoke a day, how long they have been smoking (calculate the number of packs per year), and whether they smoke at work, at home or both.

> Ask about what type they smoke (cigarettes, cigars, roll-ups or pipes).

> Ask why they started smoking (stress, social or habit).

> Ask how soon after waking they smoke their first cigarette.

> Ask if they have ever tried quitting before (what happened, if they had any support, if they have ever been smoke free, and why they started smoking again).

> Ask if they have had any cravings or withdrawal symptoms (irritability, low mood, restlessness, increasing appetite or disturbed sleep).

» Social history

> Ask whether anyone else smokes at home or at work.

> Ask about their occupation.

> Ask if they are under any stresses.

> Ask about their alcohol consumption.

> Ask if they take any recreational drugs.

» Past history

> Ask if they have made any previous attempts to try to stop smoking.

> Ask if they suffer from any medical problems (DM, CVA, HTN, cholesterol, asthma or cancer).

> Contraindications – Ask if they have had depression or any other mental health disorders, epilepsy or a pregnancy.

» Drug history – Ask if they have taken nicotine replacement therapy (NRT), bupropion (Zyban) or varenicline (Champix).

## Investigations

» Smoking-cessation clinics often monitor carbon monoxide (CO) levels every session. Anyone with a reading of <10ppm is classed as a non-smoker.

## Management

### Conservative

✓ Counselling – Refer them to a stop-smoking service (more effective than minimal support). Advise them that the best way to stop is with behavioural support and medication.

✓ Quit date – Agree a date when they should completely stop smoking. Withdrawal symptoms often get worse during the first few days but start to improve by the fourth day.

✓ Motivational – Offer quit-smoking tips tailored to the patient.

> Financial – One packet of cigarettes costs approx £7. This can save them £2,500 in one year, on average.

> They should make a list of reasons why they want to quit smoking.

> They should inform their friends and relatives that they wish to quit.

> Paraphernalia – They should discard ashtrays, lighters, pipes and cigarette boxes.

> They should avoid events and situations where there may be a large amount of other smokers (making it more difficult to cut down / stop).

> Food – Quitting smoking can cause an increased appetite. They should try to avoid fatty and sugary snacks, and eat fruit instead.

✓ Withdrawal symptoms – These can cause nausea, headaches, anxiety, irritability, cravings and insomnia. These symptoms are caused by a lack of nicotine in the blood. It is worse on the first day, but reduces after two to four weeks.

✓ Advise them to consider practising relaxation techniques; e.g. deep-breathing exercises.

✓ Distraction – Advise them to manage cravings with short bouts of exercise, talking to friends/family or go outside.

✓ Reduce cravings – Suggest chewing on sugarless gum, eating carrots or celery, or drinking water.

✓ Lapse – Explain that smoking just one cigarette could lead to a return to regular smoking. Advise them to avoid people who smoke.

✓ Stress – Consider referring them to counselling, or for cognitive behavioural therapy (CBT) if they have underlying stress.

*Medical*

✓ Medication – Enquire about and offer appropriate medication to help the patient stop smoking. If medication is unsuccessful, do not offer a repeat prescription within six months.

✓ NRT – Different forms are available; e.g. gum, inhalators, lozenges, nasal sprays and patches. The different types can be combined. NRT increases the chances of quitting by 70%. Start with higher doses in dependent patients and taper down two weeks before the end date (except for gum, which can be stopped instantly). The typical duration is eight to twelve weeks.

> Side effects – Nausea and vomiting, flushing headaches or flu-like symptoms.

> Contraindications – A CVA/TIA or MI in the last six months, or arrhythmias.

✓ Most use a combination (e.g. patches and a nasal spray, or patches and gum) to try to closely mimic the regularity of their cigarette smoking.

✓ Bupropion (Zyban) – Agree a quit date within the first two weeks of commencement. Start with 150mg for six days, then 150mg (bd) for seven to nine weeks. This doubles the chance of quitting. Initiate medication one to two weeks prior to the quit date. If there is no response after eight weeks, stop the medication.

> Side effects – Dry mouth, insomnia, GI symptoms or anxiety.

> Contraindications – Pregnancy, breastfeeding, epilepsy/ history of seizures, bipolar disorders, eating disorders or monoamine oxidase inhibitors (MAOI).

✓ Varenicline (Champix) – Agree a quit date within one to two weeks of commencement. Start treatment one week before the quit date. Take 0.5mg od for three days, 0.5mg bd for four days, then 1mg bd for 11 weeks. Cessation rates more than double using this treatment.

> Side effects – Nausea and vomiting, headaches and insomnia; stop the medication if the patient develops anxiety, depression or suicide ideation.

> Contraindications – Pregnancy, breastfeeding or psychiatric disorders (depression / suicide ideation).

✓ E-cigarettes – Acknowledge that e-cigarettes are less harmful than smoking cigarettes, and do not discourage a patient if they wish to switch.

## Safety Netting

» Review – Advice they should attend weekly for the monitoring of their CO levels. Successful quitting is defined as a CO reading <10ppm at four weeks after the quit date.

» Admission – If the patient feels suicidal, has a low mood or is anxious while on Champix, advise them to stop immediately and seek medical advice.

### References

Action on Smoking and Health (2019). *Young people and smoking.* https://ash.org.uk/information-and-resources/fact-sheets/young-people-and-smoking/

National Institute for Health and Care Excellence (2018). *Stop smoking interventions and services.* https://www.nice.org.uk/guidance/ng92

# Shortness of Breath

Dyspnoea can be quite an anxiety-provoking symptom for the patient. Some may describe a feeling of tightness or pressure in the chest, swelling over the throat, or an inability to breathe. Dyspnoea is entirely a subjective experience that may vary widely between patients. The intensity of it as described by the patient may not necessarily correlate to the severity of the underlying pathology. There are a number of different causes of SOB, including diseases of the cardiac or respiratory systems, or it may be due to other conditions such as anaemia or obesity, or it may even as be a result of a panic disorder.

## Causes of SOB Based upon Duration

- Sudden onset (minutes) – Upper airway obstruction (inhaled foreign body [FB] or anaphylaxis), PE, pneumothorax, MI or arrhythmia.

- Acute (hours) – Asthma, pneumonia or pulmonary oedema.

- Chronic (week/month) – COPD, lung cancer, HF, pleural effusion, pneumoconiosis, anaemia or panic attacks.

## *History*

» Focused questions

> Ask when they first noticed the dyspnoea, how long they have had it, whether it came on suddenly, and whether it is gradually getting worse.

> Ask if it comes and goes or is there all the time.

> Ask if there are triggers such as lying down (HF), walking (HF), exercise or allergens (asthma).

> Ask if anything makes it better, such as inhalers (asthma/COPD), being away from work, or sitting down and resting.

> Ask how far they can walk before they get breathless, how many stairs they can climb, and how far they could walk before this started.

» Associated history

> Sleep – Ask whether the SOB is mainly at night and whether it affects sleep.

> Chest pain – Ask whether it is worse when breathing in (pneumonia, pneumothorax or PE).

> Ask if there is any coughing.

> Ask if there are any palpitations (arrhythmia or panic attacks).

» Past history – Enquire about any cardiac risk factors (HTN, high cholesterol, angina, DM or MI), previous PE/DVT, any atopy, or any mental health issues.

» Drug history – Ask if they are taking any medications, including whether they have any allergies.

» Social history – Ask about their occupation and if their symptoms are affected by work, whether they smoke or drink alcohol, and whether they have taken any recent long-haul flights (PE).

» Family history – Ask if they have a family history of asthma.

## RED FLAGS

» Anaphylaxis – Acute or severe, SOB, angioedema or stridor.

» Asthma – An inability to complete sentences, or a silent chest.

» MI/ACS – Cardiac chest pain.

» PE – Haemoptysis.

## Differential Diagnosis

| PE | Sudden SOB with pleuritic chest pain. May also have haemoptysis and tachycardia. Risk factors: DVT, travel, trauma, OCP and malignancy. OE: tachypnoea with calf tenderness. |
|---|---|
| Panic attack | Stressors, perioral tingling, palpitations, hyperventilation, short-lived, anxiety, sweating or past medical history of mental health issues. |
| Pneumonia | Pleuritic chest pain associated with fever, a productive cough and dyspnoea. OE: coarse crackles with a dull percussion note and fever. |
| Asthma | Diurnal variation, wheeze and SOB, and is reversible with salbutamol/steroids. OE: reduced PF and expiratory wheeze. |
| COPD | Heavy smoker, productive cough, >35 years and lacks reversibility on spirometry. OE: cyanosis, hyperinflation and wheeze. |
| Arrhythmia | Sudden onset, pounding heart with a rapid pulse, dyspnoea, chest tightness and dizziness. OE: tachycardia. |
| Pneumothorax | Sudden onset of SOB with pleuritic chest pain. OE: hyperresonance, reduced breath sounds and chest-wall movement, tracheal deviation away, tachycardia and low BP (tension pneumothorax). |
| Lung collapse | Caused by inhaled FB, TB or enlarged LN. Acute breathlessness and cough. OE: tracheal deviation towards the lung, reduced chest-wall movement (affected side), dull percussion note, reduced breath sounds and reduced/absent VF. |

| Pleural effusion | Caused by HF, RF, liver failure, PE, pneumonia or cancer. Progressive SOB and chest pain (pleuritic). OE: reduced chest-wall movement (affected side), stony dull percussion note, absent/reduced breath sounds, reduced VF and bronchial breathing just above effusion. |
|---|---|
| Bronchiectasis | Chronic cough, daily production of mucopurulent sputum (thick and viscous), recurrent infections, wheeze, haemoptysis and fatigue. OE: coarse crackles (early inspiration) and clubbing. |
| HF | Previous MI; SOB that is worse when lying down (orthopnoea) or on exertion, and worse at night (patient may sleep sitting up); and oedema of the legs. May feel fatigued and weak. OE: Raised JVP, basal crackles, and sacral and pedal oedema. |

## Examination

» Vitals – BP, pulse, temperature, respiratory rate, oxygen saturations and weight (increased in HF and decreased in lung cancer).

» Respiratory

› Inspection – Inspect for reduced chest movements, lips (central cyanosis) and for a hyperinflated chest.

› Hands – Check for clubbing (lung cancer, bronchiectasis and interstitial lung disease) and peripheral cyanosis.

› Palpation – Palpate for tracheal deviation (towards, indicates lung collapse and away, indicates pneumothorax).

› Percussion – Hyperresonance indicates pneumothorax, dull indicates pneumonia, stony dull indicates effusion, and vocal fremitus indicates pneumonia or fluid.

› Auscultation – Listen to the chest for crepitations (pneumonia), wheezing (asthma/COPD), reduced air entry, and reduced or absent breath sounds (effusion).

» LNs – Examine the head and neck LNs (URTI, lung cancer and sarcoid).

» Cardiovascular – Listen for heart sounds (AS), palpate the legs for oedema (HF) and DVT (PE), and check JVP (HF).

## Investigations

» Bloods – FBC, U&E, LFTs, ESR and CRP.

› Others – D-dimers (PE), proBNP (CCF), TFTs (AF), troponin (MI) and radioallergosorbent test (RAST) (allergies).

- » Sputum – MCS.
- » ECG – CCF (LVH), PE (AF, RBBB and S1Q3T3) and arrhythmia.
- » CXR – To exclude chest infection, lung cancer and pneumothorax.
- » PEFR – Useful in diagnosing asthma.
- » Spirometry – COPD (lacks reversibility).
- » Echo – HF and valvular dysfunction.
- » Others (specialist) – VQ scan or CTPA, bronchoscopy, CT chest, arterial blood gas (ABG) and lung function tests.

## Management

*HF (See Heart Failure section, page 72)*

*Conservative*

✓ There are medication risk factors and comorbid conditions (BP and IHD). Advise them to lose weight and avoid alcohol.

  › Immunisation – Offer the annual flu jab and a one-off pneumococcal injection.

*Medical*

✓ Initiate an ACEi and b-blocker. Use furosemide for congestion. Second-line treatment includes aldosterone antagonist, hydralazine with nitrates, digoxin and amiodarone.

*QOF*

✓ The diagnosis is usually made by a specialist and/or echo confirmation. Ensure the patient is on an ACEi and/or b-blocker.

*Asthma (See Asthma section, page 79)*

*Conservative*

✓ Avoid allergens such as pets, pollen and dust. Provide education re inhalers.

*Medical*

✓ Consider salbutamol, inhaled steroids and LTRA. Follow the NICE guidelines. Consider oral steroids in acute exacerbation.

*COPD (See Chronic Obstructive Pulmonary Disease section, page 90)*

*Conservative*

✓ Advise them to stop smoking (most important) and offer pulmonary rehabilitation.

### Medical

✓ Consider ipratropium bromide, LABAs, LABA plus ICS, and oral steroids. Provide a rescue pack (oral steroids plus antibiotics).

### PE

✓ If this is suspected, start them on LMWH. If it is confirmed, start them on warfarin (INR 2-3) for three months (or NOACs) if there are transient risk factors (surgery, trauma, transient immobility), or for six months if there are permanent risk factors.

### Palpitations

✓ SVT – Perform an ECG and consider admitting the patient. You can try a carotid sinus massage (except if they have had IHD or a TIA, or are elderly) or the Valsalva manoeuvre. If the attack terminates, refer them to cardiology.

✓ AF – Find the cause if relevant (hyperthyroidism, pneumonia, HF, alcohol. etc.).

### LRTI

✓ Initiate antibiotics, considering doxycycline, amoxicillin or erythromycin/clarithromycin. Warn the patient about the side effects (diarrhoea/nausea).

### URTI

✓ Reassure them; explain why antibiotics are not needed; advise the use of OTC meds, paracetamol or NSAIDs, and fluid hydration; and consider delayed antibiotic prescription.

## Referral

→ Refer the patient to the speciality for the management of SOB if it is poorly controlled.

→ Consider admission if there are any red flags, MI, PE, reduced oxygen saturations (<92%), tachycardia (>130 bpm), tachypnoea (>30 breaths per minute) or a PF that is 33% of normal.

## Safety Netting

» If there are any red-flag symptoms, advise the patient to seek medical advice.

## NATIONAL EXAM TIPS

It is important to appreciate the impact that SOB has on the patient, particularly in the elderly. These patients may not be initially forthcoming in revealing their difficulties, and a more detailed social history may be required to establish whether they have assistance in the form of a carer or relative. Also determine whether they can perform simple activities of daily life – such as going to the toilet, and walking up and down stairs – and whether they can go shopping unaided. A patient may present with a low mood as they can no longer perform outdoor activities due to their symptoms.

## *References*

Global Initiative for Chronic Obstructive Lung Disease (2020). *Global strategy for the diagnosis, management and prevention of COPD.* https://goldcopd.org/wp-content/uploads/2019/12/GOLD-2020-FINAL-ver1.2-03Dec19_WMV.pdf

BMJ Best Practice (2019). *Assessment of dyspnoea.* https://bestpractice.bmj.com/topics/en-gb/862

# 4

# Gastroenterology

## Abdominal Pain

Abdominal pain is a common complaint in GP. Its aetiology may be a number of different organs within the abdominal cavity, as well as from surrounding structures that may refer to it, such as from the chest, pelvis or loin. You should always attempt to exclude as soon as possible an acute abdominal issue that may be a surgical emergency. Also consider the patient's age, gender and lifestyle when drawing up a list of differentials.

Patients presenting with abdominal pain may have very vague and nonspecific symptoms. However, it is important that a sound, focused history is performed to narrow down your list of differentials. This may be aided by examining the patient, and you must not forget to request to perform a pelvic examination on females. It may be that the patient has already had an investigation, such a USS or blood test, and you will be required to reconfirm the history before offering an explanation of the results.

### History

» Focused questions

> Ask about the site, ask the patient to point to the area affected, ask when they first noticed it, and ask how long it lasts for.

> Ask about radiation (shoulder, back or groin).

> Ask how severe the pain is on a scale of 1 (very mild) to 10 (very severe).

> Ask about the character of the pain (sharp, dull, burning sensation, cramp, gnawing, aching or boring).

> Ask if it comes and goes (colicky) or is there all the time.

> Ask if there are any triggers, such as spicy or fatty foods, alcohol or lying flat.

» Associated history – Ask if they have they had any nausea, vomiting or fever, what is their appetite is like, and how their bowels are (any constipation or diarrhoea).

» Past history – Ask if they have they ever experienced similar symptoms before, ask about their medical history (inflammatory bowel disease [IBD], gallstones or depression). Ask if they have had any surgery (adhesions).

» Drug history – Ask if they have they taken aspirin, steroids, bisphosphonates, ferrous sulphate, erythromycin or NSAIDs.

» Social history – Determine whether they smoke or drink alcohol, what their occupation is, whether they have suffered any stress, and whether they have recently travelled abroad.

» Family history – Determine whether any family have had IBD, bowel cancer or hereditary nonpolyposis colorectal cancer (HNPCC).

## RED FLAGS

» Ectopic – Pain with per vaginal (PV) bleeding or a missed period.

» Obstruction – Severe colicky pain with no bowel movements or flatus.

» Upper GI bleed – Dizziness, melaena or haematemesis.

» Ruptured abdominal aortic aneurysm (AAA) – Tearing central abdominal pain radiating to the back.

» Peritonitis – Sharp, constant pain that worsens with movement.

## Differentials

➤ Gastroenteritis

➤ Gallstones

➤ Ectopic pregnancy

| Peptic ulcer (PU) / duodenal ulcer (DU) | Burning abdominal pain associated with meals. Patients often point to the epigastric area. PU: pain typically 15 minutes after meals, relieved by vomiting and worse during the day. DU: pain one to three hours after eating and worse at night. Both may cause acid/water brash or heartburn. Milk can help with symptoms. |
|---|---|
| Pancreatitis | Commonly caused by alcohol or gallstones. Severe epigastric pain radiating to the back or chest. Constant gnawing pain for hours, worsened by drinking alcohol or eating a meal. Bending forwards provides temporary relief. Severe pancreatitis can cause fever, jaundice, a rapid pulse, nausea and vomiting. OE: jaundice, fever, epigastric pain with rigidity, Cullen's (umbilical bruising) and Grey Turner's (flank bruising) signs. |

| Biliary colic | Right upper quadrant (RUQ) pain radiating to the back and the interscapular area. Often worse at night. Associated with nausea, especially after eating a meal. The pain may be constant, but is classically colicky and often present with obstructive jaundice (pale stools and dark urine). Consider the risk factors (female, fat, 40s, fair and fertile). |
|---|---|
| Acute cholecystitis | Nagging, grumbling pain with local peritonism, fever and vomiting may indicate a biliary tract infection (acute or chronic cholecystitis). Raised inflammatory markers (WCC and CRP). OE: fever, jaundice, RUQ pain and positive for Murphy's sign (the patient stops inspiration when two fingers are placed on RUQ as the patient breaths in; absent in left upper quadrant [LUQ]). |
| Irritable bowel syndrome | Colicky abdominal pain associated with defecation, a change in bowel habits (constipation/diarrhoea) or bloating. Symptoms are made worse by eating. The patient may have urgency or incomplete evacuation. Often a diagnosis of exclusion. |
| Appendicitis | Diffuse central abdominal colic, shifting to the right iliac fossa (RIF). Worsened by movement, touch and coughing. Associated with anorexia, nausea and vomiting, and occasionally diarrhoea. OE: Low grade fever, tachycardia, tender RIF (McBurney's point) and Rovsing's sign (pain in the RIF when the left iliac fossa [LIF] is palpated). |
| Renal colic | Sudden onset of a dull ache that is colicky in nature, with the passing of blood in the urine, and often may be severe enough to cause nausea and vomiting. Pain can originate from the flank or loin area and radiate to the groin. |
| Diverticulitis | Small outpouchings of the large bowel that become inflamed or infected. Often affects females from 50–70 years. Symptoms include abdominal pain, bloating and cramps, mainly in the LIF, with fever, nausea, vomiting and constipation. Patients may also have flatulence and distension. Frank blood mixed in with the stools is a complication. Per rectum (PR): tenderness on the left side (inflamed colon). |
| Intestinal obstruction | A history of adhesions (previous surgery) or malignancy. Colicky abdominal pain, distension and absolute constipation, including wind. Bowels not opened. 'Tinkling' bowel sounds. |

## Examination

» Vitals – BP (hypotension), pulse (tachycardia) and temperature.

» General – Inspect for anaemia and jaundice in the eyes. Look at the patient's general appearance; is the patient silent, pale and still?

» Abdomen

  › Inspection – Inspect for swollen abdomen or peristalsis.

  › Palpation – Palpate the four quadrants for pain. Examine for constipation, organomegaly (liver/spleen) and pulsatile mass (AAA). Percuss for ascites if present.

  › Auscultation – Listen for bowel sounds (tingling, reduced or absent).

» PR – Perform if there is evidence of PR bleeding or melaena.

» Pelvic exam – Consider this in females with pelvic masses. Look for cervical excitation or adnexal pain.

## Investigations

» Bloods – FBC (anaemia), U&E, LFTs, ESR (IBD), CRP and calcium (pancreatitis).

  › Others – Amylase (pancreatitis), carcinoembryonic antigen (CEA) (bowel cancer) and cancer antigen 125 (CA125) (ovarian cancer).

» Urine – Leukocytes, nitrates (urinary tract infection [UTI]), blood (renal stones or infection) and pregnancy test.

» Stools – Faecal occult blood (FOB), Helicobacter pylori (H. pylori )(PU) and culture and sensitivity (C&S).

» High vaginal swab (HVS) – Pelvic inflammatory disease (PID).

» Abdominal x-ray (AXR) – Renal stones, constipation and intestinal obstruction.

» USS – Gallstones, renal stones, hepatitis and appendicitis.

» Others (specialist) – Barium meal/enema, CT abdomen, ERCP and endoscopy (oesophago-gastro-duodenoscopy [OGD] and colon/sigmoidoscopy).

## Management

*Treat the underlying cause*

### Gastric/Peptic Ulcer

#### Conservative

✓ Advise the patient to avoid chilli and spicy food, to cut down on caffeine and alcohol, to stop smoking and to avoid NSAIDs. They should eat small, regular meals, and ensure that the last meal of the day is several hours before bedtime.

*Medical*

✓ Alginates – Gaviscon.

✓ Ranitidine – 150mg bd or 300mg for four to eight weeks.

✓ PPI – Omeprazole.

✓ H. pylori – Initiate triple therapy; e.g. seven days PPI, amoxicillin 1g and clarithromycin 500mg bd.

## Gallstones

*Conservative*

✓ Advise them to lose weight, exercise, adhere to a low-fat diet and stop smoking. Offer analgesia (NSAIDs/paracetamol).

*Medical*

✓ Do not remove asymptomatic gallstones.

*Surgical*

✓ Refer the patient for consideration of a cholecystectomy if symptomatic.

## Acute cholecystitis

*Conservative*

✓ Offer the patient analgesia if it is painful.

*Medical*

✓ Admit the patient for IV fluids and antibiotics.

*Surgical*

✓ Refer the patient for a cholecystectomy, lithotripsy or ursodeoxycholic acid.

## Gastroenteritis

*Conservative*

✓ Advise them to take oral rehydration salts and fluids. They should eat lighter foods, but more regularly. They should avoid fruit juice and fizzy drinks. The patient should ensure that they wash their hands thoroughly with soap and water, and dry them well.

*Medical*

✓ Antidiarrheals (loperamide) are not usually recommended, but may help reduce the frequency of bowel motions. Do not offer this to patients with blood/mucus or high fever (dysentery). Consider antiemetics (metoclopramide 10mg intramuscular [IM]) in patients who are vomiting severely.

## Constipation

### Conservative

✓ Advise the patient to increase fluids, take regular exercise, and eat more fibre (cereals), less red meat, five portions of fruit or vegetables per day, and whole grains and fruits (and juices) that are high in sorbitol (pears, plums, peaches, prunes, apple, apricots and vegetables). *See Constipation section, page 129.*

### Medical

✓ Consider bulk-forming laxatives (ispaghula), osmotic laxatives (macrogol), then lactulose if the patient has hard stools. If the patient is suffering from opioid-induced constipation, offer macrogol or lactulose.

## Renal stones

✓ Advise them to increase fluids, reduce their salt intake, and reduce their intake of dairy products (calcium), animal protein (amino acid), and grape juice and apple juice. *See Renal Stones section, page 179.*

## Pancreatitis

### Conservative

✓ Advise them to avoid alcohol, and take a high-protein, low-fat, and high-calorie diet. Refer them to a dietician.

### Medical

✓ Acute – Admit for IV fluids, analgesia and nutrition.

✓ Chronic – Advise them to stop smoking and drinking alcohol, and to eat a low-fat diet. Offer analgesia if they are in pain.

✓ CREONs – Prescribed to help digestion if they have steatorrhoea.

### Surgical

✓ Treat the cause by removing any gallstones.

✓ Refer the patient to a specialist to consider a pancreatectomy.

## Diverticular disease

### Conservative

✓ Advise them to eat a high-fibre diet and increase fluid intake.

### Medical

✓ Admit for IV fluids, analgesia and antibiotics. Consider paracetamol for pain and mesalazine (specialist).

## References

National Institute for Health and Care Excellence (2008). *Irritable bowel syndrome in adults: diagnosis and management.* https://www.nice.org.uk/guidance/cg61

National Institute for Health and Care Excellence (2014). *Gastro-oesophageal reflux disease and dyspepsia in adults: investigation and management.* https://www.nice.org.uk/guidance/cg184

National Institute for Health and Care Excellence (2014). *Gallstone disease: diagnosis and management.* https://www.nice.org.uk/guidance/cg188

National Institute for Health and Care Excellence (2018). *Pancreatitis.* https://www.nice.org.uk/guidance/ng104

National Institute for Health and Care Excellence (2019). *Renal and ureteric stones: assessment and management.* https://www.nice.org.uk/guidance/ng118

# Diarrhoea

Diarrhoea is the passing of loose stool motions. It is defined by the World Health Organization (WHO) as the passing of three or more loose motions per day or having an increased stool frequency for that person. Gastroenteritis is thought to be the most common cause. However, persistent diarrhoea in the elderly should be taken seriously, as it could signify bowel cancer. Diarrhoea can be a debilitating and embarrassing condition, with patients soiling their undergarments. It is important to enquire about the impact the patient's symptom is having on their social or work setting. Acute diarrhoea is the presence of symptoms of less than two weeks in duration, persistent diarrhoea has a duration of more than 14 days, and chronic diarrhoea is that lasting more than four weeks.

## Bacterial Causes of Gastroenteritis

➤ If found on stool MC&S, the local Health Protection Agency should be notified.

| Time to Symptoms | Organism and Symptoms |
|---|---|
| 1–6 hours | Staphylococcus aureus presents acutely with severe symptoms, and is due to uncooked meat. Bacillus cereus is usually contracted from rice consumption. Gives rise to nausea and vomiting before diarrhoea. |
| 12–48 hours | Staphylococcus aureus presents acutely with severe symptoms, and is due to uncooked meat. Bacillus cereus is usually contracted from rice consumption. Gives rise to nausea and vomiting before diarrhoea. |
| 48–72 hours | Shigella is found on contaminated vegetables or salads. It causes bloody diarrhoea, abdominal cramps and fever. Campylobacter arises from undercooked chicken or unpasteurised milk. Patients present with a flu-like prodrome and diarrhoea. It can cause Guillain-Barré syndrome. |
| >7 days | Giardiasis is a parasite that is found in water contaminated by sewage. Its most common feature is prolonged, non-bloody diarrhoea. |

## *History*

» Focused questions

› Ask when it started and how long it has been going on for.

› Ask how often they are opening their bowels.

› Ask if their stools are loose, watery or have any mucus. Ask if there is any pain, and if so, where.

› Do not forget to ask about blood in the stools.

» Associated history – Ask if they have had any nausea, vomiting or fever, or if they have met anyone else who has had diarrhoea recently.

» Family history – Ask if there is a family history of thyroid problems, IBD, bowel issues or ovarian cancer.

» Past history – Ask about any previous episodes of diarrhoea, if they suffer from any other issues, if they have had any recent hospital admissions and about their surgical history. Also ask if they have any stress or anxiety.

» Drug history – Ask if they have recently taken any antibiotics, laxatives, etc.

» Social history – Ask if they smoke, if they have recently travelled abroad, what their recent diet has been like, and what their occupation is.

## RED FLAGS

» Any change in bowel habits (if they are >50 years old), weight loss or any blood in the stools (if they are >40 years old).

» Diarrhoea for more than six weeks in someone >60 years old, persistent diarrhoea in someone >40 years old with rectal bleeding, a right lower abdominal mass or rectal mass, a male with iron deficiency anaemia (Hb <11g/dl) or a female (non-menstruating) with iron deficiency anaemia (Hb <10g/dl).

## Examination

» Vitals – BP, weight, pulse and temperature.

» Assess stool against the Bristol stool chart (types 5, 6 and 7 are abnormal).

» Abdominal exam

  › Inspection – Inspect for signs of dehydration, anaemia or jaundice.

  › Palpation – Palpate the four quadrants for any pain or masses.

  › Auscultation – Listen for bowel sounds.

» PR – Check for fresh blood, a rectal mass or impacted faeces.

» Thyroid – Inspect outstretched hands (tremor), pulse (AF) and the thyroid gland (goitre).

## Investigations

» Bloods – FBC (anaemia and platelets), U&E, LFTs (hypoalbuminaemia), TFTs, coeliac screen (tissue transglutaminase [tTG] for immunoglobulin A [IgA] antibodies, and reintroduce gluten in the diet), ESR and CRP (IBD), vitamin B12, folate, ferritin (malabsorption screen) and HIV.

» Stools – FOB or quantitative faecal immunochemical test (qFIT), faecal calprotectin (IBD) and MC&S (ova, cysts, parasites and Clostridium difficile [C. diff]).

» Specialist – Hydrogen breath test (lactose intolerance), colonoscopy, jejunal biopsy (coeliac) and barium enema.

## Differential Diagnosis

| Food poisoning | Acute onset of diarrhoea, nausea, vomiting and cramping abdominal pain. Have recently eaten out or might have eaten uncooked foods. Contacts are also unwell. Usually associated with vomiting. Blood in diarrhoea (campylobacter or enterohemorrhagic E. coli Shiga toxin) can occur. |
|---|---|
| Traveller's diarrhoea | Has recently travelled abroad. |
| IBS | Extremely common. Most consistent features are a six-month history of abdominal pain relieved by defecation, urgency, incomplete evacuation, straining during bowel movements, bloating and a change in bowel habits between constipation and diarrhoea. Symptoms often worsen with eating. Patients may be divided into diarrhoea-predominant IBS or constipation-predominant IBS. Symptoms may be triggered by stress. |
| Coeliac disease | Autoimmune, gluten-sensitive enteropathy. Intolerance to foods containing gluten (wheat, barley and rye). Pale, fatty stools that are difficult to flush away (steatorrhoea), abdominal pain, nausea and vomiting, weight loss, fatigue, and unexplained iron, folate and vitamins K and D deficiency. Endomysium antibodies (EMA), tTG and gliadin-antibody positive. |
| Crohn's disease | Transmural chronic inflammatory disease that can affect any part of the GI tract. Crampy abdominal pains and diarrhoea (chronic or nocturnal) and, less commonly, blood in diarrhoea. Other features include perianal tags, fissures and fistulae with extra-intestinal symptoms such as arthritis, uveitis and erythema nodosum. |
| Ulcerative colitis | Ulcerating disease affecting only the mucous membrane of the large bowel starting from the anus. |
| Pancreatitis | Steatorrhoea, epigastric pain and high alcohol intake. |
| Hyperthyroidism | Overactive thyroid gland. Presents with heat intolerance, tremor, sweating, irritability, heavy periods, palpitations, weight loss despite increased appetite, and hyperdefecation. |

| Appendicitis | Pain that moves from the umbilical region to the RIF, and is worse on walking or moving. |
|---|---|
| Diverticulitis | More common in 50–70-year-olds. Small outpouchings of the large bowel that become inflamed or infected. Symptoms include abdominal pain, bloating and cramps, mainly in the LIF, with fever, nausea, vomiting and constipation. |
| Overflow | Occurs after a bout of constipation, with no control over passing stools, including soiling underwear. |
| Post antibiotics | Any antibiotic, but more so ciprofloxacin and broad-spectrum ones such as co-amoxiclav. C. diff produces offensive smelling diarrhoea, particularly after using broad-spectrum antibiotics. |

## Management

*Treat the underlying cause*

### Gastroenteritis

#### Conservative

✓ Most patients will improve within five days. Occasionally, this may last up to two weeks. Advise them to drink plenty of fluids or oral rehydration salts (dioralyte). They should follow a normal diet, but have small, light meals. They should avoid fizzy drinks, fatty or spicy foods. Children should not go to school, and should only return 48 hours after the last episode of diarrhoea and vomiting. They should not swim for two weeks. Healthcare professionals and those working with food should avoid work for 48 hours.

✓ Take paracetamol or NSAIDs for any fever, body aches or headaches.

#### Medical

✓ Antimotility – Loperamide for adults or racecadotril for up to five days, alternatives are bismuth/codeine. Do not use if diarrhoea is bloody or there is shigellosis.

✓ Antiemetics – Consider metoclopramide if the patient is vomiting severely.

✓ If an organism is grown on a culture, treat with appropriate antibiotics:

  › Amoebiasis – Metronidazole 400mg tds (five to ten days) followed by dilocadine 500mg tds (ten days).

  › Campylobacter – Erythromycin 250–500mg qds (five to seven days) or ciprofloxacin 500mg bd (five to seven days).

  › Giardiasis – Metronidazole 500mg bd (seven to ten days).

  › Salmonella – Ciprofloxacin 500mg bd (one day).

## Coeliac disease

### Conservative

✓ Suggest a lifelong gluten-free diet. Advise the patient to check labels on foods.

✓ Advise the patient to avoid wheat, bread, pastry, pasta, barley, beer and rye. Oats may be tolerated. Rice, potatoes and corn (maize) are gluten free.

### Medical

✓ Ensure the patient takes folic acid 5mg if pregnant. Directed by a dietician, consider advising the patient to take calcium and vitamin D supplements.

✓ Refer them to a dietician.

## IBD

### Conservative

✓ For Crohn's disease, advise the patient to stop smoking (to reduce the risk of relapse).

### Medical

✓ Refer the patient for a diagnosis.

✓ Treat with aminosalicylates (mesalazine, which is often started on first presentation), steroids (oral or topical), immunosuppressive drugs (azathioprine or methotrexate) or metronidazole (perianal disease).

✓ Monitor and treat for the risk of osteoporosis.

## Hyperthyroidism

✓ Propranolol for symptomatic treatment.

✓ Refer to edocrine and consider carbimazole.

## Diverticulitis

### Conservative

✓ Encourage the patient to have a high-fibre diet (30g daily) and increase fluid intake.

### Medical

✓ Admit for IV fluids, analgesia and antibiotics (augmentin, or metronidazole and ciprofloxacin).

✓ Consider paracetamol for pain relief and mesalazine (specialist).

## Overflow diarrhoea

✓ Manual disimpaction, laxatives (macrogol), suppositories (glycerine) or an enema (docusate, arachis oil or sodium phosphate).

✓ Refer the patient to a nurse-led continence clinic service if they are elderly and need pads to prevent soiling.

✓ Consider an occupational therapy (OT) assessment if they have problems using the toilet, for adaptions or the installation of a commode.

## Safety Netting

» Admit the patient if they are showing signs of severe dehydration.

» Always ask the patient to return if they become dehydrated, cannot keep fluids down, see blood in their vomit or diarrhoea, or have severe abdominal pain or a high fever.

## References

Arasaradnam, R.P., Brown, S., Forbes, A., Fox, M.R., Hungin, P., Kelman, L., Major, G., O'Connor, M., Sanders, D.S., Sinha, R., Smith S.C., Thomas, P. and Walters, J.R.F. (2018). Guidelines for the investigation of chronic diarrhoea in adults: British Society of Gastroenterology. Gut, 67(8). http://dx.doi.org/10.1136/gutjnl-2017-315909

Centres for Disease Control and Prevention. (n.d.) *E.coli (Escherichia coli)*. https://www.cdc.gov/ecoli/index.html

Joint Formulary Committee (2018). *BNF 76 (British National Formulary) September 2018*. Pharmaceutical Press.

World Gastroenterology Organisation (2012). *Acute diarrhoea in adults and children: a global perspective*. https://www.worldgastroenterology.org/guidelines/global-guidelines/acute-diarrhea/acute-diarrhea-english

# Pruritis Ani

Pruritis ani describes the sensation of an intense need to scratch around the back passage. It is an uncomfortable feeling and may lead patients to feel quite embarrassed. If left untreated, it may encourage bad hygiene habits that could promote infections via the ano-faecal route. The majority of cases are thought to be functional, due to faecal material causing itchiness and localised erythema. Other causes include skin infections, eczema, overflow diarrhoea and piles. It may also be due to depression, so it is important to screen for this.

## Pathophysiology

» Haemorrhoids – These are abnormally enlarged vascular mucosal cushions in the anal canal. It is only when they become enlarged and start to cause symptoms that they become haemorrhoids.

» Anal fissures – These are tears to anal mucosa, often posterior to the anal canal.

» Fistulas – The glands inside the anus become blocked and can form an anal abscess. If one increases in size, it can form a tunnel leading to the skin around the anus. This will create a fistula leading from inside the anus to an opening in the skin surrounding the anus. Fistulas can be seen in conditions such as Crohn's disease. This is a transmural chronic inflammatory disease that can affect any part of the GI tract from the mouth to the anus.

» Threadworms – These are spread via the faecal–oral route.

## History

» Focused questions

› Ask when it started and how long it has been going on for.

› Ask if it comes and goes, or is there all the time.

› Ask if anything makes it better or worse.

› Ask if it has affected their sleep or social life.

» Associated history

› Ask if they have had any bleeding from the back passage.

› Ask if they have experienced any pain around the back passage.

› Ask if they find themselves straining when they are opening their bowels.

› Ask if they suffer from hard stools.

› Ask if they have had any diarrhoea.

» Past history – Ask if they suffer from psoriasis, eczema or urticaria. Ask if they suffer from DM.

» Drug history – Ask if they are taking any medications (colchicine, tetracycline, erythromycin, metronidazole, steroids or peppermint oils).

» Travel history – Determine if there has been any recent travel abroad (threadworm).

» Social history – Ask what their diet is like.

» Family history – Ask whether anyone in the family suffers from any GI disorder or has recently been treated for threadworms.

## RED FLAGS

Any changes in bowel habits, tenesmus, weight loss or PR bleeding.

## Examination

» Vitals – Weight and temperature.

» Rectal examination

  › Inspection – Look for skin tags, ulcers, fissures, polyps or external haemorrhoids. Look for any skin conditions such as psoriasis, candida infection, contact dermatitis, seborrhoeic dermatitis, lichen planus, lichen sclerosis or scabies (track-like burrows).

  › Palpation – Palpate for any masses if malignancy is suspected. Ask the patient to strain downwards. Check for blood or mucus.

## Differential Diagnosis

| Anal fissure | Pain on defecation with blood on the toilet paper. Associated with constipation. |
| --- | --- |
| Haemorrhoids | May feel a lump around the back passage. A background of constipation with painless fresh blood on the toilet paper, the surface of stools or dripping into the pan. Tenesmus and pruritis ani. Soiling may occur in severe haemorrhoids. |
| Threadworms | Itching is worse at night, and patients may see worms or white eggs in the stools. Patients may have lost weight. |
| Crohn's disease | Presents with crampy abdominal pains and diarrhoea, which is occasionally bloody. Other features include perianal tags, fissures, fistulas, arthritis, uveitis and erythema nodosum. |
| Psoriasis/eczema | Ask if the patient suffers from any skin problems elsewhere. |

| Sexually transmitted infection (STI) | Ask if the patient practises anal sex. |
|---|---|
| Depression | Ask how the patient's mood has been, and whether they feel low or suffer from depression. |

## Investigations

» Sellotape test – Perform the Sellotape test if threadworms are suspected but not visible.

» Bloods – FBC and ESR (Crohn's disease).

» Stools – MC&S (ova).

» Specialist – Proctoscopy.

## Management

*Treat the underlying cause*

### Conservative

✓ Advise the patient to wash the anus after each bowel movement and before sleeping. They should avoid rubbing the anus vigorously, bubble baths, soaps and scented products. They should dry the perianal area after bowel movements.

✓ Advise them to wear loose clothing and light pyjamas, use cotton underwear, avoid any tight, synthetic clothing and avoid biological, enzyme-based detergents.

✓ Advise them to avoid scratching, and keep their nails short; advise them that they should perhaps wear gloves at night time. They should wash their hands after every bowel motion.

✓ Advise them to avoid any foods that may exacerbate the problem, and cut down on caffeine, chocolate and fizzy drinks.

✓ For constipation, advise them to drink plenty of fluids, make sure they have at least five pieces of fruit or vegetables a day, reduce their weight and ensure they have plenty of fibre.

### Medical

✓ Threadworms – Treat with mebendazole stat and repeat in two weeks if necessary. Ensure adequate hygiene measures are taken.

✓ Skin conditions – Apply barrier creams or soothing ointment (bismuth subgallate or zinc oxide). Consider a trial of hydrocortisone, such as chlorphenamine 4mg at night, which will help to reduce the itch and help them sleep.

✓ Haemorrhoids – Treat any constipation if present. Recommend a diet high in fibre and vegetables. Topical local anaesthetic agents, including Anusol and Proctosedyl, may be used for short periods. Suppositories are also available.

✓ Fissures – Treat any constipation if present (first-line treatment is bulk-forming laxatives, such as ispaghula husk), barrier cream, topical anaesthetics (Anusol) and sitz baths (remaining seated in hot water for several minutes before applying cold water for one minute) For chronic fissures, offer GTN 0.4% ointment bd for eight weeks. If there is severe pain consider, 1–2ml lidocaine, applied before passing stools, for two weeks. Alternatives include diltiazem 2%, and nifedipine oral or topical.

*Surgical*

✓ Chronic fissures – Internal sphincterotomy or fistulectomy.

## Referral

→ If they have an unresponsive skin condition, refer the patient to a dermatologist or a GPwSI in dermatology.

→ Refer the patient to a colorectal surgeon if symptoms have not improved after three months despite treatment.

→ With haemorrhoids, consider band ligation or sclerotherapy if they are persistent. Refer the patient to secondary care on the same day if haemorrhoids are extremely painful or thrombosed.

## Safety Netting

» Review the patient if the symptoms persist for more than three to four weeks or are worsening.

---

*References*

National Institute for Health and Care Excellence (2013). *Chronic anal fissure: botulinum toxin type A injection.* https://www.nice.org.uk/advice/esuom14/ifp/chapter/What-is-chronic-anal-fissure

# Dyspepsia

Dyspepsia is not a diagnosis; rather, it describes a collection of upper GI symptoms that persists for more than four weeks. Symptoms may include persistent or recurrent pain or discomfort centred in the upper abdomen. It is often associated with abdominal fullness, bloating, nausea, belching and a feeling of satiety. It is an extremely common symptom, with 40% of people suffering from it at some point in their lives. Heartburn is often confused with dyspeptic symptoms; however, it is synonymous with acid reflux (GORD). Causes of dyspepsia include GORD, PU disease, gastritis, non-functional dyspepsia, stomach cancer and oesophagitis.

## Risk Factors for Peptic Ulcer Disease

➤ **H. pylori**

› May increase gastric acid secretion (which increases the risk of mucosal ulceration) or decrease secretion, causing chronic atrophic gastritis and gastric ulceration.

➤ **Drugs**

› NSAIDs

› Aspirin

› SSRI

› Steroids

› Bisphosphonates

› Cocaine

➤ **Other**

› Smoking

› Alcohol

› Stress

› Zollinger-Ellison syndrome

## *History*

» Focused questions

› Ask about abdominal pain, nausea and bloating. Ask when it was first noticed and how long it lasts for.

› Ask about site, character (bloated, crampy or burning feeling), and whether it comes and goes or is there all the time.

› Ask about triggers (spicy or fatty foods, alcohol, coffee, chocolate or citrus fruits) and alleviating factors (Gaviscon, food and milk).

» Associated history – Nausea and vomiting, belching or burping, or any persistent cough.

» Past history – Ask if there has been any previous GORD, IBS, H. pylori, Barrett's oesophagus, depression or anxiety. Determine if there have been any previous investigations (OGD or stool tests).

» Drug history – Ask if they have taken any NSAIDs, aspirin, bisphosphonates, steroids, a-blockers or TCAs. Ask if they have tried any OTC medications (Gaviscon).

» Social history – Ask if they smoke or drink alcohol, what their occupation is, if they have any current stress and what their diet is like.

» Family history – Ask if there is a family history of PUs or stomach cancer.

## Risk Factors for Stomach Cancer

➤ Country of origin (Japan)

➤ H. pylori infection

➤ Pernicious anaemia

➤ Atrophic gastritis

➤ Stomach surgery (partial gastrectomy)

➤ Smoking

## RED FLAGS

Progressive dysphagia, persistent vomiting, iron deficiency anaemia, unintentional weight loss, upper abdominal mass, or aged >55 with persistent unexplained dyspepsia.

## Differentials

➤ GORD

➤ PU

➤ Stomach cancer

➤ Biliary colic

➤ Cardiac

## Examination

» Vitals – Weight, BMI and pulse.

» Abdomen

› Inspection – Inspect the conjunctiva for signs of anaemia.

› Palpitation – Palpate the four quadrants for any pain or masses, particularly over the epigastric area. Palpate the left supraclavicular area for Virchow's nodes (stomach cancer).

› Auscultation – Listen for bowel sounds.

» PR – Check for melaena (if there is evidence of PR bleeding/black stools).

## Investigations

» Bloods – FBC, ferritin (iron deficiency anaemia), U&Es, tTG for IgA (coeliac screen), CA125 (ovarian cancer).

» Stools – H. pylori stool antigen test (stop PPI for two weeks before the test, and no antibiotics for four weeks). For confirmation of eradication, a urea breath test is more sensitive.

» CXR – Barium swallow (hiatus hernia).

» Other specialist – OGD, barium meal and CT abdomen.

## Management

### Conservative

✓ Position – Advise the patient to raise the head of their bed by 10–15cm or sleep on more pillows.

✓ Diet – Advise them to eat smaller regular meals and make sure that last meal of the day is three to four hours before going to bed. Tailor the advice to the patient. Advise them to avoid trigger drinks or foods.

✓ Weight – Advise them to try to lose weight if they are obese.

✓ Exercise – To help them reduce their weight if needed, exercise programmes may be recommended.

✓ Food diary – Advise them to keep a food diary and see if there are any links between the food eaten and symptoms.

› Foods to avoid for those with dyspepsia – Fatty or fried foods, spicy or chilli foods, garlic, onions, tomato sauce, acid fruits (lemons, limes and oranges), and chocolate.

› Drinks to avoid – Tea, coffee, orange juice, grape juice and carbonated drinks.

✓ Smoking – Advise them to stop smoking and offer smoking-cessation advice. Refer them to a smoking clinic.

✓ Alcohol – Advise them to reduce their intake to <=14 units a week.

✓ Stress – Advise them to use relaxation or breathing techniques, speak to friends or a counsellor, and undergo CBT.

*Medical*

✓ Antacids – Offer Gaviscon or magnesium trisilicate.

✓ PPI – Give one month of PPI (lansoprazole 30mg od / omeprazole 40mg).

✓ Ranitidine – Give an H2 antagonist if there is no response to PPI (ranitidine 150mg bd) for one month.

✓ Prokinetic – Give domperidone 10mg tds if they have severe nausea.

✓ NSAIDs – If the patient is on NSAIDs, review the need to continue, and discuss the potential harm they could cause; this should be done every six months. Consider stopping them or substituting them with paracetamol or a low dose of ibuprofen (1.2g daily).

✓ Functional dyspepsia – If the patient is diagnosed with functional dyspepsia, consider tricyclic antidepressants (TCAs) (to improve anxiety/depression and improve gastric accommodation) or probiotics.

✓ Pregnancy – If they are pregnant, recommend lifestyle changes. Consider antacids or alginates (Gaviscon) as first-line treatment. Avoid medication containing sodium bicarbonate or magnesium trisilicate in pregnancy. If symptoms still persist, consider ranitidine (off label) or omeprazole.

✓ H. pylori infection – If they are H. pylori positive, determine if they are allergic to penicillin, and treat as follows. If diarrhoea develops, consider C. diff and treat.

**No penicillin allergy**

› First-line treatment for seven days – PPI bd, amoxicillin 500mg tds, and clarithromycin 500mg bd or metronidazole 400mg bd.

› Second-line treatment for seven days – PPI bd, amoxicillin 300mg tds and alternative antibiotic was not used in first-line treatment.

**Penicillin allergy**

› First-line treatment for seven days – PPI bd, clarithromycin 500mg bd and metronidazole 400mg bd.

› Second-line treatment for 10 days – PPI bd, metronidazole 400mg bd and levofloxacin 250mg bd.

# Referral

→ Refer the patient urgently to the speciality if there is evidence of chronic GI bleeding, progressive unintentional weight loss, progressive difficulty swallowing, persistent vomiting, iron deficiency anaemia, an epigastric mass or a suspicious barium meal.

→ Endoscopy – Refer them if the patient experiences recurrent or refractory symptoms, the second-line H. pylori treatment failed, or they have an allergy to a number of antibiotics. Stop PPI for two weeks before the procedure, but they can use antacids/alginates instead.

## Safety Netting

» If there is haematemesis or melaena, consider hospital admission.

---

### References

National Institute for Health and Care Excellence (2014). *Gastro-oesophageal reflux disease and dyspepsia in adults: investigation and management.* https://www.nice.org.uk/guidance/cg184

Public Health England (2017). *Helicobacter pylori in dyspepsia: test and treat.* https://www.guidelines.co.uk/infection/phe-h-pylori-in-dyspepsia-guideline/252887.article

# Constipation

The term 'constipation' may be understood differently between patients and clinicians. It is always useful to clarify with the patient what they mean by the word 'constipation'. Constipation is synonymous with the passage of hard stools. However, a health professional may define it as the infrequent passing of bowel motions or incomplete defecation. Stools are usually hard and dry, and can fluctuate from being extremely large to being small.

Constipation may be caused by a variety of problems, including poor dietary intake, reduced fluids, as a side effect of medications or due to poor mobility. In the elderly, any prolonged change in bowel habits should trigger the possibility of bowel cancer as a diagnosis. Constipation is more common in women, pregnant women and the elderly.

Faecal loading/impaction is when an immobile, solid, large bulk of faeces has developed in the rectum, preventing evacuation. Overflow diarrhoea is the leakage of liquid stools (diarrhoea) around the impacted faeces. This can occur without sensation to the patient, and happens frequently.

## Rome IV Criteria for Functional Constipation

The following symptoms suggestive of constipation must have occurred for at least the last three months with symptom onset more than six months ago. The patient must not fulfil the IBS criteria, and never or rarely has loose stools. Do *not* use the Rome IV criteria for patients with alarm symptoms (rectal bleeding, iron-deficiency anaemia, weight loss, family history of colon cancer and age of onset >50).

The patient must have two or more of the following:

➤ Straining

➤ Bristol stool type of 1 or 2.

➤ The sensation of incomplete evacuation.

➤ The sensation of anorectal obstruction/blockage.

➤ Manual manoeuvres to facilitate defecation.

➤ Fewer than three spontaneous bowel movements weekly.

## *History*

» Focused questions

› Ask when the constipation started, how long it has been for (chronic if more than three months), and if it is getting worse or better.

› Ask about the frequency, straining and pain.

› Ask about the appearance of the stools (rabbit droppings or large – use the Bristol stool chart).

› Ask if there has been any blood in the stools.

» Associated history – Ask if they have experienced overflow diarrhoea (if they have ever soiled their undergarments or had uncontrolled diarrhoea), nausea and vomiting, or loading (if they have to remove a stool). Ask about their toileting habits (if they go regularly or can hold it when they cannot go).

» Past history – Ask if they have had any fissures, diverticular disease, IBS, IBD, thyroid issue, depression or bowel cancer.

» Drug history – Ask if they have taken any OTC medications. Ask if it worsens with opioids, ferrous sulphate, SSRIs, furosemide, TCAs or risperidone. Ask if it improves with laxatives.

» Social history – Ask if they smoke or drink alcohol, ask what foods they eat (red meat, fast foods or gluten) and ask about their fluid intake.

» Family history – Ask if they have a family history of colon cancer.

## RED FLAGS

» Bowel cancer – Weight loss, PR bleeding or a change in bowel habits.

» Intestinal obstruction – Abdominal distention, absolute constipation or vomiting.

## Secondary Causes of Constipation

➤ Drugs – Analgesia (opioids and NSAIDs), antacids, supplements (iron and calcium), antimuscarinics (procyclidine and oxybutynin), antidepressants (TCAs), antipsychotics (amisulpride and quetiapine), antiepileptic (carbamazepine, gabapentin, pregabalin and phenytoin), antihistamines (hydroxyzine), diuretics (furosemide) and CCBs.

➤ Endocrine – DM (auto and neuropathy), hypothyroidism and high levels of calcium.

➤ Neurological – CVA, Hirschsprung's disease, multiple sclerosis (MS), Parkinson's disease (PD), spinal cord injury and tumours.

➤ Structural – Anal fissures, haemorrhoids, strictures (anal and colon), colon cancer, IBD and rectal prolapse.

## Differentials

➤ Diet/functional

➤ Haemorrhoids

## Differential Diagnosis

| | |
|---|---|
| Anal fissures | A tear to the anal mucosa, often posterior to the anal canal. Pain on defecation, with blood on the toilet paper. Associated with constipation. OE: fissure visible and very tender on PR exam. |
| IBS | Extremely common. The most consistent features are abdominal pain, bloating and a change in bowel habits. Patients may be divided into those with diarrhoea-predominant IBS and those with constipation-predominant IBS. Features such as lethargy, nausea, backache and bladder symptoms may also be present. |
| Colorectal cancer | Weight loss, PR bleeding and an abdominal mass (which can be in the RIF). Unexplained iron deficiency anaemia. |
| Intestinal obstruction | A history of adhesions (previous surgery) or malignancy. Colicky abdominal pain, distension and absolute constipation, including wind. Bowels not opened. 'Tinkling' bowel sounds. |
| Hypothyroidism | Underactive thyroid gland. Presents with cold intolerance, hair loss, dry skin, fatigue, heavy or irregular periods, increased weight and low mood. OE: bradycardia, hypotension, reduced skin turgor, and may have a goitre, hair loss and reduced reflexes. |

## Examination

» Vitals – BP, weight (if increased it indicates hypothyroidism), temperature, Bristol stool chart (assess the stool quality; types 1 and 2 are abnormal).

» Thyroid – Goitre, hair loss, cold peripheries and reduced skin turgor.

» Abdominal

› Inspection – Inspect for signs of peristalsis or distension.

› Palpitation – Palpate the four quadrants for any pain, faecal loading and masses (colon cancer).

› Auscultation – Listen for bowel sounds (tinkling or absence).

» PR – Inspect for anal fissures and piles. Consider PR if there are impacted stools.

## Investigations

» Bloods – FBC, ferritin (iron deficiency indicates bowel cancer), TFTs, parathyroid hormone (PTH), calcium (hypercalcaemia), and U&Es (dehydration).

» Radiography – AXR (faecal loading, obstruction) and barium enema.

» Specialist – Colonoscopy, sigmoidoscopy and CT scan.

## Management

### Conservative

✓ Water – Advise that the patient increases their oral fluid intake to 2l/day (eight cups), and that they should avoid alcohol and fizzy drinks.

✓ Diet

› Fruit – Advise that they increase their fruit and vegetable intake (at least five portions per day); e.g. apples, apricots, pears, prunes, peaches and plums. Dried fruits have a higher concentration of sorbitol. This can be via fresh fruit juice.

› Fibre – Advise that they increase their fibre consumption by eating coarse bran, wholegrain bread and flour, brown rice, and wholemeal spaghetti. The effects are often rapid, but can take as long as four weeks.

✓ Exercise – Losing weight by exercising can help constipation. Immobility can cause constipation.

✓ Routine – Advise them to try not to hurry passing a motion. They should try going to the toilet first thing in the morning and 30 minutes after a meal. They should not hold a motion.

### Medical

✓ Side effects – Review the possible side effects of medications; if any occur, stop that medication and change to one of the alternatives.

✓ Laxatives – Start with a bulk-forming laxative. If they are passing hard stools, consider adding or transferring to an osmotic agent. If the patient still struggles or complains of tenesmus, add a stimulant laxative. Be aware of overuse and titrate downwards based on the symptoms (diarrhoea):

› Bulk-forming – Increases faecal mass thereby stimulating peristalsis; e.g. ispaghula husk 3.5g bd.

› Osmotic – Increases the amount of water in the large bowel; e.g. lactulose or macrogols (Movicol), one to three sachets daily.

› Stimulant – Increases intestinal motility (avoid in cases of obstruction); e.g. senna or bisacodyl.

› Softeners – Softens the stools; e.g. docusate 100–200mg bd.

✓ In pregnancy – Avoid osmotics, except lactulose. Avoid senna when they are near to term.

✓ IBS-C – If the patient has IBS that is mostly with constipation, try Linaclotide tablets.

✓ Impaction – Consider a high dose of macrogols for hard stools. Add a stimulant (senna) if it persists. Try suppositories (for soft stools use bisacodyl, and for hard stools use glycerol and bisacodyl) or a mild enema (docusate or sodium citrate). If there is still a poor response, try a sodium phosphate enema. Enemas may need to be given several times to release the hard, impacted stools. Leave the patient on regular laxatives once cleared. The enema may need to be given by a carer / district nurse (DN).

## Referral

→ Gastroenterologist – Refer the patient if there are red flags for bowel cancer. Surgical input may be required for anal fissures that are resistant to treatment. Refer them if a possible underlying aetiology (e.g. Crohn's disease) is suspected or there is no response to treatment.

→ Psychiatrist – Psychiatry input may be required if constipation is caused by depression.

→ Dietician – A dietician can offer useful advice regarding the patient's diet.

## Safety Netting

» If they have had symptoms for more than four to six weeks, they should reattend for a review. If the patient begins to vomit or suffers abdominal distension, they should seek medical advice.

*References*

National Institute for Health and Care Excellence (2010). *Prucalopride for the treatment of chronic constipation in women*. https://www.nice.org.uk/guidance/ta211

Simren, M., Palsson, O.S. and Whitehead, W. (2017). *Update on Rome IV Criteria for Colorectal Disorders. Current Gastroenterology Reports, 19(4)*. DOI: 10.1007/s11894-017-0554-0

World Gastroenterology Organisation (2010). *Constipation: a global perspective*. https://www.worldgastroenterology.org/guidelines/global-guidelines/constipation/constipation-english?utm_source=wgofundation&utm_medium=wdhd2012&utm_campaign=guidelines

# Liver Disease

The liver is a vital organ that has a wide range of functions, including metabolism, detoxification, the production of enzymes for digestion and protein synthesis. Given its multiple functions, the liver is prone to disease and damage. It may become infected with hepatitis (hep) (A, B or C), damaged due to alcohol or a high fat intake, or diseased from an overdose of medications (paracetamol). Common symptoms of liver disease include pain, jaundice and malaise.

## History

- » Focused questions
  - › Ask the patient about jaundice symptoms, including the onset (sudden or gradual), pruritus (itchy skin), and any change in urine (dark) or stools (pale).
  - › Ask them about lethargy/malaise symptoms, if they have any blood in their stools, haematemesis or sticky, black stools (varices).
  - › Ask if they have noticed that they bleed longer than normal (from any wound).

- » Associated history – Ask if they have experienced any pain and about the onset of it (gallstones), or if they have any nausea or vomiting (acute hepatitis), weight loss (carcinoma), pregnancy (obstetric cholestasis) or fever (hepatitis and cholangitis).

- » Past history – Ask if they have had raised cholesterol, liver disease, sickle cell disease or ERCP.

- » Family history – Ask if there is a family history of Wilson's disease, haemochromatosis, gallstones, glucose-6-phosphate dehydrogenase (G6PD) deficiency or hepatitis.

- » Drug history – Ask if they have taken aspirin, paracetamol, statins, methotrexate, terbinafine or allopurinol.

- » Social history – Ask if they smoke or drink alcohol (how much and how often), if they take recreational drugs (if there is any needle use or sharing needles), if they have travelled abroad, if they have had any unprotected sexual intercourse (UPSI) abroad, and what their occupation is (sewage worker, health worker or sex worker).

## RED FLAGS

Painless jaundice, weight loss or confusion (hepatic encephalopathy).

## Risk Factors for Hepatitis

➤ Blood transfusions in the past (<1992)

➤ Needle use (IV drugs, shared needles or tattoos/body piercing)

➤ Travel abroad (hep A)

➤ Food eaten (shellfish)

➤ Sexual history (including anal sex)

## Differential Diagnosis

| | |
|---|---|
| Hep B and C | A history of a blood transfusion, IV drugs, being a sex worker or having a tattoo. Hep C may be acquired from travel to Africa, the Middle East or Asia. May have been engaged in high-risk intercourse (anal). Usually asymptomatic, but patients may present with a prodrome (two weeks) of weakness, arthralgia, malaise, fever and tiredness. Later, the disease causes jaundice (dark urine / pale stools indicates cholestasis) and weight loss. OE: jaundice and signs of liver disease. |
| Hep A | A history of travel to Africa or Asia. May get a prodrome (two weeks) of weakness, malaise, fever, joint pain and GI symptoms (nausea and vomiting, and RUQ pain). Later, it may cause jaundice, pruritus, pale stools and dark urine. OE: fever, jaundice and hepatomegaly. |
| Gallstones | Calculi formed in the gallbladder or duct. Affects females who are >40 years, obese, have DM or are on COCP/HRT. Can have a family history of gallstones. May be asymptomatic. If impacted, may cause colicky RUQ pain radiating to the shoulder tip, jaundice, nausea and vomiting, and fever. OE: fever, jaundice, RUQ pain, positive Murphy's sign seen in cholecystitis (place two fingers over the RUQ, ask the patient to breathe in, and the patient stops due to pain; repeat over LUQ). |
| Pancreatitis | Often caused by gallstones or excessive alcohol. Patients present with acute, severe epigastric pain (which becomes continuous), radiating to the back, along with nausea and vomiting. In chronic pancreatitis, patients report dull, severe pain that is often precipitated by food. They may complain of difficulty in flushing away their stools, which are paler and have an offensive smell. OE: jaundice, fever, epigastric pain with rigidity, Cullen's (umbilical bruising) and Grey Turner's (flank bruising) signs. |
| Gilbert's syndrome | An inherited condition, for which there may be a positive family history. Usually asymptomatic, but may develop jaundice from time to time, especially after an infection or excess exercise. OE: nil to find. |
| Haemochromatosis | An inherited condition from iron overload. Usually begins in those >40 years. Causes symptoms of fatigue, erectile dysfunction (men), amenorrhoea (women) and joint pain. Leads to DM, bronzing of the skin, and liver and heart failure. |

## Examination

»   Vitals – Temperature (fever), BP, pulse and BMI (anorexia).

»   Inspection – Jaundice (skin and sclera), bronzed (haemochromatosis), signs of liver disease (tremor, clubbing, spider naevi, Dupuytren's contracture, palmar erythema, gynaecomastia, caput medusae or ascites).

»   Abdominal exam

  ›   Palpation – Examine the left supraclavicular area for LN (Virchow's indicates pancreatic/gastric cancer).

  ›   Liver – Feel for tenderness (acute hepatitis), hepatomegaly (smoothly enlarged indicates hepatitis/cirrhosis, and irregularly enlarged indicates carcinoma).

  ›   Spleen – Feel for an enlarged spleen (malaria or decompensated liver failure).

  ›   Gallbladder – Check for palpable gallbladder (gallstones or pancreatic carcinoma).

## Investigations

»   Bloods – FBC (reduced platelets and increased mean corpuscular volume [MCV] indicates excessive alcohol), ferritin (haemochromatosis), CRP, hepatitis serology, TFTs (thyrotoxicosis) and lipids (gallstones or non-alcoholic fatty liver disease [NAFLD]).

  ›   LFTs – gamma-glutamyl transferase (GGT) (excessive alcohol or cholestasis), ALT, AST, alkaline phosphatase (ALP) (gallstones), bilirubin and albumin (reduced indicates chronic liver disease).

  ›   Reticulocytes (haemolysis), viral load, clotting screen and amylase (pancreatitis).

  ›   Alpha-fetoprotein (AFP) (liver cancer) and malaria screen (travel).

»   Urine – Bilirubin and urobilinogen.

»   USS – Liver USS (gallstones, fatty liver, liver cysts, liver cancer or pancreatic masses).

»   Specialist – OGD (varices), ERCP/MRCP, etc.

### Interpreting Liver Function Blood Tests

| AST > ALT | Fatty liver, alcoholic hepatitis, cirrhosis, liver cancer or haemolytic jaundice. |
| --- | --- |
| ALT > AST | Acute hepatitis (viral or drug autoimmune) or obstructive jaundice. |
| ALP > ALT | Intrahepatic cholestasis, cholangitis or extrahepatic obstruction. |

| High ALT >500IU/l | Viral hepatitis, drug induced (paracetamol overdose [OD]) or autoimmune hepatitis. |
|---|---|
| High GGT and MCV | Alcohol abuse. If ALT is raised, consider alcohol hepatitis. |
| HIGH GGT and ALP | Cholestasis. |

## Management

*Treat the underlying cause*

### NAFLD

#### Conservative

✓ Lifestyle – Advise the patient to eat a healthy, balanced diet; cut down on fried and fatty foods; exercise daily; cut down on their alcohol intake; and try to lose 10% of their weight in six months.

#### Medical

✓ Statins – Advise them to continue unless their liver enzymes have doubled in three months (even from a raised baseline).

✓ Ensure type 2 DM, BP and lipids are managed optimally.

✓ Specialist – Use the enhanced liver fibrosis (ELF) test to check for liver fibrosis.

### Alcoholic hepatitis

✓ Advise them that they should aim to stop their alcohol intake. *See Alcoholism section, page 575.*

### Hepatitis

✓ Hep A – Reassure the patient as it is self-limiting (under two months). Advise them to avoid alcohol as it resolves.

✓ Hep B & C – Refer the patient to a specialist (hepatology/gastro).

#### Conservative – Prevention

✓ Hygiene (hep A) – Advise them to wash their hands with soap and water after going to the toilet or before handling food.

✓ Advise them to not share needles, and to attend a needle-sharing programme.

✓ Advise them to avoid sharing toothbrushes, razors and scissors.

✓ Advise them to use condoms when having sexual intercourse.

✓ Advise them only to go to tattoo parlours that sterilise equipment or use disposable equipment.

✓ Ensure patients have received a hep A, diphtheria, tetanus and pertussis (DTP) vaccination.

*Medical*

✓ Pain – Treat pain with paracetamol/NSAIDs or codeine. Reduce the dose of paracetamol and avoid codeine if the patient has severe liver dysfunction.

✓ Nausea – Offer metoclopramide for a short duration.

✓ Pruritus – Advise the patient to wear loose clothing and avoid hot showers. Give Piriton, but avoid in cases of severe impairment. Give cholestyramine or ursodeoxycholic acid if they are unresponsive (specialist).

✓ Pregnancy – Infants should be immunised against hep B at birth. Breastfeeding is safe if a child is immunised.

✓ Refer the patient to genitourinary medicine (GUM), or the drugs support team for IV users. Hepatology will start antiviral treatment (peginterferon, entecavir or tenofovir).

## Haemochromatosis

### Conservative

✓ Avoid food rich in iron. Drink tea and eat non-citrus fruits.

### Medical

✓ Perform a regular (weekly) venesection until serum iron is in the normal range, then perform every three months. Consider chelation therapy (specialist) if venesection contraindication.

## Cirrhosis

### Medical

✓ Refer the patient to a specialist to monitor. Conduct an urgent medical team admission if there are signs of encephalopathy.

✓ Immunisation – Advise them to get the yearly influenza and a one-off pneumococcus vaccination.

✓ Specialist – Perform 6–12 month bloods for LFTs and AFP (carcinoma). Place on the waiting list for a liver transplant.

✓ Diet – High-protein and high-calorie diet. Consider thiamine replacement.

✓ Ascites – Treat with salt and fluids.

✓ Varices – B-blocker for medium-sized varices and OGD for ligation.

✓ Palliative – Refer them to palliative care if their prognosis is <12 months.

## Pancreatitis

### Conservative

✓ Advise the patient to avoid alcohol, and adhere to a high-protein, low-fat diet. Refer them to a dietician.

✓ Chronic – Advise them to stop smoking and drinking alcohol, to eat a low-fat diet and to take analgesia if in pain (paracetamol, NSAIDs or codeine phosphate).

*Medical*

✓    Acute – Admit the patient for IV fluids, analgesia and nutrition.

✓    CREONs – Offer to prescribe these to help digestion if they have steatorrhoea.

*Surgical*

✓    Treat the cause by removing any gallstones.

## Gallstones

*Conservative*

✓    Advise the patient to lose weight, stop smoking, exercise and adhere to a low-fat diet.

*Medical*

✓    Asymptomatic gallstones do not need surgery.

>    Acute cholecystitis – Admit the patient (IV antibiotics). Offer analgesia if they are painful.

>    Chronic - Refer them routinely for a cholecystectomy. Consider a more urgent admission if the patient is acutely unwell, cholangitis is suspected or bilirubin >100.

---

## References

National Institute for Health and Care Excellence (2013). *Hepatitis B (chronic): diagnosis and management.* https://www.nice.org.uk/guidance/cg165

National Institute for Health and Care Excellence (2016). *Non-alcoholic fatty liver disease (NAFLD): assessment and management.* https://www.nice.org.uk/guidance/ng49

National Institute for Health and Care Excellence (2016). *Cirrhosis in over 16s: assessment and management.* https://www.nice.org.uk/guidance/ng50

# Irritable Bowel Syndrome

IBS is a chronic (more than six months) relapsing and remitting bowel disorder that presents with gastrointestinal symptoms. It is a functional disorder with no known organic cause. It mainly affects people who are 20–30 years of age, with females suffering twice as commonly as men. Approximately 10–20% of people suffer from it in the general population. Symptoms typically include abdominal bloating, pain and discomfort, often associated with bouts of diarrhoea and/or constipation. There can be an overlap of symptoms with other GI disorders, such as coeliac disease or non-ulcer dyspepsia. However, patients often present with symptom profiles that are diarrhoea predominant (IBS-D), constipation predominant (IBS-C) or a mixed type (IBS-M).

## Diagnosing IBS by History

Consider IBS if the person reports the following symptoms for at least six months:

- » Abdominal pain or discomfort
- » Bloating
- » Change in bowel habits

A diagnosis of IBS should be considered if the person has the following:

- » Abdominal pain or discomfort that is relieved by defecation; or
- » Altered bowel frequency or stool form.

  **This should be accompanied by at least two of the following four symptoms:**

  - Altered stool passage (straining, urgency or incomplete evacuation).
  - Abdominal bloating (more common in women than men), distension, tension or hardness.
  - Symptoms made worse by eating.
  - Passage of mucus.

- » Other features such as lethargy, nausea, backache and bladder symptoms are common in people with IBS, and may be used to support the diagnosis.

## History

- » Focused questions
  - › Ask the patient to describe the diarrhoea/constipation and abdominal discomfort.
  - › Ask them about the abdominal pain (site, timing, onset, etc.) and bloating.
  - › Ask if there has been any change in bowel habits (diarrhoea, constipation or a bit of both).

> › Ask if there has been any faecal incontinence, urgency, tenesmus, straining, stool consistency or mucus.

> › Ask if the pain is relieved after defecation.

> › Ask about stress and if there is anything that exacerbates the symptoms (after eating, any foods that trigger symptoms, such as alcohol, caffeine, or spicy or fatty foods).

» Associated history – Ask if they experience fatigue, nausea or vomiting.

» Past history – Ask if they have had IBD, hypothyroid/hyperthyroid, generalised anxiety disorder (GAD) or depression, or recent surgery.

» Drug history – For constipation, ask if they have taken SSRIs, TCAs, codeine, steroids, loperamide or ferrous sulphate; for diarrhoea, ask if they have taken antibiotics or laxatives. Ask if they have taken NSAIDs.

» Social history – Ask if they smoke or drink alcohol, ask what their occupation is, and ask about their diet.

» Family history – Ask if there is a family history of bowel problems (IBD or IBS), bowel cancer or ovarian cancer.

## Differential Diagnosis

| | |
|---|---|
| Coeliac | Steatorrhoea, related to gluten. Weight loss. |
| Diverticulitis | Cramping pain on the left side of the abdomen, bloating, fever or blood in the stools. |
| IBD | Mucus or blood in the stools, ulcers in the mouth, fever, weight loss or eye symptoms. |
| Ovarian cancer | Always feeling bloated, continuous pelvic or abdominal pain, feeling full all the time or feeling sick when eating. |

## RED FLAGS

» Colon cancer – Unintentional weight loss, rectal bleeding, or a change in bowel habits to looser or frequent stools for more than six weeks in a >60-year-old.

» A family history of bowel cancer or ovarian cancer.

## Rome IV Criteria for Diagnosing IBS (Lacy et al., 2016)

Recurrent abdominal pain, for at least one day/week on average in the last three months, associated with two or more of the following:

» Related to defecation.

» A change in stool frequency.

» A change in the form (appearance) of the stools.

## Examination

» Vitals – Weight, BMI and use the Bristol stool chart to assess the stools.

» Abdominal

> Inspection – Inspect for anaemia in the eyes.

> Palpation – Palpate for pain and masses. Examine for organomegaly (liver/spleen).

> Auscultation – Listen for bowel sounds.

» Perform PR for rectal masses, impacted stools or melaena.

» Consider pelvic exam in females to exclude pelvic masses (ovarian cancer).

## Investigations

» Bloods – FBC (anaemia), ESR/CRP (IBD), coeliac disease screen, CA125 (ovarian cancer) and TFTs (hypothyroidism/hyperthyroidism).

» Stools – If the diagnosis is in doubt, perform MC&S, ova, cysts, parasites, FOB and faecal calprotectin.

» Request a referral for an AXR if an intestinal obstruction is suspected.

## Management

*Conservative*

✓ Food diary – Offer the patient a food diary for them to complete over two weeks to establish any food triggers.

✓ Reassure – Explain the diagnosis and reassure the patient that it is not life-threatening.

✓ Fluids – Advise them to drink plenty of fluid (eight cups/day), restrict tea and coffee, and avoid alcohol and fizzy drinks.

✓ Diet – Offer them dietary advice depending on symptoms (i.e. constipation/diarrhoea). Signpost them to the low fermentable oligo-, di-, mono-saccharides and polyols (FODMAP) diet (which identifies foods to avoid that may not be absorbed in the gut properly, causing bloating, diarrhoea and cramping pains) via a dietician. Also advise them of the following:

> They should eat regularly and slowly, not miss meals and avoid long gaps between meals. If the experience bloating and diarrhoea, they should try taking probiotics for four weeks, and restrict intake of fruit and vegetables.

> › They should consider limiting their fibre intake (bran, brown rice and wholemeal bread) and monitor the impact.

> › If they are bloated, they should try eating oats or linseeds (one tablespoon/day).

> › If they have diarrhoea, they should avoid sorbitol (artificial sweetener).

✓ Exercise – Encourage them to exercise for 30 minutes five times/week.

✓ Relaxation – Suggest they employ relaxation techniques and ways to reduce stress.

*Medical*

✓ Bloating – Mebeverine, hyoscine and peppermint oils. Rotate through the agents separately if there is no response. If there is improvement, then leave the patient on an as needed (pro re nata [PRN]) dose.

✓ Constipation – Ispaghula husk is the first-line treatment. They should avoid lactulose, but consider Movicol or senna.

✓ Diarrhoea – Loperamide is the first-line treatment. They should avoid codeine phosphate.

✓ People with IBS should be advised how to adjust their doses of laxative or antimotility agent according to the clinical response. The dose should be titrated according to stool consistency, with the aim of achieving soft, well-formed stools (Bristol stool chart type 4).

✓ TCAs/SSRI – Consider a low dose of amitriptyline (5–30mg) as the second-line treatment if laxatives, loperamide or antispasmodics have not helped. If there is no response, consider SSRIs (citalopram or fluoxetine). If there is no response after one year of treatment, refer the patient for CBT.

# Referral

→ Refer the patient urgently if there is evidence of unexplained anaemia, raised ESR/CRP, an abdominal or rectal mass, or symptoms in a >60-year-old.

→ Routinely refer them to gastroenterology if symptoms persist.

→ Refer them to a dietician for single food exclusion diets (FODMAP).

→ Refer them for CBT for depression or a low mood.

# Safety Netting

» Review the patient if their symptoms persist for more than four to six weeks. Assess for the presence of depressive symptoms.

## References

Lacy, B.E., Mearin, F., Chang. L, Chey, W.D, Lembo, A.J., Simren, M. and Spiller, R. (2016). *Bowel disorders. Gastroenterology, 150,* 1393–1407.

National Institute for Health and Care Excellence (2008). *Irritable bowel syndrome in adults: diagnosis and management.* https://www.nice.org.uk/guidance/cg61

# Obesity

Obesity is rapidly becoming a worldwide pandemic. A patient is classified as obese when they have a BMI >30. It increases the relative risk of a whole range of different conditions, including type 2 DM, IHD, gallbladder disease, BP, OA, sleep apnoea, cancer (breast, endometrial and colon), polycystic ovarian syndrome (PCOS) and back pain, among others. Over 50% of people are considered to be overweight or obese in the UK, and it requires remedial advice or exercise interventions to buck this trend. Life expectancy drops by two to four years in patients with a BMI of 30–35, and by eight to ten years if they have a BMI of 40–50.

### Classification of Obesity

| BMI | Classification |
| --- | --- |
| 18.5–24.9 | Healthy weight |
| 25–29.9 | Overweight |
| 30–34.9 | Obesity I |
| 35–39.9 | Obesity II |
| >40 | Obesity III |

## Causes of Obesity

➤ Common – Lifestyle (food and drink consumption), physical inactivity, social/psychological factors or genetic predisposition.

➤ Conditions – Genetic (e.g. Prader-Willi syndrome), hypothyroidism, PCOS, growth hormone deficiency (GHD) or Cushing's syndrome.

➤ Medication – Steroids, b-blockers, lithium, antipsychotics (atypical), anticonvulsants (valproate or gabapentin), antidepressants (TCA or mirtazapine), or oral hypoglycaemic drugs (sulphonylureas or glitazones).

## History

» Open questions

› Motivation – Ask them to tell you why they want to lose weight. Ask if anything has happened recently that made them want to lose weight now.

› Thoughts about weight – Ask them how confident they are of losing weight. Ask what their thoughts are.

» Focused questions:

› Diet – Ask what they eat, and let them talk through a typical day. Ask them about the types of food they eat in a day, including fatty foods (pizza or burgers), sugary foods (snacks and fizzy drinks) and snacks before bedtime.

› Exercise – Ask how much exercise they do in a week, and if they do any intense exercise (football, swimming, cycling or jogging).

› Previous attempts – Ask if they have made any previous attempts to lose weight, what happened, and if they have tried any diet plans or weight-loss programmes (Weightwatchers or Slimfast).

» Associated history – Ask if they have any breathing problems (asthma), joint pains (OA), difficulty breathing at night (sleep apnoea) or chest pain (IHD).

» Past history – Ask if they have had IHD (high BP, DM, strokes or high cholesterol).

» Drug history – Ask if they have taken any steroids, COCP, antipsychotics, sulphonylurea, insulin, HRT, TCAs, sodium valproate or gabapentin.

» Social history – Ask if they smoke or drink alcohol, and ask what their occupation is.

» Family history – Ask if there is a family history of obesity, IHD or DM.

## Differentials

➤ Hypothyroidism
➤ PCOS

## Examination

» Vitals – Height, weight, BMI, weight circumference and BP.

## Investigations

» Bloods – U&Es, LFTs, lipids and HbA1c

› Others – Follicle stimulating hormone (FSH) and luteinizing hormone (LH) (PCOS), TFT and cortisol (Cushing's syndrome).

» Urine – Glucose and protein.

## Management

*Conservative*

✓ Target – Advise them to aim to lose 5–10% of their original weight at a rate of around 0.5–1kg/week.

✓ Diet – Suggest that they eat food slowly. They should chew each morsel of food 20 times. They should spread the food thinly over the plate and not stack it up. They should have small portions. They should grill or steam rather than fry.

✓ Alcohol – Advise them to minimise the calories they get from drinking alcohol by cutting down.

✓ Exercise – Advise them to do 30 minutes exercise a day, five days a week, and enough to get slightly breathless or to increase the rate at which the heart pumps. They should consider using a pedometer / fitness tracker.

> They should make enjoyable activities part of everyday life (walking, cycling, swimming, going to the gym and gardening).

> They should minimise sedentary activities (watching television, using the computer and playing video games).

> They should build activity into the working day (taking the stairs instead of the lift, and taking a walk at lunchtime).

✓ Motivational – Stress the health benefits of losing weight and that it should be achieved over a period of time.

✓ Support – Suggest support groups such as Weight Watchers. Consider counselling therapies if obesity is affecting the patient's mood.

**Diet Advice Regarding Obesity**

> Advise the patient to do the following:

- Eat five portions of fruit or vegetables each day, in place of foods higher in fat and calories.

- Do not base their meals on starchy foods (potatoes, bread, rice or pasta), but choose wholegrain versions if possible.

- Eat fibre-rich foods.

- Avoid drinks and snacks that are high in fat and sugar (takeaway and fast foods), and consider drinking water.

- Eat breakfast, watch the portion size of meals and snacks, and watch how often they are eating.

*Medical*

✓ Orlistat – Offer orlistat as an adjunct to lifestyle advice. Take 120mg tds before or with meals (30 minutes before or up to one hour after). If they miss a meal or the meal lacks fat, omit the dose. It can be taken with vitamin tablets (with reduced absorption of fat-soluble vitamins – K A, D and E).

✓ Initiate – Consider if patient has a BMI >28 with associated risk factors (HTN, DM or cholesterol), or a BMI >30 without risk factors.

✓ Target weight loss – Advise them to aim for 5% weight loss after three months before continuing. Provide treatment for >12 months if the pros and cons have been discussed with the patient.

✓ Side effects – Wind, diarrhoea, faecal urgency and faecal incontinence.

✓ Contraindications – Malabsorption, breastfeeding or cholecystectomy.

*Surgical*

✓ Consider surgery (banding/gastric bypass) in patients with severe obesity (e.g. BMI >40, BMI >35 plus risk factors, or where non-surgical measures have been attempted for six months and failed). The patient is to receive intensive follow up with a specialist team, including a dietician and counsellors. The patient must be physically fit for surgery. There are often long waiting lists.

## Referral

→ Refer the patient to a local exercise programme, if appropriate.

→ Refer them to a dietician for diet advice and support.

## Safety Netting

» Follow up and monitor weight, initially fortnightly and then monthly. Consider referral to a nurse run obesity clinic.

---

*References*

National Institute for Health and Care Excellence (2014). *Obesity: identification, assessment and management.* https://www.nice.org.uk/guidance/cg189

# Dysphagia

Dysphagia, also known as difficulty in swallowing, affects a large number of patients, particularly those who are elderly. It can be quite a distressing symptom to suffer from, especially as a result of the choking sensation felt when trying to swallow. It is estimated that in the general population around 6% suffer with dysphagia, increasing to 30% in patients with mental health problems. There are a number of different causes that may present with dysphagia, particularly oesophageal or pharyngeal disorders; however, you should also consider neurological conditions such as strokes and achalasia. Patients suffering with learning disabilities often have associated dysphagia, and this should be enquired about.

## History

- » Focused questions
  - › Dysphagia – Ask when they first noticed it, and how long it lasts for.
  - › Onset – Ask if it was sudden or gradual.
  - › Nature – Ask if it comes and goes (intermittent), or is there all the time (persistent).
  - › Site – Ask if there is a particular level at which they feel the food gets stuck.
  - › Character – Ask if they have difficulty swallowing solids, liquids or a combination.

- » Associated history – Ask if they experience odynophagia (pain swallowing), coughing (bothersome, worse after eating or drinking, or a recurrent chest infection), aspiration (voice change), choking, vomiting or weight loss.

- » Past history – Ask if they have had any swallowing issues, medical issues (iron deficiency anaemia, GORD, PU, or calcinosis, Raynaud phenomenon, oesophageal dysmotility, sclerodactyly, and telangiectasia [CREST]), steroid inhalers for asthma, any camera tests (OGD) or a barium swallow.
  - › For CREST – Ask if they have had any tightening or thickening of the skin of the hands or feet, and whether they have noticed their hands changing colour from white to blue or red.

- » Drug history – Ask if they have taken any NSAIDs or SSRIs.

- » Social history – Ask if they smoke or drink alcohol, ask what their occupation is, and ask about their diet.

- » Family history – Ask if there is a family history of ulcers, stomach cancer or throat cancer.

## RED FLAGS

Progressive dysphagia, persistent vomiting, unexplained iron deficiency anaemia, weight loss, upper abdominal mass, >55 years with unexplained dyspepsia, haematemesis, persistent vomiting, epigastric mass or stroke.

## Differential Diagnosis

| | |
|---|---|
| Oesophagitis | A burning sensation radiating from the stomach to the neck, related to meals or retrosternal discomfort, with an acidic taste in the mouth (acid brash) or water brash (excessive saliva). Odynophagia. Absence of weight loss. Relieved by antacids. Risk factors: smoking, diet, coffee, pregnancy, big meals or hiatus hernia. |
| Oesophageal spasm | Intermittent dysphagia with chest pain. GORD-like symptoms with regurgitation. |
| Achalasia | The neuromuscular failure of the relaxation of the lower oesophageal sphincter (LOS). Typically affects 30–40-year-olds. Dysphagia is more marked for solids than liquid. Gradual insidious onset over several years. Associated with heartburn, the regurgitation of food and foul belching. Regurgitation can lead to a night cough and the risk of aspiration pneumonia. |
| Oesophageal cancer | Rapid progressive dysphagia of solids then liquids. The regurgitation of foods and haematemesis. A feeling of food stuck at a certain level. Pain is a late feature. Associated with weight loss and appetite change. Risk factors: Barrett's oesophagus, GORD, smoking, excessive alcohol, and a lack of fruit and vegetables. |
| Oesophageal candidiasis | Retrosternal pain or dysphagia (foods or fluids). Consider in HIV-positive patients or from steroid inhaler use in asthmatics. |
| Pharyngeal pouch | Seen more often in elderly men (>70 years). Patients complain that the first morsel of food is swallowed easily while later mouthfuls are progressively more difficult. Associated with halitosis (food decay in the pouch) and the regurgitation of foods. Risk of aspiration (chronic cough) and weight loss. OE: a lump protruding to one side (L>R) that gurgles on palpation. |
| Globus pharyngeus | Common in middle age; men and women are equally affected. Past history of anxiety/depression. Patients report feeling a lump in their throat (front), that moves up and down, with no difficulty swallowing. Symptoms are intermittent. All investigations will be normal. OE: nil to find. |

## Examination

» Vitals – Weight (loss), BMI, pulse and oxygen saturation.

» Hands – Inspect for calcinosis, telangiectasia and sclerodactyly (CREST).

» Neck – Inspect for masses. Palpate the thyroid gland.

» Abdominal

› Inspection – Inspect the conjunctiva for signs of anaemia. Look in the throat for signs of candidiasis.

› Palpitation – Palpate the upper epigastric area for masses.

» Neurological – Perform a cerebellar or focused cranial nerve assessment (bulbar palsy), inspect for muscle fasciculations (motor neurone disease [MND]) and examine the power of the limbs (CVA).

## Investigations

» Bloods – FBC, ferritin, U&E, TFTs and ESR.

» X-ray – Barium swallow (achalasia or oesophageal spasm) and CXR (mediastinal tumour).

» USS – Thyroid gland.

» Endoscopy – OGD (oesophageal web or cancer).

» Other (specialist) – MRI, oesophageal manometry (achalasia) or oesophageal pH monitor.

## Management

*Conservative*

✓ Eating habits – Advise them to eat several small meals regularly instead of large meals. After eating, they should wait two hours before lying down. They should avoid any late-night snacks.

✓ Dysphagia – Advise them to alter the consistency of the foods consumed (thickeners). They should adhere to speech and language therapy (SALT) and dieticians' advice.

✓ Tablets – Consider substituting tablet preparations with liquids, orodispersible formulas, patches, rectal medications and buccal sublingual tablets.

*Dry mouth*

*Conservative*

✓ Advise them to ensure a good fluid intake (>2l daily). They should stop smoking and reduce their alcohol intake. They should sip cold drinks frequently or consider sucking ice cubes. Chewing gum helps increase salivation, or they could eat partly frozen melon/pineapple chunks. They should apply petroleum jelly to lips to prevent dryness and cracking.

*Medical*

✓     Advise them to stop medications that cause xerostomia. Prescribe artificial saliva (bioXtra gel or Saliva) or pilocarpine 5mg.

## Globus pharyngeus

### Conservative

✓     Perform a diagnosis of exclusion. Advise them to stop smoking. Reassure them.

### Medical

✓     Some respond to empirical PPI or treatment for postnasal drip (nasal spray).

✓     It is often precipitated by anxiety or a recent life event. Offer talking (CBT) or hypnosis therapies.

✓     Refer the patient to ear, nose and throat (ENT) department if it is persistent. Consider a SALT referral.

## GORD

### Conservative

✓      Advise the patient to reduce their weight, and avoid chilli and spicy food. They should cut down on caffeine and alcohol. They should stop smoking. They should eat small, regular meals and ensure that the last meal of the day is at least three hours before bedtime. They should avoid hot drinks.

### Medical

✓      Alginates(Gaviscon), H2 antagonist (ranitidine) or PPI (omeprazole).

## Achalasia/Spasm

✓     Usually under specialist care for management.

### Medical

✓     Consider nitrates or nifedipine to relax the LOS for symptomatic relief.

### Surgical

✓     May require a balloon dilatation.

## Oesophageal Candidiasis

### Medical

✓      Treatment is under secondary care, and consider admission. Treat with oral fluconazole 200–400mg od.

## Pharyngeal pouch

✓     Refer the patient to ENT for further investigations.

## Referral

→   Patients with dysphagia who show signs of aspiration or choking of unknown cause should be kept NBM and referred to hospital. Patients with red flags should be referred urgently. Patients with a possible CVA should be admitted.

→   Dietician – Consider referring them to a dietician for tailored nutritional advice to prevent dehydration and malnutrition.

→   SALT – Refer them to SALT for swallowing retraining, as well as to grade the severity of the dysphagia. They may need assessment for nasal or percutaneous endoscopic gastrostomy (PEG) feeding.

---

*References*

National Institute for Health and Care Excellence (2015). *Suspected cancer: recognition and referral.* https://www.nice.org.uk/guidance/ng12

Scottish Intercollegiate Guidelines Network (2010). *SIGN 119 Management of patients with stroke: identification and management of dysphagia.* https://www.sign.ac.uk/media/1057/sign119.pdf

# Per Rectum Bleeding

PR bleeding is blood passed per rectum. It includes bleeding that can occur anywhere along the GI tract. It is often classified as upper or lower GI bleeding based upon the appearance of the blood. Usually, the higher the site of the bleed, the darker the appearance of the blood. Conversely, the closer the site of the bleed is to the anus, the brighter the colour will be. The most common cause of PR bleeding is haemorrhoids; however, more serious conditions (such as bowel cancer) must always be considered, particularly in older persons.

## History

- » Focused questions
  - › Ask when they first noticed the PR bleeding and how long it has been going on for.
  - › Ask if it is fresh (seen on toilet paper), has turned the toilet bowl red, or is mixed in with stools or separate.
  - › Ask how much blood they passed (measured in cupfuls).
  - › Ask about the colour (bright red, or black and tarry).

- » Associated history – Ask if they experience abdominal pain, diarrhoea or constipation, fever, feeling bloated or any weight loss.
- » Past history – Ask if they have had rectal bleeding in the past or bowel problems.
- » Drug history – Ask if they have taken NSAIDs, aspirin or warfarin.
- » Social history – Ask if they smoke or drink alcohol, what their occupation is, if they have travelled abroad, and what their diet is like.
- » Family history – Ask if there is a family history of bowel cancer, HNPCC, familial adenomatous polyposis (FAP) or IBD.

## Different Colours of Stools

- ➤ Dark and tarry (melaena) – Upper GI bleed (peptic or oesophagus), iron or bismuth treatment.
- ➤ Blood red – Diverticulitis (large volume), colorectal cancer (mixed with stools), ulcerative colitis and colitis (blood and mucus mixed in the stools), haemorrhoids (painless, fresh blood on the stools and in the pan), anal fissure (painful, fresh blood on the toilet paper and the stools).
- ➤ Pale and bulky (steatorrhoea) – Fat malabsorption (coeliac) or pancreatic disease.

## RED FLAGS

» Colon cancer – >40 years, weight loss, change in appetite, change in bowel habits for more than six weeks or a rectal mass.

» Upper GI bleed – Melaena, haematemesis or persistent vomiting.

» Iron deficiency – Dizziness and fatigue.

» IBD – More than four to six episodes of bloody diarrhoea with fever.

## Differential Diagnosis

| | |
|---|---|
| Anal fissures | Tear to the anal mucosa, often posterior to the anal canal. Pain on defecation, with bright-red blood on the toilet paper. Associated with constipation. Patients may develop a fear of defecation or sitting. OE: visible fissure or sentinel pile, and very tender on PR exam. |
| Haemorrhoids | Background of constipation with fresh blood on toilet paper, the surface of the stools or dipping into the pan. The patient sometimes experiences soiling. Tenesmus, mucus discharge and pruritus ani. OE: piles are often visible on PR (grades two to four). |
| Crohn's disease | Transmural chronic inflammatory disease that can affect any part of the GI tract from the mouth to the anus. Crampy abdominal pains (may mimic appendicitis) and diarrhoea. OE: mouth ulcers and a mass in the RIF; other features include perianal tags, fissures, fistulas and extra-intestinal symptoms, such as arthritis, uveitis and erythema nodosum. |
| Ulcerative colitis | Ulcerating disease affecting only the mucous membrane of the large bowel, starting from the rectum. There may be some relief from passing stools. Bloody diarrhoea, rectal bleeding (more than Crohn's disease), urgency, tenesmus, nocturnal defecation and weight loss. |
| Diverticulitis | Small out outpouchings of the large bowel that become inflamed or infected. Often affects females from 50–70 years. Symptoms include abdominal pain, bloating and cramps, mainly in the LIF, with fever, nausea, vomiting and constipation. Frank blood mixed in with the stools is a complication. OR: tenderness on the left side (inflamed colon). |
| Polyp | Common benign growth of the lining of the colon/rectum. Causes PR bleeding. Can turn cancerous. |
| Colorectal cancer | Suspect if there is weight loss, a change in bowel habits (diarrhoea or constipation) or stools with mucus (secreting tumour). PR bleeding and abdominal mass. Unexplained iron deficiency anaemia. |

| Angiodysplasia | Caused by a small vascular malformation of the colon. Produces painless rectal bleeding and iron deficiency anaemia. |
|---|---|

# Examination

» Vitals – BP (hypotension), pulse (tachycardia), temperature and weight (loss).

» Request a chaperone.

» Abdominal

  › Inspection – Inspect the conjunctiva for signs of anaemia.

  › Palpation – Palpate for hepatomegaly, masses or tenderness.

» Rectal exam

  › Inspection – Look for skin tags, ulcers, fissures, polyps, piles or external haemorrhoids.

  › Palpation – Palpate for any masses. Ask the patient to strain downwards. Check for blood or mucus.

## Grading of internal haemorrhoids

» Grade I – Do not prolapse out of the anal canal.

» Grade II – Prolapse on defecation but reduce spontaneously.

» Grade III – Can be reduced manually.

» Grave IV – Cannot be reduced.

# Investigations

» Bloods – FBC (anaemia), ferritin (iron def), U&E (acute bleed) and LFTs (oesophageal varices).

  › Other – ESR, CRP (IBD), CEA (bowel cancer), coeliac screen and clotting screen.

» Stools – FOB / faecal immunochemical test (FIT), H. pylori, MC&S and faecal calprotectin.

  › Offer qFIT for people without rectal bleeding but with unexplained symptoms that do not meet the criteria for a suspected cancer pathway referral.

» Specialist – Barium enema, CT abdomen and endoscopy (OGD, colonoscopy and sigmoidoscopy).

# Management

*Treat the underlying cause*

## IBD

### Conservative

✓ Offer an elemental diet for a patient with Crohn's disease (particularly in flare ups, which settles within four weeks) and advise them to quit smoking. Suggest probiotics for ulcerative colitis.

### Medical

✓ Refer the patient to a specialist for a colonoscopy and diagnosis.

✓ Crohn's disease – Specialists use aminosalicylates (mesalazine), steroids or immunosuppressants (azathioprine or methotrexate). Consider surgery. Patients are sometimes given prolonged courses of antibiotics.

✓ Ulcerative colitis – Rectal mesalazine or steroids for distal colitis. Oral mesalazine or steroids if severe. Can be offered azathioprine or tacrolimus. Surgery for stoma.

## Diverticulitis

### Conservative

✓ Encourage the patient to have a high-fibre diet, fluids and exercise.

### Medical

✓ If severe, refer them for admission and IV antibiotics. Can give augmentin or metronidazole in hospital. Avoid NSAIDs (due to the risk of perforations). For chronic diverticular disease, consider laxatives (ispaghula husk or lactulose) and antispasmodic agents.

## Haemorrhoids/Fissures

### Conservative

✓ Treat constipation by giving dietary advice: they should eat at least five portions of fruit or vegetables a day, encourage increased fluid intake and more fibre, they should lose weight, and they should decrease their alcohol and red meat intake. Advise them to try not to strain when passing a motion, and to not delay passing stools when they feel they have to go. They should keep the anal area clean and dry.

### Medical (haemorrhoids)

✓ Prescribe a stool softener (ispaghula or lactulose). Oral analgesics such as paracetamol. Avoid codeine (which worsens constipation) or NSAIDs if they have a PR bleed. Consider Anusol haemorrhoid cream or topical local anaesthetic (LA) for symptomatic relief. Give a low dose topical steroids if anal inflammation or eczema is present.

✓ Admit those with acutely thrombosed external piles <72 hours from onset.

*Surgical (haemorrhoids)*

✓ Refer the patient to a colorectal surgeon for banding, sclerotherapy (injecting) or haemorrhoidectomy.

*Medical (fissures)*

✓ Consider topical GTN or diltiazem ointment for fissures. Warn the patient about headaches as a common side effect. They may be referred for trial of botulinum toxin injections if they are not keen on surgery.

## Referral

→ Ulcerative colitis – Refer the patient to hospital if they are producing more than six stools/day, have blood in their stools, or have a systemic illness (fever, tachycardia, abdominal pain, distension or reduced bowel sounds).

→ Colon cancer – Refer the patient according to NICE guidance, under 2WW.

**Colon cancer referrals – NICE guidance**

A referral should be made for one of the following:

- Patient >40 years with unexplained weight loss or abdominal pain.

- Patient >50 years with unexplained rectal bleeding.

- Patient >60 years with iron deficiency anaemia or a change in bowel habits.

- Positive qFIT/FOB test of faeces.

- Patient with a rectal or abdominal mass.

- Patient <50 years with rectal bleeding plus any of these: abdominal pain, change in bowel habits, weight loss or iron deficiency anaemia.

### Safety Netting

» Admission – Refer the patient for hospital admission if there are signs of shock.

» Follow-up – Review the patient if their symptoms worsen or persist for more than three to four weeks.

*Reference*

National Institute for Health and Care Excellence (2015). *Suspected cancer: recognition and referral.* https://www.nice.org.uk/guidance/ng12

National Institute for Health and Care Excellence (2019). *Ulcerative colitis: management.* https://www.nice.org.uk/guidance/ng130

National Institute for Health and Care Excellence (2019). *Crohn's disease: management.* https://www.nice.org.uk/guidance/ng129

# Lactose Intolerance

Lactose intolerance is a type of malabsorption of carbohydrates, which is a result of lactase deficiency. Typically, lactose is hydrolysed by lactase in the intestinal mucosa.

The symptoms result from the reduced absorption of lactose, which is then broken down by intestinal bacteria, leading to gas and short-chain fatty acids.

*There are three different types of lactase deficiency:*

1. Congenital – A rare disorder in which there is no lactase activity.

2. Primary – A gradual reduction in lactase production as you grow from infancy into adulthood.

3. Secondary – A deficiency in lactase due to another cause, such as immune disorders, gastroenteritis, cystic fibrosis or bowel surgery.

## History

» Symptoms occur from one to a few hours after the intake of milk or dairy products.

» Infants may also present with abdominal distension and vomiting.

» Ask about these symptoms of gas build up:

  › Bloating

  › Flatulence

  › Abdominal discomfort

» Ask about the acidic and osmotic effects of undigested lactose:

  › Loose, watery stools with a degree of urgency an hour or two after the ingestion of milk.

  › Perianal itching due to acidic stools.

## Differentials

➤ IBS
➤ An allergy to milk proteins
➤ Infantile colic
➤ Diverticular disease
➤ Ulcerative colitis
➤ Coeliac disease

## Examination

» In children, there may be malnutrition and a failure to thrive, but this is uncommon.

» In adults, the examination is usually normal.

## Investigations

» The use of an exclusion diet (low lactose) is the simplest diagnostic method (it should show an improvement in symptoms), followed by reintroduction (should cause symptom recurrence). The symptoms usually improve within 48 hours of exclusion.

» Breath tests are used. When colonic bacteria acts upon undigested lactose, hydrogen forms. Breath hydrogen analysis is useful in the diagnosis of lactose intolerance.

» A biopsy of the small intestinal mucosa by endoscopy is taken to test for lactase activity.

## Management

*Conservative*

✓ For infants, the treatment of documented lactose intolerance is the removal of lactose from the diet in the form of lactose-free formulas.

✓ Lactose-free formulas have a greater potential to cause dental cavities because the non-cariogenic sugar lactose is replaced with cariogenic glucose. Therefore, parents must follow proper dental hygiene.

✓ Advise the patient to exclude any milk or food containing cows' milk, even though a few individuals may tolerate some with low lactose. If it is the secondary type, this should resolve within six weeks.

✓ Children with suspected lactose intolerance do not usually require any testing and should improve within 48 hours of being on a low-lactose diet.

*See flowchart on following page,* (source: GP Notebook [n.d.b])

*References*

GP Notebook (n.d.a). *Lactose intolerance.* https://gpnotebook.com/simplepage.cfm?ID=1999962119

GP Notebook (n.d.b). *Management.* https://gpnotebook.com/simplepage.cfm?ID=x20090624153451398225

# Flowchart for managing SECONDARY LACTOSE INTOLERANCE

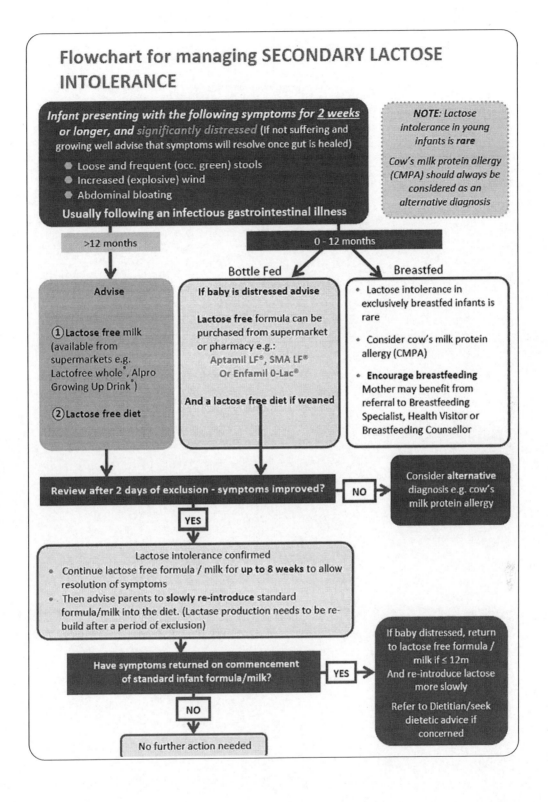

**Infant presenting with the following symptoms for _2 weeks_ or longer, and** *significantly distressed* (If not suffering and growing well advise that symptoms will resolve once gut is healed)

- Loose and frequent (occ. green) stools
- Increased (explosive) wind
- Abdominal bloating

**Usually following an infectious gastrointestinal illness**

*NOTE: Lactose intolerance in young infants is **rare***

*Cow's milk protein allergy (CMPA) should always be considered as an alternative diagnosis*

**>12 months**

**0 - 12 months**

Bottle Fed

Breastfed

**Advise**

①**Lactose free** milk (available from supermarkets e.g. Lactofree whole°, Alpro Growing Up Drink°)

②**Lactose free diet**

**If baby is distressed advise**

**Lactose free** formula can be purchased from supermarket or pharmacy e.g.:
Aptamil LF®, SMA LF®
Or Enfamil 0-Lac®

**And a lactose free diet if weaned**

- Lactose intolerance in exclusively breastfed infants is rare
- Consider cow's milk protein allergy (CMPA)
- **Encourage breastfeeding** Mother may benefit from referral to Breastfeeding Specialist, Health Visitor or Breastfeeding Counsellor

**Review after 2 days of exclusion - symptoms improved?** → **NO** → Consider **alternative** diagnosis e.g. cow's milk protein allergy

**YES**

Lactose intolerance confirmed
- Continue lactose free formula / milk for **up to 8 weeks** to allow resolution of symptoms
- Then advise parents to **slowly re-introduce** standard formula/milk into the diet. (Lactase production needs to be re-build after a period of exclusion)

**Have symptoms returned on commencement of standard infant formula/milk?** → **YES** → If baby distressed, return to lactose free formula / milk if ≤ 12m And re-introduce lactose more slowly

Refer to Dietitian/seek dietetic advice if concerned

**NO**

No further action needed

# 5

# Renal and Genitourinary

## Testicular Problems

Testicular problems often create the greatest anxiety and angst in male patients, probably more than any other symptom. Males are particularly sensitive to testicular problems, as there is a social perception that masculinity and virility are linked to the health of their testicles. Unfortunately, as a result, men often present symptoms late to the GP and can find it embarrassing to discuss. It is important to remember that a scrotal lump does not automatically equate to cancer of the testes, nor does it have to originate from the scrotum. When examining the patient, consider where the lump arises from and whether it is solely confined to the testes. Doing so will help you distinguish between a mass and a hernia.

### Pathophysiology

*Testicular*

- » Testicular torsion – Usually occurs in young adults.

- » Epididymo-orchitis – An infection of the epididymis that can spread to the testicle (orchitis). Usually caused by E. coli from UTIs / anal intercourse. STIs or mumps can also cause it.

- » Testicular cancer – There are two types: seminoma (common in older patients) and teratoma (common in younger patients).

*Extra-testicular*

- » Hydrocele – A collection of fluid within the. Primary (idiopathic) or secondary (trauma, cancer - may be presenting feature of testicular cancer, infection) or haematocele.

- » Varicocele – A collection of dilated veins in the tunica vaginalis pampiniform plexus due to problems in the valves. Typically found on the left (the testicular vein drains into the renal vein). It can be linked to subfertility.

- » Epididymal cyst or spermatocele – This is a fluid-filled swelling in the epididymis and may contain sperm (spermatocele); it is often bilateral. It is associated with polycystic kidney disease of CF.

- » Indirect inguinal hernia.

## Risk Factors for Testicular Cancer

➤ Family history of the same (brother or father)

➤ Infertility

➤ Undescended testicle

➤ Young (25–35-year-olds)

➤ Caucasian males

## *History*

» Always reassure the patient; for example, say something like this: *'I just want to let you know that while you feel embarrassed to talk about your problem, it is something that we see and treat every day.'*

» Focused questions

› Testicular pain – Ask when they first noticed the pain, how long it lasts for, if it come on suddenly (torsion) or gradually (epididymo-orchitis), whether the pain moves anywhere, whether it comes from their tummy going into their groin or it moves from the groin upwards, and if it is severe or a dull ache.

› Swelling – Ask when they first noticed it, how they noticed it, if it affects one side or both, if it came on suddenly or gradually built up (epididymo-orchitis), whether the swelling goes when they lie down (inguinal hernia), and if it is red, hot or painful.

» Associated symptoms – Ask if there is any nausea or vomiting, or any recent injury to the scrotum.

» Sexual history, if relevant – Ask when was their last UPSI, was their partner male or female, have they had any anal sex, do they have any history of STI, or have they had any unusual discharge from their penis.

» Past history – Ask if they have any previous history of testicular problems or STIs. Ask if they have had any previous surgeries on their testes (orchidopexy or a vasectomy).

» Social history – Ask if they smoke.

» Family history – Ask if there is any family history of testicular cancer.

## RED FLAGS

Haematuria, Acute pain, weight loss, vomiting or lethargy.

## Differential Diagnosis

| Testicular | |
|---|---|
| Testicular torsion | Sudden onset of severe pain (unilateral), swelling and vomiting. OE: the affected testis is held transversely and at a higher position compared with the other testicle; the testicle is hard, tender and enlarged, which is not eased by elevation. |
| Epididymo-orchitis | Unilateral pain and swelling to the testes, including fever, scrotal erythema, dysuria, urethral discharge and sometimes vomiting. There may be pain on ejaculation. The pain is usually in one of the testicles. Haematospermia. Ask if they had the measles, mumps and rubella (MMR) vaccination when they were younger. Ask if they have any pain or swelling around the side of the face under the ears (parotid glands), or any fevers. |
| Testicular cancer | Often painless and non-tender, sometimes may have a dragging sensation. Weight loss, no pain, growing in size or gynaecomastia. Can present as a painless swelling of the testis. OE: a firm, solid lump limited to the scrotum, which is irregular, nodular and hard with no evidence of transillumination. |
| Extra-testicular | |
| Hydrocele | Often a non-painful, unilateral, non-tender scrotal swelling. The testicle may be impalpable (must exclude testicular cancer). There may be a fluid thrill and it can transilluminate. It is usually possible to 'get above the swelling'. Haematoceles do not transilluminate as well. |
| Varicocele | They appear tortuous and distended on standing, and are often described as a 'bag of worms'. Classically, on lying down, they disappear and become impalpable. The patient may describe a dragging or an aching feeling in the scrotum. |
| Epididymal cyst or spermatocele | Often painless and seen in >40-year-olds. OE: often a smooth, bilateral, multilocular cyst located above and behind the testis, clearly distinct and separate to it. It is usually possible to 'get above the lump'. |

## Examination

» Always request a chaperone.

» Vitals – BP and pulse.

» Abdominal exam – Palpate for generalised tenderness (obstruction), as well as for pain and swelling in the inguinal region (inguinal hernia). Check for a cough impulse if a hernia is suspected.

» Testicular exam

> Examine from the standing position.

> Inspection – Observe the size (enlarged indicates testicular cancer), the position of the testicles (transverse and high riding indicates torsion) and look for any swelling.

> Palpation – Palpate the testes for any lumps (testicular cancer), epididymis (pain indicates epididymitis) and spermatic cord (varicocele or spermatocele) for tenderness.

> LNs – If cancer is suspected, palpate the inguinal and para-aortic LNs.

> Transilluminate – Shine a light such as a pen torch through the scrotum and over from the other end. Check for the illumination seen in a hydrocele.

> Specialist

- Prehn's sign (pain is relieved by raising the testes in epididymitis).

- Cremasteric reflex (stroking the superficial aspect of the medial thigh near the testes causes the testicle to rise on the respective side). This is absent in testicular torsion.

## Investigations

» Urine – Dipstick urine / midstream specimen of urine (MSU) to check for UTI and/or urine STI screen.

» Swabs – Urethral swabs to exclude STIs (chlamydia and gonorrhoea – epididymitis).

» Bloods – AFP, beta human chorionic gonadotropin (BHCG) and lactate dehydrogenase (LDH) for testicular cancer.

» USS – Consider a scrotal USS if a lesion is suspected.

### Indications for Urgent USS

» Unclear if scrotal swelling is testicular or extra-testicular.

» Testicle cannot be distinguished from the swelling.

» Hydrocele noted in a young male adult (20–40 years) at risk of testicular cancer.

» Haematocele that is chronic and not caused by trauma.

» Trauma associated with scrotal pain or ongoing testicular symptoms.

» There is diagnostic uncertainty.

## Management

*Treat the underlying cause*

### Conservative

✓ Self-examination – Recommend that the patient practices self-examination or gets their partner to examine them to monitor for testicular cancer.

✓ Support – Advise them to wear supportive undergarments when engaged in contact sports.

✓ Trauma – Advise them to apply pain relief and ice packs to the area.

✓ Contraception – Advise them to use condoms to prevent STIs.

✓ MMR – Recommend that all children have their MMR vaccination to prevent mumps.

*Medical*

✓ Epididymo-orchitis – Advise the patient to wear supportive underwear and take analgesia. Refer them to an STI clinic if they are found to have an STI, including gonorrhoea, or treat with ceftriaxone 500mg IM or oral cefixime 400mg and doxycycline 100mg bd for 10–14 days. Alternatives include the use of ofloxacin 200mg bd for 14 days or levofloxacin 500mg od for 10 days. If there is a contraindication to quinolones, consider co-amoxiclav 500/125mg tds for 10 days.

✓ Epididymal cyst – Reassure them, as this rarely needs treatment. If symptoms persist, refer them routinely to a urologist.

✓ Testicular torsion – Refer them immediately for surgical review (specifically within six hours).

✓ Hydrocele – Infantile hydrocele should be repaired if it has not resolved by age two. Monitor in adults, unless it is severe, in which case it would need to be drained.

✓ Varicocele – Usually only conservative treatment is required, but consider surgery if it is causing pain. Refer them urgently if appears suddenly, is painful, does not drain when lying down, or is unilateral to the right side.

✓ Haematocele – The patient should be admitted following acute trauma or USS if chronic.

## Safety Netting

» If the symptoms do not improve within two to four weeks, review with the GP.

## Referral

→ If cancer is suspected, then refer the patient to a specialist under 2WW.

*References*

National Institute for Health and Care Excellence (2020). *Scrotal pain and swelling.* https://cks.nice.org.uk/topics/scrotal-pain-swelling/

Street, E.J., Justice, E.D., Kopa, Z., Portman, M.D., Ross, J.D., Skerlev, M., Wilson, J.D., and Patel, R. (2017). The 2016 European guideline on the management of epididymo-orchitis. *International Journal of STD & AIDS, 28(8)* 744–749. doi: 10.1177/0956462417699356

# Erectile Dysfunction

Erectile dysfunction or impotence is defined as the inability to attain or maintain an erection for satisfactory sexual performance. It is an acutely embarrassing problem for patients, which affects almost 40% of 40–70-year-olds. The vast majority of patients are too embarrassed to seek medical advice regarding their problem. It can be due to psychological problems, but a large percentage of patients have an underlying condition. When presenting, it is useful to screen for CVD, HTN, hypercholesterolemia, PVD and DM. Be aware that erectile dysfunction is also an independent marker of increased CVD risk.

## History

» Reassure the patient; for example, say something like this: *'I just want to reassure that, while you may feel embarrassed talking about your problem, it is something that we see and treat every day.'*

» Open questions

  › *'Please can you tell me a little more about your problems maintaining an erection?'*

» Focused questions

  › Ask when the problem started, and how long it has been going on for.

  › Ask about consistency (are there problems initiating or maintaining, and has there been a gradual onset).

  › Ask if there are any issues with masturbation and difficulty getting erections when doing so.

» Associated history (if relevant) – Ask about their sexual history (libido, partners and STIs / penile discharge).

» Past history – Ask if they have had depression, CKD, DM, prostate cancer, spinal cord injury, Parkinson's disease, Cushing's disease, MS, or any surgery (pelvic, prostatectomy or transurethral resection of the prostate [TURP]).

» Drug history – Ask if they take (antihypertensives such as thiazides), antidepressants, finasteride, b-blockers, methotrexate, carbamazepine, spironolactone or steroids, which can worsen symptoms.

» Social history – Ask about their relationship(s) and if there are any issues, what their occupation is, if they cycle for more than three hours/week, or if they smoke, drink alcohol, or take any recreational drugs (cannabis or cocaine).

» Family history – Ask if there is family history of cardiac issues (IHD, DM or PVD).

## RED FLAGS

Chest pain and disc prolapse.

# Examination

» Vitals – BP, weight, BMI (obesity) and waist circumference.

» Genitalia – There is no need to perform this routinely. It is only required if structural problems are being considered: hypogonadism or secondary sexual characteristics (gynaecomastia or hair distribution).

» PR – If prostate problems (enlargement or irregular) are being considered or there are obstructive symptoms.

» Spinal exam – Check for lumbar spine tenderness, reduced straight leg raise (SLR), sensation and reflexes.

» Cardiovascular – Consider a peripheral vascular exam as well as cardiovascular if the patient has risk factors.

# Investigations

» Bloods – U&Es, lipid profile, HbA1c, prostate-specific antigen (PSA), testosterone (morning), SHBG, FSH, LH, prolactin, LFTs and TFTs.

» Urine – Dipstick urine (DM).

» ECG – Consider performing a routine ECG (IHD and left ventricular hypertrophy [LVH]).

» Determine the 10-year QRISK score.

# Management

*Conservative*

✓ Smoking – Recommend the patient stops smoking. Refer them to the smoking-cessation clinic.

✓ Alcohol – Advise them to reduce their intake to <=14units/week.

✓ Exercise – If they are overweight, advise them to lose weight and increase their exercise.

✓ Cycling – If they cycle more than three hours/week, then advise they cease to see if the symptoms improve. Advise them to use a comfortable, padded bike seat that is placed at the correct height.

✓ Psychogenic – Offer counselling such as psychosexual counselling or couples counselling (Relate).

*Medical*

✓ Medication review – Substitute medications that can cause impotence with alternatives.

✓ PDE5 inhibitor – Consider sildenafil (via a private prescription unless they fulfil exemption criteria) or a second-line treatment of vardenafil or tadalafil. Try a daily dose of tadalafil if there is a poor response.

› Viagra (sildenafil) taken one hour before planned sexual intercourse with their partner engaged in foreplay. The onset is delayed if taken with food.

Does not initiate an erection, but requires sexual stimulation to facilitate. Diabetics may need to take the maximum dose. Patients can get Viagra Connect 50mg OTC without a prescription.

› Contraindications – Avoid if they have unstable angina, strokes, recent MI, low BP or if on nitrates.

› Side effects – Flushing, headaches and GI (acid reflux).

› NHS prescriptions – Generic sildenafil has no NHS restrictions. Viagra, Cialis, Levitra and Spedra are only available on the NHS if the patient is being treated for prostate cancer, CKD, spinal cord injury, DM, MS, Parkinson's disease, radical pelvic surgery, a prostatectomy (not TURP) or they have already received medication for impotence before 14/09/1998. A prescription can be issued if it is initiated from specialist services for men suffering severe distress due to erectile dysfunction.

### Complications

- They must seek medical advice if the erection lasts more than four hours, they have chest pain or the sudden loss of vision.

## Referral

→ If there is a poor response to PDE5 inhibitors, then refer them to a specialist to consider vacuum erection devices, intracavernous injection and prothesis.

→ Refer them to endocrine if they have low testosterone or high prolactin. Specialists can offer testosterone replacement (oral, transdermal or depot) or SHBG. For hyperprolactinemia, the treatment is usually cabergoline 500mcg twice weekly.

→ Refer them to the cardiologist if they have severe IHD; likewise for any young person who has always had difficulty sustaining an erection.

## Safety Netting

» Review the patient if their symptoms persist for more than four to six weeks. Assess them for the presence of depressive symptoms. Consider bringing their partner in for a joint consultation.

*References*

Hackett, G., Kirby, M., Wylie, K., Heald, A., Ossei-Gerning, N., Edwards, D. and Muneer, A. (2018). British Society for Sexual Medicine Guidelines on the Management of Erectile Dysfunction in Men—2017. *Journal of Sexual Medicine, 2018,* 1–28. doi: https://doi.org/10.1016/j.jsxm.2018.01.023

Joint Formulary Committee (2017). *BNF 74 (British National Formulary) September 2017.* Pharmaceutical Press.

# Prostate-Specific Antigen

PSA is a glycoprotein that is produced specifically from both healthy and malignant prostate cells. It is often used as a screening tool to diagnose prostate cancer, even before symptoms have begun. A single PSA result is usually insufficient to make a diagnosis, and a repeat blood test is needed when considering cancer. While it may be a sensitive test, it lacks the specificity for prostate carcinomas and can be raised in prostatitis, benign prostatic hyperplasia (BPH), following urinary catheterisation and after a PR exam.

## Features of Prostate Cancer

➤ Risk factors – Age (>65 years), family history of first-degree relatives with prostate cancer or breast cancer, Afro-Caribbean heritage, diet (low fruit intake, and high fat and meat intake) and obesity.

➤ History – Often symptomless. Hesitancy, post-void dribbling, urinary retention and haematuria.

➤ Examination – A hard, asymmetrical, irregular, non-tender prostate with central sulcus loss.

➤ Metastatic indicators – Weight loss, back pain, fractures and spinal cord compression.

### Prostate Cancer Symptoms

Suspect prostate cancer if there is unexplained lower back pain/bone pain (metastasising is often the first symptom), lethargy, erectile dysfunction, haematuria, weight loss, lower urinary tract symptoms (LUTS) (frequency, urgency, dribbling and an overactive bladder), hard nodular prostate on PR, or raised PSA (after UTI has been excluded).

## History

» Open questions

&gt; 'Will you tell me more about why you would like to have a PSA test?'

&gt; Understanding – 'Will you tell me what you already know about it?'

&gt; Concerns – 'Is there anything in particular that worried you for you to want the test today?'

&gt; Introduction – 'Before I begin explaining what the PSA test is about, may I ask you a few questions about your health?'

» Focused questions

&gt; Ask about any problems passing urine, urine frequency, urine stream (hesitancy), dribbling, nocturia or erectile dysfunction.

» Past history – Ask if they have had DM, BPH or prostate cancer.

» Drug history – Ask if they have taken finasteride or dutasteride.

» Social history – Ask if they smoke or drink alcohol.

» Family history – Ask if there is a family history of prostate or breast cancer.

## RED FLAGS

Metastasis (back pain, weight loss and haematuria).

## Examination

» Vitals – BP, weight and BMI.

» General – Observe the patient to check if they are cachectic.

» PR – Consider performing this after a blood test or if the patient has haematuria, back pain, weight loss or erectile dysfunction, to exclude prostate cancer.

## Investigations

» Urine – Dipstick urine or MSU to exclude infection.

» MRI – Consider the spine for bone metastasis.

» Questionnaire – The severity of the symptoms of prostatism can be assessed by using the International Prostate Symptom Score (IPSS).

» Bloods – U&E, PSA and HbA1c.

**When to offer a PSA test:**

› Offer to men >50 years requesting a PSA test.

› Consider if the patient has LUTS (nocturia, frequency or dribbling), erectile dysfunction, visible haematuria or unexplained symptoms (lower back / bone pain or weight loss).

### Pros and Cons of the PSA Tests

» Advantages – Provides reassurance if the blood test is normal; raises awareness of the cancer before symptoms occur; finds the cancer early, permitting treatment to be started earlier; and prevents one death from prostate cancer for every 1,000 tests.

» Disadvantages – It can occasionally falsely reassure the patient and miss cancer, it provides unnecessary worry and invasive testing if falsely positive, and it cannot distinguish between fast- and slow-growing cancers.

It is important to bear in mind that certain things – such as exercise, sex or a UTI – may affect the results.

## Referral

→ Initiate a cancer referral via 2WW if the PSA is >2.5 in 45–50-year-olds or >3.0 in 50–70-year-olds, or if the prostate feels malignant on digital rectal exam (DRE).

→ Specialist – Prostatic biopsy. The treatment includes surveillance, radical prostatectomy, radiotherapy or brachytherapy.

---

### References

National Institute for Health and Care Excellence (2015). *Suspected cancer: recognition and referral.* https://www.nice.org.uk/guidance/ng12

National Institute for Health and Care Excellence (2019). *Prostate cancer: diagnosis and management.* https://www.nice.org.uk/guidance/ng131

# Haematuria

Haematuria signifies the presence of blood in the urine. It can be an incidental finding on a dipstick (microscopic – non-visible), or with frank haematuria (macroscopic – visible) it can be an alarming and frightening experience for the patient. It is often difficult to quantify the severity of haematuria, as the amount of blood passed may not strictly correlate with the significance of the underlying disorder. However, its presence should warrant a thorough investigation.

Haematuria could be due to dysfunction at any point of the urinary tract, from the molecular level at the kidneys, down to trauma or damage to the urethra. Non-renal causes should also be considered, and include bleeding disorder, trauma, infarction and anticoagulants.

## History

» Open questions

› Clarify what the patient means by blood in the urine.

» Focused questions

› Ask when it started and how long it has been going on for.

› Ask what colour the urine is: bright red, pink or brown.

› Ask when in the stream the blood is noticed (beginning indicates urethral, middle indicates renal/ureter, towards the end indicates the neck of the bladder.)

› Ask if there have been any clots.

» Associated history – Ask about the frequency, and if there has been any fever, rigors, pain (bladder or loin) or dysuria.

» Past history

› Medical – Ask if they have had sickle cell disease, blood disorders, recurrent UTIs, renal stones, a recent illness or a sore throat.

› Surgical – Ask if they have had TURP, cystoscopy, prostatectomy or a recent urinary catheter.

» Drug history – Ask if they have taken aspirin, warfarin, NSAIDs, rifampicin (orange urine) or nitrofurantoin (brown urine).

» Social history – Ask what their occupation is (dye or rubber industry may indicate bladder cancer), if they smoke or drink alcohol, what their diet is like (beetroot may cause red urine and fava beans may cause orange urine), what their water intake is, and whether they have meat or spinach in their diet (renal stones).

» Travel history – Ask if they have been to the tropics or subtropics, or swimming in any rivers, canals or lakes (schistosomiasis).

## RED FLAGS

Frank haematuria, painless haematuria (>50 years), microscopic haematuria (>40 years), weight loss and night sweats.

## Differential Diagnosis

| | |
|---|---|
| Bladder cancer | Primarily papillary transitional cell carcinoma. Around a 50% association with smoking or an occupation in the dye, textile or rubber industries. Presents with painless macroscopic haematuria in the absence of fever. |
| UTIs | Affects females more than males. E. coli is the most common organism. LUTS include abdominal pain, frequency, dysuria, urgency and haematuria. Suprabladder infections (i.e. renal) may also cause fever, vomiting and general malaise. Confirmed with a positive dipstick for leucocytes and nitrates. Urine is often offensive smelling and cloudy. |
| Renal stone | The most common type is calcium stones. It is more common in males and is associated with medication (e.g. loop or thiazide diuretics) and diet. Presents with sudden onset of loin or flank spasmodic pain radiating to the groin. Often with very severe, colicky pain, nausea, vomiting and haematuria. The patient is often restless and has UTI features. |
| Prostate cancer | Usually adenocarcinoma. It is the second most common cancer in men. Symptoms include urgency, frequency, hesitancy and nocturia. Metastatic spread is often characterised by weight loss and bone pain. |
| Pyelonephritis | It is more common in females. The patient may have underlying structural abnormalities. Presents with unilateral or bilateral loin pain, fever, rigors, nausea and vomiting. Lower UTI symptoms of frequency, dysuria and haematuria may also be present. |

## Causes of Haematuria

➤ Transient microscopic – UTI, periods, intensive exercise or intercourse.

➤ Persistent microscopic – Cancer (bladder, kidney or prostate), renal stones, BPH, prostatitis, urethritis (chlamydia) or renal (IgA nephropathy).

➤ Common – UTI or renal stones.

➤ Less common – BPH, glomerulonephritis, malignant HTN or ulcer.

➤ Uncommon – Polycystic disease or transitional cell carcinoma.

➤ Rarer – SLE, infective endocarditis, vasculitis or AF.

## Examination

» Vitals – BP (raised) and pulse.

» Abdominal exam – Palpate the abdomen for any pain (loin, flank or suprapubic area).

» PR – If prostate problems are being considered.

## Investigations

» Bloods – FBC, haematinics, U&E, estimated glomerular filtration rate (eGFR), ESR/CRP, PSA (prostate), creatine kinase (CK) (rhabdomyolysis), clotting screening and serum bilirubin.

» Urine – Dipstick urine to confirm blood, nitrates (UTI) and protein (glomerulonephritis). MC&S, cytology, urine albumin to creatinine ratio (ACR), 24-hour urine protein and urine red cell morphology (specialist).

» Kidneys, ureters and bladder (KUB) x-ray – Renal stones.

» USS – Renal pathology (polycystic kidney) or prostate.

» Specialist – CT scan, cystoscopy, blood cultures and renal biopsy.

*Interpretation of Urine Dipstick Tests in People with Urinary Tract Symptoms*

| Probability | Nitrates | Leucocytes | Information |
|---|---|---|---|
| Highly likely | +ve | +ve or -ve | >90% will have UTI |
| Moderately likely | -ve | +ve | 50% will have a UTI |
| Unlikely | -ve | -ve | 5% will have a UTI |

» If a woman has typical symptoms of a UTI, a dipstick should not be done. Treat with antibiotics regardless of symptoms.

» Send for an MSU when it is important to know sensitivities; e.g. persistent symptoms of UTI, pregnancy, impaired renal function, abnormal tract (reflux or stone) or immunosuppression.

## Management

*Treat the underlying cause*

*UTI (women)*

*Conservative*

✓ Encourage fluids, probiotics and cranberry juice (prevention, not treatment); urinating often when feeling the urge; wiping from front to back; wearing cotton and loose-fitting undergarments; and avoiding nylon, tight jeans and bubble baths.

*Medical*

✓ Initiate empirical antibiotics and await sensitivity. Consider trimethoprim as first-line treatment (200mg bd for three days for women and seven days for men), nitrofurantoin (50mg qds for three days for women and seven days for men) or cephalexin. Alternate between antibiotics if the previous one has been given in the past year. Give for 10 days if it is a complicated UTI.

> Pregnant – First-line treatment is nitrofurantoin (50mg qds).

> Recurrent – Offer a stand-by course of antibiotics if they suffer with recurrent UTIs. If more than three UTIs a year, consider offering prophylaxis.

> Sex – If UTIs occur post sexual intercourse, advise the patient to wash their genitals before and after sex. Post sex, advise them to empty their bladder. Consider stat antibiotics less than two hours prior to intercourse. Advise them to stop using a spermicide and to use condoms.

> Pain – Simple analgesia (paracetamol or codeine) or NSAIDs. Ensure no contraindications for NSAIDs (PU or asthma).

## Pyelonephritis

✓ Consider admission if there are signs of dehydration or sepsis.

✓ Antibiotics – Ciprofloxacin 500mg bd for seven days or co-amoxiclav 500/125mg tds for 14 days as an alternative. If the patient is pregnant, consider cephalexin 500mg bd for 10–14 days.

✓ Pain – Paracetamol only, as NSAIDs have a risk of renal impairment with acute pyelonephritis.

## Renal stones

### Conservative

✓ Advise the patient to increase their fluid intake (3l/day). Depending on type, offer dietary advice (avoid spinach and red meat). *See Renal Stones section, page 179.*

### Medical

✓ Offer NSAIDs (diclofenac) for pain and antiemetics (metoclopramide/cyclizine).

## Prostatitis

✓ Treat with antibiotics for up to four weeks (ciprofloxacin 500mg bd or ofloxacin 200mg bd). Can use trimethoprim 200mg bd if contraindication to quinolone.

## Bladder cancer

✓ Advise the patient to stop smoking, and to avoid exposure to occupations manufacturing dyes and rubber. Refer as follows.

## Referral

→ For patients with suspected bladder cancer within two weeks:

› >45 years – Unexplained visible haematuria (to exclude UTI) or visible haematuria that persists/recurs after UTI treatment.

› >60 years – Unexplained non-visible haematuria with either dysuria or raised WCC.

→ Non urgent – >60 years with recurrent or persistent unexplained UTI:

› Endometrial cancer – Consider USS for women aged >55 years with visible haematuria and reduced Hb, thrombocytosis, raised blood glucose, or unexplained vaginal discharge.

→ Renal cancer – Refer the patient within two weeks if they are aged >45 years with unexplained visible haematuria (UTI excluded), or a visible haematuria that persists or recurs after treatment for UTI.

→ Routine – Refer to urology all patients with visible haematuria, all patients with symptomatic non-visible haematuria, and all patients with asymptomatic non-visible haematuria >40 years.

## Safety Netting

» Review the patient if their symptoms persist for more than four to six weeks or sooner if there are red-flag symptoms. Assess them for the presence of depressive symptoms.

---

### References

National Institute for Health and Care Excellence (2020). *Urological cancers – recognition and referral.* https://cks.nice.org.uk/topics/urological-cancers-recognition-referral/

# Renal Stones

Urinary tract or kidney stones are common, with one in 20 suffering from a stone at some point in their life. Although stones are commonly associated with dehydration or dietary intake, they can also be caused by a number of medical conditions, including gout, hyperparathyroidism and renal tubular acidosis, and by inherited metabolic conditions, including cystinuria and hyperoxaluria. Renal stones usually present with sudden onset, colicky abdominal pain with the passing of blood in urine, and they may be severe enough to cause nausea and vomiting. Around 80% of stones are made from calcium salts, the remaining ones are struvite (8%), uric acid (10%) or cystine (<2%).

## Features of Renal Stones

➤ Risk factors – Family history of renal stones, male, obesity, dehydration, chronic UTI, gout, hypercalcaemia, abnormal kidneys (horseshoe) and drugs (diuretics).

➤ History – Acute, colicky abdominal pain, but can be constant, and is often described as a dull ache. It has been described as the worst pain experienced. Loin pain (kidney), suprapubic pain (bladder) and pain that radiates to the groin (ureteric).

➤ Examination – Tender flank or loin area. The patient may be writhing in pain. Haematuria on the dipstick.

## History

» Focused questions

› Ask when the pain started and how long it has been going on for.

› Ask about the site (loin or flank), radiation (to groin, labia or testes), severity, character (colicky), triggers and alleviating factors.

» Associated history – Ask if they experience haematuria.

» Past history – Ask if they have had renal stones, abnormal kidney (horseshoe kidney or medullary sponge kidney), or metabolic problems (gout, hypercalcaemia, hyperparathyroidism or cystinuria).

» Drug history – Ask if they have taken Adcal (calcium plus Vitamin D), steroids, NSAIDs or diuretics (loop or thiazide).

» Social history – Ask what their occupation is, if they smoke or drink alcohol, what their diet is like (meat, spinach, rhubarb and chocolate), and how much water they drink.

## RED FLAGS

» Obstruction – Urinary hesitancy, poor stream or oliguria.

» Haematuria, intolerable severe abdominal pain (aortic aneurysm), pain not responding one hour after taking medication, pregnant or CKD.

## Differential Diagnosis

| | |
|---|---|
| Renal stones | The most common type is calcium stones. More common in males, and associated with medication (e.g. loop or thiazide diuretics) and diet. Presents with sudden onset of spasmodic pain in the loin or flank, radiating to the groin. Often with very severe (described as more intense than childbirth) and colicky pain, nausea, vomiting and haematuria. The patient is often restless and has UTI features. |
| UTIs | Affects females more than males. E. coli is the most common organism. LUTS include abdominal pain, frequency, dysuria and haematuria. Suprabladder infections (i.e. renal) may cause fever, vomiting and general malaise. Confirmed with positive dipsticks for leucocytes and nitrates. |
| Pyelonephritis | Most common in females. The patient may have underlying structural abnormalities. Presents with unilateral or bilateral loin pain, fever, rigors, nausea and vomiting. Lower UTI symptoms of frequency, dysuria and haematuria may also be present. |
| Appendicitis | Diffuse central abdominal colic, shifting to the RIF. Worsened by movement, touch and coughing. Associated with anorexia, nausea, vomiting and, occasionally, diarrhoea. OE: Low-grade fever, tachycardia, tender RIF and Rovsing's sign (pain in the RIF when the LIF is palpated). |
| Diverticulitis | Small outpouchings of the large bowel that become inflamed or infected. Often affects females from 50–70 years. Symptoms include abdominal pain, bloating and cramps, mainly in the LIF with fever, nausea, vomiting and constipation. Patients may also have flatulence and distension. Frank blood mixed in with the stools is a complication. PR: tenderness on the left side (inflamed colon). |
| Ruptured AAA | Triad of shooting abdominal or back pain, hypotension and pulsatile abdominal mass. Patients often have risk factors (family history, CVD, male, >50 years, a smoker, HTN, obesity and high cholesterol). |
| Ectopic pregnancy | Missed period, PV bleeding and generalised abdominal pains. |

## Examination

- » Vitals – BP, pulse and temperature (coexisting UTI / pyelonephritis).
- » Abdominal exam – Palpate the abdomen for any pain (loin, flank or suprapubic area). Exclude aortic aneurysm.

## Investigations

- » Bloods – FBC, U&E, calcium and phosphate (if calcium >2.6mmol/l, check PTH which indicates hyperparathyroidism), CRP, uric acid and LFTs (albumin and ALP).
- » Urine – Dipstick (ph-urate stones, haematuria [positive suggests a stone], proteinuria and nitrates), MSU and pregnancy test (ectopic).
- » KUB USS – Renal stones (75% radio-opaque).
- » USS – Underlying renal pathology.
- » Specialist – Intravenous urography (IVU), spiral CT scan and cystoscopy.

## Management

### Conservative

- ✓ Reassure the patient; most stones that are <5mm pass spontaneously.
- ✓ Fluid intake – Advise them to increase fluids to >3l/day, reduce salt intake (<3g/day), and avoid tea (calcium oxalate) and alcohol (particularly binges).
- ✓ Diet – Recommend a balanced diet with lots of fruit and vegetables. Advise them to avoid grapefruit juice, but drink cranberry juice or add lemon juice to water. Offer specific dietary advice depending on the type of stone:
  - › Calcium oxalate – Advise them to avoid tea, rhubarb, cocoa, chocolate, nuts, spinach, strawberries, beetroot and wheat bran.
  - › Calcium phosphate – Advise them to avoid calcium and vitamin D supplements. Dietary calcium should not be restricted due to inverse proportional relationship with stone formation.
  - › Urate – Advise them to avoid liver, kidney, sardines, anchovies, herring with skin on, and fructose-containing drinks.
  - › Cystinuria – Advise them to avoid animal meat (<1g/kg body weight).

### Medical

- ✓ Analgesia – If they are in severe pain, offer diclofenac 75mg IM or diamorphine 5mg in hospital. Otherwise, consider oral or rectal NSAIDs (diclofenac) or paracetamol / weak opioid (codeine/tramadol).
- ✓ Antiemetics – Metoclopramide or cyclizine IM.
- ✓ Expulsive therapy – Can offer tamsulosin or nifedipine to facilitate stone passage (if stones are <10mm).

✓ UTI – Initiate antibiotics, depending on sensitivity. Common antibiotics include trimethoprim, nitrofurantoin and cephalexin.

✓ Preventative – Consider thiazide diuretics (for calcium), allopurinol (uric acid stones) or calcium citrate (oxalate).

*Surgical*

✓ On occasion, stones persist. These need to be reduced and broken to prevent complications. Procedures such as extracorporeal shock wave lithotripsy and percutaneous nephrolithotomy may be employed by secondary care.

## Referral

→ Urology – Refer the patient as per red-flag symptoms, or for chronic renal stones that need surgical input or lithotripsy.

→ Dietician – Can refer them to a dietician for tailored advice for the patient.

→ Admit – If the patient has shock, fever, a systemic infection or acute kidney injury (AKI), is pregnant or has dehydration.

## Safety Netting

» If symptoms recur, the patient may need to be referred for more investigations (recurrence is high).

*References*

National Institute for Health and Care Excellence (2019). *Renal and ureteric stones: assessment and management*. https://www.nice.org.uk/guidance/ng118

Türk, C., Knoll, T., Petrik, A., Sarica, K., Skolarikos, A., Straub, M. and Seitz C. (2015). *Guidelines on urolithiasis. European Association of Urology*. https://uroweb.org/wp-content/uploads/22-Urolithiasis_LR_full.pdf

# Urinary Incontinence (Female)

Urinary incontinence (UI) is the involuntary passage of urine. It can be an acutely embarrassing and distressing problem that can significantly impact the patient's quality of life. Broadly speaking, there are three different types of UI including stress, urge (with or without overactive bladder) or mixed. Risk factors include age (50–70 years), vaginal delivery, increased parity, obesity, constipation and a family history of UI.

## Types and Definitions of UI

➤ Stress UI – Involuntary urine leakage on effort or exertion, or on sneezing or coughing.

➤ Urge UI – Involuntary urine leakage accompanied or immediately preceded by urgency (a sudden compelling desire to urinate that is difficult to defer).

➤ Mixed UI – Involuntary urine leakage associated with urgency and exertion, effort, sneezing or coughing.

➤ Overactive bladder (OAB) – Urinary urgency that occurs with or without urge UI. Often associated with frequency and nocturia.

➤ Overflow UI – The patient cannot empty their bladder completely, becoming distended (chronic urinary retention). Results in the continuous or frequent leaking of small quantities of urine.

## History

» Ensure understanding by asking the patient what they mean when they say the urine leaks.

» Focused questions

› Ask when the incontinence started, how long it has been going on for, and if it occurs during certain activities.

› Ask about the frequency, volume of urine passed and severity (if there is any use of incontinence pads, how often they are changed, and if they have had to change garments because of any leakage).

» Associated history

› Stress – Ask if it occurs when sneezing, coughing, lifting, bearing down or exercising.

› Urge – Ask if they sometimes get a sudden urge to go to the toilet and pass urine, and if they have had any accidents.

› Overflow – Ask if they struggle to pass urine when trying (hesitancy), and if there is any staining when going, a poor stream or dribbling at the end.

› Bowels – Ask if there is any leakage with stools.

» Past history

> Medical – Ask if they have had strokes, MS, DM, spinal cord lesions, Parkinson's, dementia or bladder cancer.

> Surgical – Ask if they have had pelvic, hysterectomy or spinal surgery.

> Obstetrics – Ask if they have had a recent delivery or parity.

» Drug history – Ask if they take diuretics, a-blocker, TCAs, hypnotics/sedatives, antihistamines, opioids or ACEi, which can worsen symptoms.

» Social history – Ask what their occupation is, if they smoke or drink alcohol, and what their diet is like (tea, coffee and cola).

## RED FLAGS

Visible or microscopic haematuria (>50 years), recurrent UTI, weight loss or pelvic mass.

## Differential Diagnosis

| | |
|---|---|
| Stress incontinence | The passage of small amounts of urine related to coughing, sneezing, lifting or exercise. Risk factors: childbirth, menopause and obesity. Rare in men (usually after prostatectomy). |
| Urge incontinence | Urgency and frequency with an overwhelming sensation to void. Passage of a large volume and nocturia. Risk factors: stress, neurological (spinal injury, PD, stroke or MS) and bladder (stones or cancer). |
| Overflow incontinence | The intermittent leaking or dribbling of urine throughout the day. Can be due to constipation. Can also occur in men (BPH, prostate cancer or stricture). Anticholinergic medication (oxybutynin) can worsen symptoms. |
| UTI | Abdominal pain, dysuria, frequency and urgency, with cloudy urine and a positive dipstick. |
| Prolapse | Symptoms depend on the type. Can include incontinence, frequency, urgency and incomplete bladder emptying (cystocele or cystourethrocele), constipation (rectocele or enterocele), heaviness or a dragging sensation in pelvis (e.g. 'my insides are falling out' [uterine prolapse]). OE: bulge in the posterior (enterocele or rectocele) or anterior (cystocele or urethrocele) vaginal wall. |

# Examination

»   Vitals – BP, pulse and temperature.

»   Abdominal exam – Palpate the abdomen for any pain (suprapubic area), masses (enlarged bladder) or constipation.

»   Pelvic exam

  ›   Inspection – Inspect for vulva atrophic vaginitis, fistula, prolapse or the leakage of urine when coughing.

  ›   Palpation – Palpate the vaginal wall, cervix and both adnexae for pelvic masses (ovarian or endometrial). Before withdrawing the digits, ask them to squeeze down, feeling for the tone of the pelvic muscles.

# Types of Pelvic Organ Prolapses

➤   Cystocele – Bulging of the bladder into the upper two-thirds of the anterior vaginal wall.

➤   Urethrocele – Bulging of the urethra into the lower one-third of the anterior vaginal wall. Often occurs together with a prolapse of the bladder (cystourethrocele).

➤   Enterocele – Herniation of the pouch of Douglas into the upper posterior vaginal wall.

➤   Rectocele – Prolapse of the rectum into the lower posterior vaginal wall. This is different to a rectal prolapse (rectal prolapse out of the anus).

➤   Uterine – Uterus drops down into the vagina. Graded according to the level of descent.

➤   Vaginal vault – The top of the vagina (vault) sags or bulges down into the vaginal canal. Often secondary to a hysterectomy.

# Investigations

»   Bloods – U&E, eGFR and HbA1c.

»   Urine – Dipstick urine (DM and UTI) and MSU.

»   Diary – Urinary diary for at least three days (amount and types of fluids, volume and frequency of the passage of urine and activity – normal is four to eight times a day and once at night).

»   USS – Bladder residual volume (outflow obstruction).

»   Specialist – Cystoscopy and urodynamic studies.

## Management

*Conservative*

✓ Weight loss – Advise them to lose weight and get their BMI <30, and encourage exercise.

✓ Smoking – Advise them to stop smoking, as it is associated with a chronic cough causing stress incontinence.

✓ Fluid restriction – Advise them to reduce their caffeine, alcohol and high fluid intake.

✓ Constipation – Encourage them to eat at least five portions of fruit or vegetables per day, to increase their water intake, increase their fibre intake and reduce their red meat intake.

✓ Pads – Offer absorbent pads or bed covers. Incontinence pads are not available on FP10, and are only supplied by local NHS trusts (DN/continence nurse).

✓ Bladder retraining (urge) – Over six weeks, gradually increase the interval between voiding.

✓ Pelvic-floor exercises (stress) – Recommend pelvic-floor exercises (eight contractions three times a day) or use vaginal cones.

*Medical*

✓ Stress – If the pelvic-floor exercises fail, consider referral to surgery (e.g. synthetic mid-urethral tape, colposuspension, autologous rectus fascial sling, intramural urethral bulking agents or artificial urinary sphincter). If the patient declines surgery, consider using duloxetine 40mg bd (can titrate up from 20mg bd).

› Duloxetine should not routinely be used as a second-line treatment for women with stress UI, although it may be offered as second-line therapy if women prefer pharmacological to surgical treatment or are not suitable for surgical treatment.

› Side effects of antimuscarinic drugs – Dry mouth, blurred vision, abdominal discomfort, drowsiness, nausea and dizziness. Urinary retention is a potentially serious but less common side effect.

✓ Urge (with or without OAB) – Offer oxybutynin immediate release 5mg tds (titrate upwards, avoid in the frail) as a first-line treatment. If this does not help, consider alternative antimuscarinic drugs (solifenacin or tolterodine) or oxybutynin transdermal if oral is not tolerated. Advise the patient that they must try it for at least four weeks before seeing any relief.

✓ Mirabegron – Consider 50mg od (relaxes the bladder detrusor muscle and improves urine storage) if antimuscarinic is contraindicated. Avoid in cases of severe liver dysfunction and an eGFR <15. Reduce the dose (25mg od) in cases of moderate liver dysfunction and an eGFR of 15–30.

✓ Vaginal atrophy – Consider intravaginal oestrogen therapy.

✓ Nocturia – Consider desmopressin 200mcg oral at bedtime (off label), increase to 400mcg.

✓     Overflow – Refer them to a specialist if you are able to palpate their bladder on examination, bimanual or evidence of chronic urinary retention.

✓     Prolapse – Consider a ring pessary or surgery (refer them if appropriate).

✓     UTI – Treat depending on the organism; use empirical therapy (trimethoprim, nitrofurantoin or cefalexin).

✓     Catheter – For severe incontinence, refer them for catheterisation.

## Referral

→     Physiotherapy – Refer them to physiotherapy for a bladder retraining programme or pelvic-floor exercises for incontinence.

→     Incontinence nurse – Refer them to an incontinence nurse for the further evaluation of the patient or if needing specialised incontinence pads.

→     Surgery – Refer them to urogynaecology for consideration of botulinum toxin, operations (urogenital fistula) or severe pelvic prolapse.

## Safety Netting

»     If the patient does not improve within four weeks, request for them to be reviewed by the GP or refer as appropriate.

### References

National Institute for Health and Care Excellence (2013). *Urinary incontinence in women: management.* https://www.nice.org.uk/guidance/cg171

National Institute for Health and Care Excellence (2013). *Mirabegron for treating symptoms of overactive bladder.* https://www.nice.org.uk/guidance/ta290

# Chronic Kidney Disease

CKD is a common condition that is often symptomless, and it is usually picked up on in routine blood tests or from a urine dipstick. Around 10% of the population are believed to suffer from it, which increases with age. It is diagnosed using the eGFR as a guide to the degree of renal dysfunction or damage. It is defined as an abnormality of renal function (eGFR <60ml/min) on at least two occasions separated by at least 90 days. There are five stages, ranging from mild (stage 1) to severe (stage 5).

Patients who cross an eGFR of <60 are classified as stage 3 and require medical input with closer monitoring to prevent further deterioration, possibly leading to dialysis, or transplantation in severe cases. Patients with CKD may progress, requiring renal transplant therapy, or develop CVD (HTN, PVD, HF, MI or CVA) or anaemia. They are at risk of developing AKI, falls, frailty and mortality.

## Causes of CKD

➤ Intrinsic – DM and HTN.

➤ Obstructive – BPH, recurrent renal stones and bladder voiding dysfunction (neurogenic bladder).

➤ Multisystem – SLE, vasculitis, myeloma, polycystic kidney disease and familial glomerulonephritis.

➤ Drugs – Lithium, mesalazine, cyclosporine, tacrolimus and aminoglycosides.

## *History*

CKD is usually asymptomatic, and hence it is difficult to elicit from the history alone. However, when taking a history, you should include a cardiovascular risk-factor assessment, as there is an association with IHD. Ensure that you read the notes thoroughly, and note if the patient has previously had low eGFR readings, anaemia or evidence of proteinuria.

» Focused questions

› Ask how long they have had kidney problems.

› Ask about fatigue and urinary symptoms (polyuria and nocturia).

› Ask about nausea and vomiting.

› Ask about fluid retention (any swelling of legs/ankles, SOB or puffiness around the face/eyes).

» Associated history – Ask if they experience pruritus, anorexia or sexual dysfunction.

» Past history – Ask if they have had HTN, CVA, DM, recurrent UTIs or glomerulonephritis.

» Drug history – Ask if they take NSAIDs, ACEi (renal stenosis), CCBs, diuretics, lithium or metformin.

» Social history – Ask what their occupation is, and if they smoke or drink alcohol.

» Family history – Ask if they have a family history of CKD or polycystic kidneys.

## RED FLAGS

Haematuria, proteinuria, eGFR <30, rapid deterioration in eGFR, anaemia, nephritic syndrome (panda face), weight loss, malignant HTN, hyperkalaemia or pulmonary oedema.

## Examination

» Vitals – BP (raised), weight (fluid retention) and temperature.

» Abdominal exam

  › Inspection – Inspect for a yellow 'lemon' tinge (uraemia).

  › Palpation – Palpate the abdomen for ascites, a palpable bladder or enlarged kidneys.

» Respiratory exam – Auscultate the lung bases for pleural effusions or signs of peripheral oedema.

## Investigations

» Routine bloods – U&E (creatinine, sodium or potassium), eGFR and urine ACR.

  › Others – FBC, ESR, HbA1c, cholesterol, calcium, phosphate and PTH concentrations in people with stage 4 or 5.

» USS – Offer if there is an accelerated drop in eGFR (>15/ml/min/year or 25% drop plus a drop in eGFR category), visible/persistent haematuria, obstructive symptoms, family history of polycystic kidney disease (aged >20 years) or eGFR <30.

» Patients should not eat any meat 12 hours before an eGFR as it can increase creatinine by 50%.

» Urine – Dipstick urine to exclude UTI, ACR or protein-creatinine ratio (PCR) (morning sample).

### Screening for CKD

Offer people testing for CKD if they have any of the following risk factors:

» DM, HTN, CVD (IHD, HF, PVD or CVA), structural renal tract disease, renal calculi or prostatic hypertrophy, multisystem diseases with potential kidney involvement (e.g. SLE), a family history of stage 5 CKD, hereditary kidney disease, haematuria or proteinuria.

How to test for CKD

» Perform serum creatinine (eGFR is estimated from this) and ACR (early morning urine sample):

› eGFR <60ml/min – Repeat eGFR in under two weeks (if not tested before, to rule out AKI). If the repeat test remains <60 with no deterioration, repeat in three months.

› Urinary ACR – If 3–70mg/nmol, repeat in three months. If >70mg/nmol (significant proteinuria), refer them to a nephrologist.

## Management

### Conservative

✓ Smoking – Encourage them to stop smoking. Refer them to a smoking-cessation clinic.

✓ Alcohol – Advise them to reduce their alcohol intake to <=14 units/week.

✓ Exercise/weight loss – Encourage them to exercise, so that they can lose weight.

✓ Diet – Consider advising protein restriction (dietician) if their CKD is 4 or above. Recommend salt restriction.

✓ Self-management – Offer a personalised care plan.

✓ Immunisation – Offer the annual flu vaccination and a one-off pneumococcal injection.

✓ QoF – Maintain a register of patients with CKD stages 3–5. Monitor their BP (<140/85) yearly and perform urine ACR. Ensure patients with concurrent BP and proteinuria are on ACEi.

### Medical

✓ Avoid drugs – Avoid nephrotoxic drugs (e.g. NSAIDs, even OTC). Exercise caution with drugs utilising renal clearance (stop metformin if GFR <30).

✓ BP target

› In people with CKD, aim for BP <140/90.

› In people with DM or ACR >70, aim for BP <130/80.

✓ ACEi – Initiate ACEi or ARB as per NICE guidelines. Start with a low dose then titrate up by doubling the dose every one to two weeks.

**When to initiate ACEi:**

- Diabetic ACR >3mg/mmol

- Non-diabetic ACR >70mg/mmol

- HTN with ACR >30mg/mmol

- HTN with ACR <30mg/mmol, treat BP according to NICE HTN guidance. There is no need for ACEi if not indicated

✓ Monitor – After two weeks, monitor eGFR and urine (urine dipstick and ACR). If there is evidence of proteinuria, exclude UTI. If potassium >6mmol, stop ACEi.

✓ CVD disease – Treat HTN (target 130/80), cholesterol and DM.

✓ Antiplatelets – Start antiplatelets for the secondary prevention of CVD.

✓ Anaemia – Monitor for anaemia (Hb>110g/l). If low, consider referring them for erythropoietin injections.

## Referral

→ Dietician – Refer them to a dietician if they have mildly raised potassium levels.

→ Nephrologist – Refer them to a nephrologist if eGFR <30, ACR >=70 (unless diabetic), ACR >=30 plus haematuria, a sustained decrease in eGFR (25% plus a change in GFR category or >15ml/min drop in one year), CKD and poorly controlled HTN (four agents), or suspected renal artery stenosis.

## Safety Netting

» Monitor U&Es regularly. Refer them urgently for any red flags.

---

### References

National Institute for Health and Care Excellence (2014). *Chronic kidney disease in adults: assessment and management.* https://www.nice.org.uk/guidance/cg182

National Institute for Health and Care Excellence (2015). *Chronic kidney disease: managing anaemia.* https://www.nice.org.uk/guidance/ng8

# Inguinal Hernia

A hernia is a protrusion of an organ through its cavity into another space. They may be present at birth, but may develop later in life due to weaknesses of the abdominal wall. Inguinal hernias are hernias of abdominal contents that pass through the inguinal canal, and they are more common in men (eight-to-one ratio of men to women). They are classified as direct or indirect. The majority of hernias are indirect, arising from the internal ring and exiting through the superficial ring. Direct hernias pass through a defect in the posterior wall of the inguinal canal and out into the abdominal cavity. Hernia repair is one of the most commonly performed surgical operations, with 80% of operations being performed as day cases.

## History

» Focused questions

> Ask when they first noticed or felt the lump, and what they were doing (lifting something or coughing).

> Ask about the site (groin or scrotum), size (any change), character/timing, triggers (coughing, bending or standing) and anything that makes it go away (lying down or pushing it back).

» Associated history – Ask if they are experiencing any pain or tenderness, erythema, vomiting, bowel issues (constipation), signs of obstruction (severe pain, vomiting, distention or the inability to pass flatus).

» Past history – Ask if they have had a chronic cough (COPD or asthma) or previous operations (appendicectomy or hernia repair).

» Drug history – Ask if they have taken codeine, iron or calcium.

» Family history – Ask if there is a family history of inguinal hernias or similar problems.

» Social history – Ask what their occupation is (builder, bricklayer or in delivery), what hobbies they have (weightlifting, golf or football), and if they smoke or drink alcohol.

## RED FLAGS

Signs of strangulation (severe pain, vomiting or an irreducible mass) or obstruction (absence of flatus or faeces, vomiting, pain or distention).

## Examination

» Vitals – BP and BMI.

» Inspection – Have the patient stand. Look for obvious lumps. Observe any cough impulse and the lump's location (above the inguinal ligament indicates an inguinal hernia, and below indicates a femoral hernia).

» Palpation – Feel from the side with one hand on the patient's back. Feel the lump and note its location, size, shape, and whether it is hard or soft. Check its temperature. Ask the patient to cough away from you, and feel for an impulse.

> Reduce – Request that the patient reduces the hernia, then place two fingers over the deep ring (1.5cm above the midpoint of the anterior superior iliac spine [ASIS] to the pubic tubercle). Ask them to cough. If you see the hernia appear, then it is likely a direct hernia. If it does not appear, then it is likely an indirect hernia.

» Auscultation – Listen over the hernia with a stethoscope for bowel sounds.

» Scrotum – Feel the scrotum for any lumps or swellings.

## Investigations

Often performed by secondary care.

» USS/MRI – May be performed to confirm the presence of a hernia.

» Herniography – An injection of x-ray contrast may be used for diagnostic uncertainty.

## Differential Diagnosis

| Inguinal hernia | Men are 10 times more likely to get this than women. Risk factors: chronic cough, prolonged heavy lifting, obesity and constipation. OE: Inguinal swelling that lies above the inguinal ligament, which may pass into the scrotum; often has a cough impulse; and is reducible. If it is red, hot and tender, and there is absolute constipation, it may be strangulated. |
|---|---|
| Femoral hernia | More common in elderly females. Located below the inguinal ligament. Does not disappear when the patient lies flat. |
| Saphena varix | Dilatation of the saphenous vein. OE: Cough impulse over the saphenofemoral junction demonstrates valve importance. Disappears when they lie down. |
| Scrotal mass | Hydrocele, spermatocele and lumps in the testes. If you can 'get above it', then it is a scrotal mass. If you cannot, then it is probable it is a hernia. |

## Management

### Conservative

✓ Reassurance – Reassure the patient if the hernia is small, asymptomatic and not strangulated; in which case you can watch and wait.

✓ Lifestyle – Recommend that they exercise and eat healthily to lose weight. Advise that they take plenty of fibre through fruit and vegetables, and drink fluids to reduce constipation.

✓ Smoking – Advise them to cut down or stop smoking.

✓ Lifting – Advise them to be careful when carrying heavy objects or bending down to lift something. They should try lifting with the knees rather than with the back, and should not carry objects that need more than one person to carry them.

### Medical

✓ Constipation – Use bulk-forming (ispaghula), osmotic (lactulose) or stimulant (senna) laxatives.

✓ Pain – Simple analgesia or NSAIDs. Ensure no contraindications for NSAIDs (ulcers or gastritis).

✓ Cough – Rationalise treatments for asthma or COPD.

### Surgical

✓ Hernia repair – This is often a day case with laparoscopic guidance. This may be under LA or general anaesthetic (GA). The surgeon locates the hernia and places a mesh to allow tissue to grow and strengthen the weakness.

✓ Risks – Local pain, infection and haematoma. Approximately one in 200 have a recurrence (more common in females than males) and one in 20 suffer with post herniorrhaphy pain syndrome.

✓ Post-operative (post-op) – Advise the patient to remain active and take OTC pain relief. For the next 10 days, they should only take a shower, but may take a bath after that. They should return to work within two weeks unless it involves heavy lifting, in which case they should return at six weeks post-op. They may drive after one to two weeks.

## Referral

→ Refer them to a specialist if there is a poor response, or according to the guidelines referenced as follows.

## Safety Netting

» Follow-up – Review the patient in four weeks for their response to treatment.

» If there are any red flags, seek emergency advice.

## References

Royal College of Surgeons (n.d.). *Groin hernia repair.* https://www.rcseng.ac.uk/patient-care/recovering-from-surgery/groin-hernia-repair/

Simons, M. P., Aufenacker, T., Bay-Nielsen, M., Bouillot, J. L., Campanelli, G., Conze, J., de Lange, D., Fortelny, R., Heikkinen, T., Kingsnorth, A., Kukleta, J., Morales-Conde, S., Nordin, P., Schumpelick, V., Smedberg, S., Smietanski, M., Weber, G. and Miserez, M. (2009). European Hernia Society guidelines on the treatment of inguinal hernia in adult patients. *Hernia,* 13(4), 343–403. doi: https://dx.doi.org/10.1007%2Fs10029-009-0529-7

# Vasectomy

Vasectomies are a near permanent form of contraception for men that result in sterilisation. It is usually performed as a day-case procedure under LA, whereby the two ends of the vas deferens are severed and tied, so that no sperm can pass into the ejaculate. While the initial sterilisation procedure is freely available on the NHS, if the patient has a change of heart, any subsequent reversal procedure must be privately funded. While it is good practice for both partners to be actively involved in the decision-making process, informed consent should only be sought from the male partner, and there is no legal requirement for the female partner's opinion or wishes to be considered.

## History

» Reassure the patient; for example, say something like this: *'I just want to reassure that while you may feel embarrassed talking about your problem, it is something that we see and deal with every day.'*

» Open questions

 › Ask them to tell you more about why they would like to have a vasectomy.

 › Understanding – Ask what they already know about vasectomies.

» Focused questions

 › Ask them about their relationship status, if they have any children with their current/previous partner, and if so, how many.

 › Ask if they use any contraception and if they have any problems with it.

 › Counselling – Ask if the decision has been discussed with their partner; if not, ask them why. Ask how their partner feels.

 › Life events – Ask if they have any new changes in their life (new baby, mortgage or a miscarriage).

 › Concerns – Ask if anything is worrying them about having the operation.

» Past history – Ask if they have any medical problems or previous surgery (scrotal or genital).

» Social history – Ask what their occupation is, about their home life, if they have any financial worries, and if they smoke or drink alcohol.

## YELLOW FLAGS

Young (<20 years), have not previously fathered children or have only fathered one child, are in an unhappy relationship, are experiencing pressure from their partner, are not in a relationship, or have suffered the death of a child.

## Examination

» Vitals – BP and BMI.

» Genital – Not usually performed.

## Risks Associated with Vasectomies

➤ Pain – Temporary pain or an ache in groin post-op.

➤ Post-vasectomy pain syndrome (PVPS) – This occurs in one in 20 cases post-op. The patient may experience a chronic, dull ache in the groin, or pain when ejaculating that persists for more than three months post-op.

➤ Inflammation, infection and skin abscesses (treat all with antibiotics).

➤ Haematoma - Bruises or blood clots. These often settle with time.

➤ Adhesion – There is a risk of fistula developing between the skin and vas. This may require surgery.

➤ Hydrocele – Fluid collection in the scrotum. This often resolves itself, but may need draining.

➤ Spermatic granuloma – Swelling caused by the seeping of sperm from the vas deferens, forming a lump. This may cause pain. It often resolves spontaneously, but may need draining.

➤ Recanalisation – The reconnection of the two ends of the vas deferens. This is very rare. Fertility may return.

➤ Reduced libido – Reduced sex drive or impotence (four in 1,000). This is usually psychological.

### Post-op

» Sex – Advise the patient it will not affect their sex drive or ability to enjoy sex. They will still be able to ejaculate and have erections, but there will be no sperm. Advise them that condoms should be used if they decide to have sex before being given the all-clear from the surgeon.

» All-clear – Advise the patient that, once the vasectomy has been done, they still have a small chance of being fertile up to three months after procedure. For this reason, their sperm count will be checked at 12 and 16 weeks after the operation.

» Reversibility – Although this is possible, it is not done on the NHS. The chances of reversal are only 50% in the first 10 years, dropping down to 30% after 15 years.

» STI risk – It is important to remember that a vasectomy does not protect against catching an STI.

## Post-op Vasectomy Care Advice

Advise the patient of the following:

- » They should use NSAIDs if there is any pain or discomfort after the operation.
- » They should ensure they rest following the procedure and avoid any strenuous activity.
- » They should avoid any sexual activity for seven days.
- » They should wear tight underwear for at least 48 hours after the procedure.

---

### References

FSRH Clinical Effectiveness Unit (2014). *FSRH clinical guideline: male and female sterilisation summary of recommendations (September 2014).* https://www.fsrh.org/standards-and-guidance/documents/cec-ceu-guidance-sterilisation-summary-sep-2014/

# Bladder Carcinoma

Bladder cancer is the seventh most common cancer in the UK. It is three to four times more common in men than women. Approximately 70–80% of bladder cancers don't involve the bladder muscle wall. Carcinoma in situ is potentially aggressive and may occur anywhere in the urinary tract. Malignant changes are confined to the bladder mucosa, and tumours of the upper urinary tract often present late.

## Risk factors

> ➤ Tobacco exposure
> ➤ Exposure to chemical carcinogens; these are often found in the rubber, dye and roofing industries
> ➤ Age of >55 years
> ➤ Pelvic radiology
> ➤ Male sex
> ➤ Chronic bladder inflammation
> ➤ Family history of bladder cancer

## History

> » Bladder cancer almost always presents with gross or microscopic haematuria.
> » Gross haematuria is often intermittent. It is essential to be aware of this to avoid the incorrect conclusion that this is from an infective cause.
> » Burning on urination and increased frequency is not uncommon in bladder carcinoma, although passing urine is often painless.
> » It is also essential to ask about any fatigue, loss of appetite, or back and flank pain.

## Examination

> » The examination is often unremarkable in patients in the early stages of the disease.
> » Abdominal exam – palpate for any masses
> » Urine dipstick – This usually finds haematuria.

## Investigations

> » Refer for cystoscopy. This is key for diagnosis.
> » FBC can show microcytic anaemia in bladder cancers.

» Urine cytology can be positive in patients with carcinoma in situ or high-grade tumours.

» CT KUB with contrast is beneficial imaging for detecting bladder cancer.

## Differentials

➤ BPH

➤ Prostatitis

➤ UTI

➤ Renal cell carcinoma

➤ Renal urothelial carcinoma

## Management

» Refer the patient via the 2WW pathway if you suspect bladder cancer. The criteria include the following:

› Patients who are >45 years with visible haematuria without a UTI, or haematuria that persists despite treatment of a UTI.

› Patients aged >60 years who have microscopic haematuria and a raised WCC on a blood test, or dysuria.

» Consider a non-urgent referral for bladder cancer in patients aged >60 years with recurrent or persistent unexplained UTIs.

» If there is no muscle involvement, then transurethral resection is the first-line treatment, followed by post-op intravesical chemotherapy and delayed intravesical Bacillus Calmette-Guerin (BCG) immunotherapy.

» For more invasive tumours, radical or partial cystectomy with pelvic LN dissection can be an effective method.

---

### References

National Institute for Health and Care Excellence (2020). *Urological cancers – recognition and referral.* https://cks.nice.org.uk/topics/urological-cancers-recognition-referral/

# 6

# Endocrine

## Diabetes Mellitus

DM is characterised by a disordered metabolism syndrome that results in hyperglycaemia. Type 2 DM is extremely common, with over 3.5 million people being diagnosed with it in the UK. Type 2 DM is usually due to a combination of insulin resistance and deficiency, whereas type 1 DM is due to absolute insulin deficiency.

Persistently raised blood-glucose levels can cause a person to suffer acutely with symptoms of thirst, tiredness, polyuria and weight loss. DM can cause quite serious long-term complications, including CVD, chronic kidney failure, retinopathy, neuropathy, peripheral arterial disease (PAD), erectile dysfunction and poor wound healing, and it reduces life expectancy by 10 years. The long-term complications of DM can be reduced with tight blood-glucose control, which can be measured through HbA1c. The tighter the HbA1c control, the less likely it is that the patient will develop complications.

### Risk Factors

➤ Overweight – Obesity worsens insulin resistance (e.g. acanthosis nigricans).

➤ Ethnicity – Asians and Afro-Caribbeans are two to four times more likely to have type 2 DM.

➤ Family history – A family history of DM increases the risk two to six times.

➤ Medications – Long-term corticosteroids, concomitant thiazide plus b-blocker, and statins.

➤ History of gestational DM – This increases the risk seven times.

➤ Diseases – High BP, PCOS and metabolic syndrome.

### *History*

» Focused questions

  › Ask about polydipsia (thirst), polyuria, nocturia, tiredness and weight loss.

  › Complications – Ask about recurrent infections (bacterial or fungal), visual changes, pins and needles in the hands or feet, and erectile dysfunction.

» Past history – Ask if they have had IHD, CVA, PVD, CKD, cholesterol, PCOS or gestational DM during pregnancy.

» Drug history – Ask if they have taken steroids, thiazides, b-blockers or olanzapine. Ask about drug compliance and blood-sugar measurement (BM) monitoring.

» Social history – Ask what their occupation is, if they smoke or drink alcohol, what their diet is like, what exercise they take, and how their mood is.

» Family history – Ask if there is a family history of DM.

## RED FLAGS

Abdominal pain, nausea and vomiting, SOB (diabetic ketoacidosis [DKA] / hyperglycaemic hyperosmolar non-ketotic coma [HONK]), or chest pain (cardiac).

## Depression Screening in DM

» Patients with DM or heart disease should be screened on one occasion during the year using two screening questions for depression. Ask the following:

› *During the past month, have you often been bothered by feeling down, depressed or hopeless?'*

› *During the past month, have you often been bothered by little interest or pleasure in doing things?'*

» A positive answer to both questions is suggestive of depression, and a Patient Health Questionnaire module 9 (PHQ-9) should be undertaken.

## Differential Diagnosis

| DKA | Defined by marked hyperglycaemia, acidosis and ketonuria. |
|---|---|
| Hypoglycaemia | Blood-glucose levels <3.5 mmol/l. Commonly caused by insulin or some oral agents such as gliclazide. |

## Examination

» Vitals – BP, pulse and BMI.

» Eyes – Assess visual acuity and fundoscopy.

» Foot – Examine the feet for ulcers and Charcot foot.

» Skin – Check for ulceration or infections.

» Neurological – Check for peripheral neuropathy, assessing sensation (vibration and touch) and reflexes.

» Pulse – Check peripheral pulses.

## Categorising Foot-Ulcer Risk

➤ Low – No risk factors present except callus.

➤ Moderate – One risk factor present, such as a deformity, neuropathy or non-critical limb ischaemia.

➤ High – Previous ulceration, amputation or more than one risk factor.

➤ Active problem – Ulceration, infection, critical ischaemia, gangrene or Charcot arthropathy.

## Investigations

» Bloods – FBC, U&E, eGFR, thyroid function tests (TFT), HbA1c and lipid profile.

## Diagnosing DM

» Screening – A diagnosis should not be made from a reading from a BM test or urine dipstick. These should only be used for screening for DM.

» Diagnosis – Requires one abnormal HbA1C (polyuria, polydipsia and weight loss) or two abnormal tests on separate dates (four weeks apart) if asymptomatic.

› Random >11.1

› Fasting >7.0

» HbA1c – A value of 48mmol/mol is the maximum cut-off point for diagnosing DM. It requires one abnormal result in symptomatic and two abnormal results if asymptomatic.

## Management

*Conservative*

✓ Diet – Recommend a high-fibre, low-fat and low-glycaemic-index foods (brown rice, boiled potatoes and pulses) diet, with at least five portions of fruits and vegetables, and oily fish. Advise them to avoid processed foods, ready meals, alcohol and refined sugars (sweets and cakes).

✓ Weight loss – Advise an obese patient to aim to lose 5–10%, which can help reduce blood-glucose levels.

✓ Exercise – Recommend they take 30 minutes exercise five times a week. Encourage brisk walking and hobbies such as cycling.

✓ Alcohol – Advise that they reduce their intake to <=14 units/week. They should not drink on an empty stomach.

✓ Smoking cessation – Offer smoking-cessation advice.

✓ Self-management – Offer a personalised care plan.

✓ DVLA – Those with diet-controlled DM need not inform the DVLA. Advise drivers to avoid hypoglycaemia, and inform them of the warning signs and actions to take. The patient should notify the DVLA if they require insulin, develop complications (polyneuropathy, vision), have more than one episode of hypoglycaemia in a year or have impaired awareness of it.

*Medical*

✓ Prescription – Diabetics on hypoglycaemic agents are offered free prescriptions for all their medications.

✓ Initial treatment – Offer slow release (SR) metformin unless contraindicated. If contraindicated, consider gliptin, sulphonylurea or pioglitazone. Metformin works by decreasing hepatic glucose production and the intestinal absorption of glucose, and it improves insulin sensitivity by increasing the peripheral glucose uptake and utilisation. Initiate if HbA1c is >48 despite lifestyle modifications. Monitor U&E and LFTs.

> Dose – 500mg od, titrate up to max 1g bd gradually over several weeks to minimise side effects.

> Side effects – Diarrhoea, GI symptoms (nausea and vomiting) and lactic acidosis (rare).

> Contraindications – CKD 4 (eGFR <30), liver disease, excessive alcohol or a recent MI.

> Monitor – Monitor U&Es annually. If eGFR <45, reduce the dose to 500mg bd.

✓ Sulfonylurea (gliclazide) is a metformin alternative or second-line treatment. An alternative to sulphonylureas is sodium-glucose co-transporter-2 (SGLT-2i) (Flozins). Sulphonylurea stimulates pancreas beta cells to release insulin. It increase insulin release (basal and mealtime insulin) and peripheral glucose utilisation, and it decreases hepatic gluconeogenesis.

> Dose – Start at 40–80mg od with food (ideally 30 minutes before) and increase by 80mg according to the response. Max dose is 160mg bd.

> Side effects – Hypoglycaemia, increased appetite and weight gain, mild GI symptoms and impaired LFTs.

> Contraindications – Avoid in cases of severe renal failure, liver impairment, breast feeding and pregnancy.

> Monitor the frequency of hypoglycaemia.

SGLT-2 works on the renal tubes to reduce glucose resorption and increase excretion (e.g. canagliflozin and dapagliflozin). Advise the patient to increase their fluid intake by 500ml a day to compensate for the loss.

> Dose – Canagliflozin 100mg od if eGFR >60.

> › Side effects – GI effects, UTIs, thrush and increased risk of AKI.

> › Contraindications – DKA and eGFR <60.

✓ Gliptins (sitagliptin)

Gliptins work by the action of dipeptidyl peptidase-4 (DPP-4), increasing the amount of incretin, and thus increasing the release of insulin. There is a low risk of hypoglycaemia and no weight gain.

> › Dose – Sitagliptin 100mg od. Reduce to 50mg if eGFR 30–50, or 25mg od if eGFR <30. If they are on insulin or gliclazide, the dose may need to be reduced (hypoglycaemia).

> › Side effects – Pancreatitis, GI symptoms (constipation), URTI and peripheral oedema.

> › Contraindications – Avoid in DKA and pancreatitis.

✓ Pioglitazone

## HbA1c Targets

Personalise the targets with the patient:

» 48mmol/mol – If diet-controlled or on a single drug not associated with hypoglycaemia (metformin).

» 53mmol/mol – If on a drug associated with hypoglycaemia (gliclazide).

» 58mmol/mol – If the duration of the disease is more than 10 years, and the patient is >60 years. If they have CVD, CKD or are on dialysis.

» 69mmol/mol – If they are frail, >80 years or suffer from dementia.

» Consider offering self-monitor devices if the patient is on insulin, taking long-term steroids or on agents that may cause hypoglycaemia during driving.

## Diabetics and the DVLA

» Insulin – Drivers should carry a glucometer and strips when driving. They should check their BM less than two hours before driving and every two hours while driving. They should aim for >5mmol/l while driving.

> › If BM falls to <5mmol/l, a snack should be eaten (fast-acting carbohydrate).

> › If BM <4mmol/l or there are warning signs of hypoglycaemia, the driver should not drive. If they are already driving, the driver should stop the vehicle safely, switch off the engine, remove the keys and move from the driver's seat, eat or drink a suitable source of sugar, then wait for 45 minutes until their BM returns to normal before continuing.

> › Drivers must not drive if their hypoglycaemia awareness has been lost, and the DVLA must be notified.

## Referral

→ DM eye screening – All diabetics should be referred to a local diabetic eye-screening programme.

→ Structured education – Refer all new patients with DM to structured programmes, such as Diabetes Education and Self-Management for Ongoing and Newly Diagnosed (DESMOND) (type 2 DM) or Dose Adjustment For Normal Eating (DAFNE) (type 1 DM).

→ Chiropody – Refer a patient with increased-risk and high-risk feet for assessment by a foot specialist.

## Complications

» Macrovascular

› CVD (angina and MI)

› TIA/CVA

› PVD (intermittent claudication)

» Microvascular

› Nephropathy (CKD)

› Retinopathy

› Neuropathy (chronic and painful)

» Metabolic

› Hypercholesterolaemia

› DKA (more common in type 1 DM)

» Psychological

› Anxiety and depression

» Infections

› UTI

› Folliculitis

› Fungal infections

## Managing Complications

» Consider initiating medication to prevent modifiable risk factors:

› Do not give aspirin or clopidogrel unless CVD is present.

› Aim for a BP <140/80 or <130/80 if the patient has end-organ damage (eye, kidney or CVA).

> › ACEis are the first-line treatment, then CCBs (amlodipine). If they are a woman of childbearing age, give CCBs.

> › Give atorvastatin 20mg if type 1 DM, or type 2 DM >40 years and a CVD risk >10% over 10 years. Follow up at three months, aiming for >40% reduction in non-HDL cholesterol.

» Offer the flu vaccination each autumn and also a single pneumococcal vaccination.

» Offer the patient contact details of appropriate support groups.

» Seek medical advice if any red-flag symptoms occur.

## References

National Institute for Health and Care Excellence (2013). *Neuropathic pain in adults: pharmacological management in non-specialist settings*. https://www.nice.org.uk/guidance/cg173

National Institute for Health and Care Excellence (2015). *Diabetic foot problems: prevention and management*. https://www.nice.org.uk/guidance/ng19

National Institute for Health and Care Excellence (2015). *Type 1 diabetes in adults: diagnosis and management*. https://www.nice.org.uk/guidance/ng17

National Institute for Health and Care Excellence (2015). *Type 2 diabetes in adults: management*. https://www.nice.org.uk/guidance/ng28

# Hypoglycaemia

Hypoglycaemia is defined as having a BM that is less than 2.5mmol/l. There are many possible causes for a hypoglycaemic episode, including adrenal insufficiency, tumours, medications, poor diet, excessive alcohol intake and poor use of insulin therapy. Hypoglycaemia occurs due to excessive amounts of insulin (which can be caused by any of the aforementioned). Sympathoadrenal symptoms – such as sweating, anxiety, tremors and palpitations – are caused by increased secretions of glucagon, adrenaline, cortisol and growth hormone. These symptoms tend to arise when blood glucose drops below 3.0mmol/l. Neuroglycopenic symptoms – such as blurred vision, dizziness and coma – occur solely due to an insufficient glucose supply to the brain. These symptoms tend to occur when blood-glucose concentrations are around or below <2.8mmol/l.

## Risk Factors

➤ DM

➤ Poor diet

➤ Diarrhoea and vomiting

➤ Infants who were born prematurely

➤ Impaired renal function

## Examination

» Vitals – HR (tachycardia) and BP (hypotension).

» Neurological – Altered consciousness or a visible tremor.

» The patient may appear sweaty, as well as being aggressive or displaying off behaviour.

## Differentials

➤ Substance abuse

➤ Alcohol abuse

➤ Cardiac dysrhythmia

## Investigation

» BM – <2.5mmol/l.

» Bloods – Routine tests (FBC, U&Es, LFTs, etc.) to determine the cause of a hypoglycaemia episode if it is not clear.

## Management

- ✓ If they are conscious, give a simple carbohydrate such as three glucose tablets, 100ml of milk, Lucozade, five sweets or Glucogel.

- ✓ If they are unable to take oral carbohydrates, give IM glucagon 1mg (Remember that there is a different dose for children!). This takes around five minutes to be effective.

- ✓ If the patient is starved or intoxicated, and you have IV access, you may give IV glucose 50–250ml of 10% solution in 50ml aliquots.

- ✓ If the patient was previously unconsciousness and has now regained consciousness, give a simple carbohydrate (this can be repeated one to three times if necessary).

- ✓ In a patient who was previously conscious, give complex carbohydrates as their symptoms improve, such as biscuits (this can be repeated one to three times if necessary).

- ✓ Repeat glucose testing in <15 minutes, then monitor hourly bloods every four hours over the next 24 hours..

- ✓ Maintain a high glucose intake for several hours if the hypoglycaemia was due to a sulfonylurea.

- ✓ Review why the patient had hypoglycaemia; do routine bloods (FBC, U&Es, LFTs, etc.) to exclude infections, liver disease, dehydration, etc.

---

*References*

National Institute for Health and Care Excellence (n.d.). *Hypoglycaemia*. https://bnf.nice.org.uk/treatment-summary/hypoglycaemia.html

# Hypothyroidism

Hypothyroidism is a condition caused by the underactivity of the thyroid gland, producing less of the thyroid hormones T4 and/or T3. It is believed that 1–2% of the population are hypothyroid, and it affects women 10 times more than men. The commonest form is Hashimoto's thyroiditis, which is an autoimmune disease affecting middle-aged women. Other causes include damage to the thyroid gland due to treating an overactive gland using radioactive iodine or following surgery. Internationally, a lack of dietary iodine is a common cause of hypothyroidism.

## Common Complications of Primary Hypothyroidism

➤ Iodine deficiency (commonest worldwide)

➤ Autoimmune thyroiditis (Hashimoto's thyroiditis, which is associated with goitre)

➤ Post-ablation surgery (i.e. treatment of hyperthyroidism)

➤ Drugs (iodine, amiodarone and lithium)

➤ Transient thyroiditis (de Quervain's thyroiditis, which is a painful swelling caused by viral infection)

➤ Postpartum thyroiditis

## *History*

» Focused questions

› Ask when symptoms started and how long they have been going on for.

› Ask about cold intolerance, tiredness, weight gain and constipation.

» Associated history – Ask if they have a low mood, dry skin, myalgia (muscle aches), hoarse voice, menorrhagia or menstrual irregularity, pregnancy or carpal tunnel symptoms.

» Past history – Ask if they have had type 1 DM, Addison's disease, pernicious anaemia, Down's syndrome or vitiligo. Ask if they have been pregnant.

» Surgery – Ask if they have had a thyroidectomy or radioiodine.

» Drug history – Ask if they have taken amiodarone, lithium, rifampicin or carbimazole. Ask about drug compliance.

» Social history – Ask what their occupation is, and if they smoke or drink alcohol.

» Family history – Ask if there is a family history of hypothyroidism.

## RED FLAGS

Myxoedema (a deterioration in their mental state, late presentation, hypothermia, psychosis and ataxia).

## Differentials

➤ Pituitary mass – Change in vision (diplopia) or headaches.

## Examination

» Vitals – Pulse (bradycardia), BP (hypotension), BMI (obesity) and temperature (hypothermia).

» Inspection – Inspect for dry skin, the thinning of temporal hair and eyebrows, and inspect the neck for goitre.

» Palpation – Stand behind the patient. Offer them a glass of water to drink to see if their goitre moves up and down with swallowing. Feel for a goitre (tenderness indicates thyroiditis), as well as assessing its size and nodularity.

» Percussion – Can percuss down for retrosternal extension if the patient has SOB or dysphagia.

» Reflexes – Slowly relaxing reflexes.

» Neurology – Paraesthesia (carpal tunnel syndrome) and reduced peripheral vision (pituitary mass).

## Investigations

» Bloods –TFTs (thyroid stimulating hormone [TSH], T3 and T4), FBC (anaemia), CRP (thyroiditis), cholesterol (raised), thyroid antibodies if an autoimmune disease is suspected, and HbA1c (type 1 DM).

» USS – Thyroid gland USS if the mass or goitre is palpable.

» TFT screening – Asymptomatic patients should not routinely be tested for hypothyroidism. Measuring the TSH is indicated in patients with a goitre, DM, AF, high cholesterol, congenital hypothyroidism, Down's or Turner's syndromes, postpartum depression or dementia, or if they have had radioactive iodine or surgery.

*Interpreting TFTs*

| TSH | T4 | Interpretation |
|---|---|---|
| ↑ | ↓ | Hypothyroidism – Initiate medication. |
| ↑ | normal | Subclinical hypothyroidism – If TSH is 5–10, check peroxidase antibodies. If it is positive, monitor TSH annually. If it is negative, then check TSH every three years. If the patient is symptomatic or TSH >10, initiate levothyroxine. If the patient is on medication, there is likely poor compliance. |
| ↓/N | ↓ | Hypothyroidism caused by pituitary failure. |
| ↑ | N | If a patient is on treatment, check their medication compliance. |

## Management

### Conservative

✓ Prescription – Hypothyroid patients are offered free prescriptions.

### Medical

✓ Levothyroxine – Initiate levothyroxine 100mcg-125mcg od (preferably before breakfast). Recheck TFTs after one month and titrate dose accordingly. Aim to get TSH within the normal range. Once stable, monitor annually. In the elderly, start with low dose of 25-50mcg, and titrate upwards monthly depending on TFTs. Low TSH levels are associated with AF and osteoporosis. Avoid taking levothyroxine with milk, coffee or soya products.

✓ Pregnancy – Aim for a TSH of 0.4–2.5 and increase the dose by 30% once pregnant. Monitor TSH each trimester if the obstetrician is not already doing so.

✓ Subclinical – Often does not require treatment, and if it is required, use levothyroxine. Aim for a stable TSH (in the lower half of the reference range, 0.4–2.5).

## Referral

Refer the patient to an endocrinologist if they are/have any of the following:

→ Under 16-years-old

→ Subacute thyroiditis

→ Pituitary disease

→ Pregnant

→ Persistent raised TSH despite increased medication

## Safety Netting

> » If the symptoms have not improved after four to six weeks with medication, then review.

---

### *References*

Royal College of Physicians (2011). *The diagnosis and management of primary hypothyroidism.*

# Hyperthyroidism

Hyperthyroidism or thyrotoxicosis is a condition that is caused by the overactivity of the thyroid gland due to an overproduction of the thyroid hormones T4 and T3. It affects 1% of women and 0.1% of men. Symptoms include sympathetic overactivity (tremors, tachycardia and sweating), onycholysis (separation of the nail from the nail bed), palmar erythema, proximal myopathy and lid retraction.

The most common form of thyrotoxicosis is Graves' disease. It is a condition that commonly affects young people, and it presents with an enlarged, smooth goitre, eye changes (exophthalmos and ophthalmoplegia) and pretibial myxoedema. It is also associated with myasthenia gravis and pernicious anaemia.

## Common Causes of Hyperthyroidism

- ➤ Graves' disease
- ➤ Multinodular goitre
- ➤ Solitary toxic adenoma
- ➤ Thyroiditis
- ➤ Drug-induced (amiodarone and lithium)

## Common Complications of Hyperthyroidism

- ➤ Graves' ophthalmopathy
- ➤ Thyrotoxic crisis
- ➤ AF
- ➤ Pregnancy complications (miscarriage, pre-eclampsia, preterm delivery and low birth weight)

## *History*

- » Focused questions:
  - › Ask when their symptoms started and how long they have been going on for.
  - › Ask about heat intolerance, weight loss, palpitations and diarrhoea.

- » Associated history – Ask if they have experienced any tiredness, sweating, tremors, irritability, periods or goitre (SOB, pressure in the neck and dysphagia).
- » Past history – Ask if they have had myasthenia gravis, type 1 DM or a pregnancy (postpartum thyroiditis).
- » Drug history – Ask if they have taken amiodarone, excessive levothyroxine or lithium.

» Social history – Ask what their occupation is, and if they smoke or drink alcohol.

» Family history – Ask if there is a family history of hyperthyroidism.

## Features of de Quervain's (Subacute) Thyroiditis

➤ Presents with a painful swelling of the thyroid gland, and it is caused by a viral infection. It is commonly seen in women (20–50 years) causing fever and pain in the neck (jaw/ear). It is associated with features of hyperthyroidism, including palpitations and anxiety. It often settles after a few weeks or months.

## RED FLAGS

» Thyrotoxic crisis – Fever, agitation, confusion, diarrhoea and vomiting, acute abdomen and tachycardia.

» Graves' disease – Thyroid-related eye disease (double vision, lid lag, eye discomfort and eye protrusion).

## Examination

» Vitals – Fever, pulse (tachycardia and AF), BP (HTN) and BMI (low).

» Thyroid exam

› Inspection – Get the patient to outstretch their hands (fine tremor), also inspect for clubbing (Graves' disease), acropachy, onycholysis, palmar erythema and sweaty palms.

› Eyes – Look for exophthalmos, loss of hair at the outer one-third of the eyebrow, lid/lag retraction and ophthalmoplegia.

› Neck – Inspect the neck for the presence of a goitre.

› Palpitation – Stand behind the patient. Offer them a glass of water to drink to see if the goitre moves up and down with swallowing. Feel the goitre (tenderness, irregular and asymmetrical indicates thyroiditis) and determine its size and nodularity (non-tender nodules indicates toxic multinodular goitre, and a unilateral non-tender nodule indicates toxic adenoma).

› Percussion – Can percuss for retrosternal extension if the patient has SOB or dysphagia.

› Auscultation – Listen for thyroid bruit.

» Legs – Palpate the legs for evidence of pitting oedema

» Inspect muscles (wasting), assess power (proximal myopathy) and check reflexes (hyperreflexia).

## Investigations

» Bloods – TFT (TSH – if it is normal, hyperthyroidism is unlikely; if it is low, then T3 and T4 should be checked), FBC (anaemia indicates Graves' disease), thyroid antibodies (Graves' disease), ESR and CRP (subacute thyroiditis).

» USS – Thyroid gland USS if there is a mass or the goitre is palpable.

### Interpreting TFTs

| TSH | T4 | Interpretation |
|-----|-----|----------------|
| ↓ | ↑ | Hyperthyroidism – Initiate medication. |
| ↓ | normal | Subclinical hyperthyroidism. Observe and monitor every three to six months. Provide treatment if it converts into frank hyperthyroidism. |
| ↑ | ↑ | Suspect pituitary microadenoma or erratic levothyroxine compliance. |

## Management

### Medical

✓ B-blocker – Can start this (propranolol 10–40mg qds or metoprolol 50mg qds) to control the symptoms (palpitations, anxiety and tremors) until antithyroid medication is initiated.

✓ Carbimazole – Inhibits the synthesis of thyroid hormones. Often given for 12–18 months, but there is a high risk of relapse (50%).

✓ Side effects – Alopecia, jaundice, pruritus, rash and a bitter taste.

✓ Complications – Agranulocytosis. Advise the patient to look for a fever, sore throat, mouth ulcers or feeling generally unwell; if these occur, they should seek urgent medical advice.

✓ Propylthiouracil – Advise the patient to seek urgent advice if they develop the features of liver disease. Organise urgent LFTs.

✓ Radioiodine – This may be offered for the patient by a specialist. Contraindicated in pregnancy, breastfeeding or thyroid eye disease.

✓ Eye symptoms – Consider Lacri-Lube or artificial tears to lubricate dry eyes. If there is periorbital oedema, elevating the head of the bed often helps reduce symptoms.

✓ Subclinical hyperthyroidism – Repeat TFT after 6–12 months, and refer the patient once it becomes hyperthyroidism.

*Surgical*

✓ A partial or total thyroidectomy can be performed, especially for a large goitre. There is the risk of hypothyroidism with lifelong thyroxine if too much is excised.

**Side effects**

› Recurrent laryngeal nerve palsy and damage to the parathyroids post-surgery.

# Referral

→ Refer the patient or seek advice from an endocrinologist if dose reduction or withdrawal may be required, if T4 is raised for six months or more after radioiodine treatment, or if TSH >20 for more than one month.

→ Refer them to ophthalmology if there is evidence of thyroid eye disease.

→ Refer them under 2WW if the patient has a thyroid nodule or goitre and malignancy is suspected.

→ Refer them urgently if they present with the symptoms of a thyroid storm.

→ Refer them to endocrinology if the patient wants to get pregnant and suffers from subclinical hyperthyroidism or hyperthyroidism. Refer them urgently if they are currently pregnant.

## Safety Netting

» If their symptoms have not improved after four to six weeks of medication, then review.

*References*

National Institute for Health and Care Excellence (2020). *Hyperthyroidism: scenario: management.* https://cks.nice.org.uk/topics/hyperthyroidism/management/management/

# Galactorrhoea

Galactorrhoea refers to the inappropriate secretion or discharge of milk from the breasts that is not associated with breastfeeding or pregnancy. The most common cause (>90%) is due to raised prolactin levels, which can originate from a prolactin-secreting tumour. However, a number of drugs have also been implicated. While galactorrhoea may be physiological in women, it is more likely to be pathological in men. It can also be seen in neonates (along with breast enlargement) who have been impacted by the temporary effects of the maternal oestrogen.

## History

» Focused questions

› Ask when the symptoms started and how long they have been going on for.

› Ask about the region (whether it affects both breasts or just one).

› Ask about discharge, and if there is any blood or pus.

› Ask if it occurs spontaneously or has to be expressed.

› Ask about the volume of discharge, breast pain and any triggers.

» Associated history (in men) – Ask about impotence, libido loss and gynaecomastia.

» Gynaecology history (in women) – Ask about menstrual disturbance, infertility (problems getting pregnant) and contraception.

» Past history – Ask if they have had hypothyroidism, acromegaly, CKD or liver cirrhosis.

» Drug history – Ask if they have taken anything OTC.

» Social history – Ask what their occupation is, if they suffer from stress, and if they smoke, drink alcohol or take illicit drugs.

» Family history – Ask if there is a family history of any thyroid problems or multiple endocrine neoplasia.

## Drugs That Can Cause Galactorrhoea

» Antipsychotics (prochlorperazine is the most common)

» Antidepressants (SSRIs and TCAs)

» Prokinetics (metoclopramide and domperidone)

» H2 antagonists (ranitidine)

» Certain antihypertensives

It is important to remember that galactorrhoea does not cause a rise in prolactin levels >2,500mU/l. Such levels warrant a full examination and further investigation to exclude pituitary pathology.

## RED FLAGS

Visual disturbances, severe headaches (pituitary adenoma) and breast cancer (unilateral, bloody discharge and a lump).

## Differential Diagnosis

| Physiological | Breast feeding, pregnancy, stress, puberty and menopause. |
|---|---|
| Prolactinoma | Can be caused by pituitary adenoma or craniopharyngioma. Presents with a headache, visual disturbances (bitemporal hemianopia), irregular periods (amenorrhoea), infertility and reduced libido. OE: reduced peripheral vision. |
| Hypothyroidism | The patient complains of tiredness, weight gain, cold intolerance, constipation and menstrual irregularities. OE: dry skin, hair thinning, reduced reflexes and a goitre may be present. |
| Acromegaly | Rare condition due to increased growth hormone. Causes large hands and feet, a prominent jaw and facial features, and an enlarged tongue. The patient may have oily, coarse skin and complain of low libido, impotence (men) or menstrual disturbances (women). |
| PCOS | Hirsutism, obesity, acne, irregular periods and fertility problems. |

## Physiological Causes of Galactorrhoea

➤ Galactorrhoea can occur during pregnancy and post-lactation from the second trimester and continue for up to two years after breastfeeding has stopped. It can also occur during puberty and the menopause, due to fluctuating hormone levels. It is commonly seen in neonates after exposure to maternal hormones in the uterus, causing gynaecomastia and galactorrhoea (witch's milk), which resolves rapidly after birth. Galactorrhoea may also occur from suckling or nipple stimulation.

## Examination

» Vitals – BP (hypothyroidism) and weight (hypothyroidism, acromegaly and pregnancy).

» General – Examine the skin for signs of hirsutism, hair loss or acne.

» Breast – Observe for any skin changes (*peau d'orange*) and palpate to exclude any breast lumps. Request that the patient expresses any milk from their nipples.

» Neurology – Assess the visual fields if a pituitary lesion is suspected. Map the visual fields and observe for bitemporal hemianopia (pituitary adenoma and craniopharyngioma).

## Investigations

» Bloods – Prolactin levels (hyperprolactinemia >500 requires investigation, >4,000 is pathological and a prolactin-secreting pituitary tumour should be suspected). A single test should not be used to diagnose this, as stress, disturbed sleep and pregnancy can cause a raise in the prolactin level. TFTs (hypothyroidism) and U&Es (Cushing's disease).

» MC&S – Breast discharge.

» Urine – Pregnancy test.

» Imaging – MRI / CT head (pituitary adenoma and craniopharyngioma) and mammography.

## Management

*Treat the underlying cause*

### Conservative

✓ Advise the patient to void repeated breast stimulation to reduce the discharge. Wear breast pads to absorb any leakage.

### Medical

✓ Identify the precipitating drug, and stop it or change it to an alternative.

✓ Hyperprolactinemia

› Microadenoma – Monitor for pituitary adenomas with MRI scans and prolactin blood tests.

› Cabergoline – Refer them to a specialist for initiation (this is the first-line treatment for prolactinomas).

› Bromocriptine – Refer them to a specialist for initiation.

› Hormone – Consider testosterone in men, and COC/HRT in women to prevent osteoporosis.

✓ Idiopathic

› Treat symptomatic galactorrhoea with bromocriptine/Cabergoline.

✓ Hypothyroidism

› Start levothyroxine, depending on TFTs. *See Hypothyroidism section, page 210.*

## Referral

→   Refer the patient to endocrinology if there is suspicion of a brain lesion causing the galactorrhoea.

## Safety Netting

»   If symptoms are not improving, or the patient has visual disturbances, headaches or dizziness while taking bromocriptine then stop driving, using power tools or machines.

*References?*

Vroonen, L., Daly, A.F., and Beckers, A. (2019). Epidemiology and management challenges in prolactinomas. *Neuroendocrinology*, 109(1), pp. 20–27. https://pubmed.ncbi.nlm.nih.gov/30731464/

Huang, W. and Molitch, M.E. (2012). Evaluation and management of galactorrhea. *American Family Physician.* 85(11), pp. 1073–80. https://pubmed.ncbi.nlm.nih.gov/22962879/

Patel, B.K., Falcon, S. and Drukteinis, J. (2014). Management of nipple discharge and the associated imaging findings. *The American Journal of Medicine, 128*(4), pp. 353–60. https://pubmed.ncbi.nlm.nih.gov/25447625/

# Gynaecomastia

Gynaecomastia describes the abnormal enlargement and development of breasts in males. Although it may be present physiologically in newborns, adolescents and the elderly, it usually causes much distress and angst in the male sufferer; particularly at the time of puberty, where up to 60% of boys may suffer from it, and it can last for up to 12 months.

## Causes of Gynaecomastia

➤ **Physiological**

› Newborns (maternal hormones persists for several months).

› Adolescents.

› The elderly (low testosterone).

› Those with obesity.

➤ **Pathological**

› Increase in oestrogen – Adrenal carcinoma, congenital adrenal hyperplasia or testicular cancer.

› Decrease in testosterone – Klinefelter syndrome, viral orchitis or trauma.

➤ **Drug-induced**

› Oestrogen (female partner's vaginal creams with oestrogen).

› Drugs that inhibit testosterone synthesis (spironolactone and metronidazole).

## History

» Focused questions

› Ask when the symptoms started and how long they have been lasted for.

› Ask about the region (unilateral or bilateral) affected.

› Ask if there has been any discharge or breast pain, and ask about sexual function.

» Past history – Ask if they have had hyperthyroidism, adrenal cancer, liver disease (cirrhosis), renal failure or hypogonadism.

» Drug history – Ask if they have taken any anabolic steroids, any spironolactone, digoxin, antipsychotics, furosemide or finasteride.

» Social history – Ask if they smoke, drink alcohol or take illicit drugs, and ask about their mood.

» Family history – Ask if there is a family history of breast cancer.

## RED FLAGS

A family history of breast cancer, a rapidly growing lesion, breast(s) >5cm, an irregular firm mass, unilateral (breast cancer), testicular cancer (testicular mass) or liver disease (jaundice or weight loss).

## Differentials

➤ Testicular cancer

➤ Hyperthyroidism

➤ Hyperprolactinemia

## Examination

» Vitals – BMI (obesity).

» Breast(s)

› Inspection – Inspect for the enlargement of the breasts. Check for unilateral or bilateral presentation. Check if there are any skin changes (*peau d'orange* or nipple retraction).

› Palpation – Place the thumb and forefinger (in a pinching movement) over the counter and inner breast margins. Palpate the disc of breast tissue under the nipple and the areola area (>2cm indicates gynaecomastia and <2cm is normal). Palpate the four quadrants for masses. Ascertain the size and shape of any masses. Feel for axillary lymphadenopathy.

» Abdomen

› Inspection – Inspect for signs of liver disease (spider naevi, jaundice and palmar erythema).

› Palpation – Palpate the liver for signs of hepatomegaly or an irregular edge (cirrhosis).

» Testicular exam

› Inspection – Inspect for hypogonadism and Klinefelter syndrome (secondary sexual characteristics).

› Palpation – Palpate the testicles for any masses.

» Thyroid exam

› Palpate the thyroid for signs of a goitre.

### Differences Between Malignancy and Gynaecomastia

» Gynaecomastia – Usually bilateral; often painless, but occasionally painful; central subareolar; and a smooth, firm, mobile, normal nipple with normal skin and axilla.

» Malignancy – Usually unilateral, often painless, and a central (70–90%) or eccentric, irregular, rubbery/hard fixed lesion. Associated with nipple deformity, or ulcerated, red skin and axillary adenopathy.

## Investigations

These are not routinely recommended for boys in puberty or men taking oral agents known to cause gynaecomastia.

» Bloods – TFTs, LFTs and U&Es. If these are normal, then LH and FSH, testosterone, oestradiol, prolactin and BHCG (testicular cancer).

» Karyotype (Klinefelter syndrome), dehydroepiandrosterone (DHEA) (testicular tumour), AFP and SHBG.

» USS – Testes or breast tissue.

» CXR – Lung cancer.

### Interpreting LH and Testosterone Levels in Gynaecomastia

| LH | Test | Interpretation |
|---|---|---|
| N | N | Idiopathic gynaecomastia. |
| N | ↓ | Pituitary or hypothalamic disease. |
| ↑ | ↓ | Testicular failure (hypogonadism) or Klinefelter syndrome. |
| ↑ | ↑ | Androgen resistance or neoplasm-secreting gonadotropins. |
| ↓ | ↓ | Increased oestrogen (testicular/adrenal cancer, liver failure, hyperthyroidism or obesity). |

## Management

### Medical

✓ Identify the precipitating drug and stop it. This often improves within one month, but if the drug has been taken for more than one year, then significant improvements are less likely (fibrosis).

### Physiological

✓ This is the most common form, which is seen in the elderly, neonates, teenagers and those with obesity. Reassure the patient.

✓ Obesity – Encourage them to lose weight. Refer them to an exercise programme to get their BMI <25.

✓ Adolescents – For the majority, it resolves within two years.

## Treatment

### Medical

✓ A specialist may initiate anti-oestrogens or consider testosterone replacements in hypogonadal men.

### Surgical

✓ Mammoplasty if the gynaecomastia does not get better or the patient cannot tolerate their appearance.

## Referral

→ Refer the patient to counselling for therapy or support.

→ Refer them to a urologist if testicular cancer is suspected.

→ Refer them to an endocrinologist if there is suspicion of a brain lesion causing the galactorrhoea.

→ Refer them to a breast surgeon, as per cancer guidelines.

### Referral Guidance for Gynaecomastia 2WW

» Unilateral enlargement

» Hard or irregular breast tissue

» Enlarging rapidly

» Recent onset

» Fixed mass

» Nipple or skin abnormalities

» Painful

» Breast(s) >5cm

» Axillary lymphadenopathy

*References*

Thiruchelvam, P., Walker, J.N., Rose, K., Lewis, J. and Al-Mufti, R. (2016). Gynaecomastia. *The BMJ, 354.* doi: https://doi.org/10.1136/bmj.i4833

# Tired All the Time

Tiredness and fatigue are extremely common symptoms that a wide range of patients present with. In the UK, it is believed that up to 20% of people suffer with tiredness lasting more than one month, with women suffering twice as much as men. Tiredness and fatigue may be caused by psychological problems (such as stress, insomnia or depression), physical problems (such as manual labour) or a number of physiological conditions (obesity, thyroid dysfunction, DM, etc.). However, fatigue that persists may suggest that something more sinister is at play, such as cancer or inflammation. It is important to take an extensive history of the patient's complaint before examining them and tailoring the investigations to locate the root cause.

## History

- » Focused questions
  - › Onset and frequency – Ask when it started, how often they are tired, and whether it is all the time or it comes and goes.
  - › Triggers – Ask if they have any stress, are taking any new tablets, or have had a recent illness.
  - › Function – Ask if it has affected their ability to carry out activities; e.g. walking, cooking, climbing stairs or getting dressed.

- » Associated history
  - › Ask how they are sleeping, what time they go to sleep and wake up, and if they take any naps during the day.
  - › Cognitive function – Ask if they have the ability to concentrate or get distracted easily.
  - › Ask if they have any dizziness, have been feeling sick or have vomited.
  - › Ask if they have had a sore throat, fever or other flu-like symptoms.
  - › Ask if they have had any change in weight.
  - › Life events/stress – Ask if they have moved house, had a new baby, changed their job or undergone any other stressful life events.

- » Past history – Ask if they have had cancer or tuberculosis (TB).

- » Drug history – Ask if they have taken any b-blockers, SSRIs, TCA, BDZs, antihistamines or opioids.

- » Family history – Ask if there is anyone else in the family with similar symptoms.

- » Social history
  - › Ask if they have travelled anywhere (malaria, hepatitis or Lyme disease [from ticks]).
  - › Ask about their relationships and support network.
  - › Ask what their occupation is (shift patterns).
  - › Ask what their diet is like.

> Ask if they smoke, drink alcohol or take recreational drugs.

## RED FLAGS

Weight loss, night sweats, persistent fevers, haemoptysis, PR bleeding, postmenopausal PV bleeding, dysphagia or swollen LNs.

## Differential Diagnosis

| | |
|---|---|
| Anaemia | Hair loss, headaches and feeling light-headed (menstruation is heavy). |
| Thyroid | Weight gain, and feel cold when others feel hot. |
| DM | Thirsty and has polyuria. |
| Sleep apnoea | Snoring at night, choking or stopping breathing when sleeping. |
| Malabsorption | Any diarrhoea related to food (coeliac), or mucus or blood in the stools (IBD). |
| Myositis | Pain or weakness of muscles (shoulder or pelvis). |
| Polymyalgia rheumatica (PMR) | Pain or tenderness in both shoulders, painful muscles or joint stiffness, which is worse in the morning. |
| Psychological | Positive depression screen, a recent bereavement, or fatigue after carrying out any activity (chronic fatigue syndrome [CFS]). |

## Examination

» Vitals – Temperature, BP, weight and pulse.

» General – Observe how they appear.

» Examination – Conduct a complete examination, focusing on systems where symptoms may be present:

> Inspection – Look at their general health and for signs of anaemia (pale conjunctiva, atrophic glossitis and tachycardia).

> Palpation – Perform a focused thyroid examination. Feel for lymphadenopathy.

» Questionnaires – Offer PHQ-9 if they are showing symptoms of depression, and complete the Epworth Sleepiness Scale (ESS) if obstructive sleep apnoea (OSA) is suspected.

## Investigations

» Bloods – FBC (anaemia), ESR, CRP, TFT and fasting glucose.

> › Others (if clinically indicated) – ferritin, U&Es, LFTs, Vit D, calcium and tissue transglutaminase antibody (TTGA).

> › Myeloma screen – Consider urine Bence-Jones protein and protein electrophoresis.

> › Viral screen – HIV, hep B and C, and monospot test (glandular fever).

» Urine – Dipstick for protein, blood and glucose. MC&S for infection.

» Stools – MC&S if they have travelled recently and have chronic diarrhoea.

» CXR – To exclude infection, TB, sarcoid and lung cancer.

## Management

*Treat the underlying cause*

*Conservative*

✓ Lifestyle changes

> › Exercise – Advise the patient to take regular exercise (e.g. walking and stretching).

> › Diet – Advise them to cut down on alcohol, and eat a balanced diet, including red meat.

> › Sleep hygiene – Advise them to relax in a dark room with minimal distractions. They should go to sleep at the same time every night and have a light snack beforehand. There should be no sleeping during the day.

> › Rest – Advise them to ensure that rest periods are not for more than 30 minutes.

> › Relaxation – Advise them to use breathing techniques or guided visualisation to help them relax during rest periods.

> › Weight – Advise the patient to reduce their weight to a BMI <25 to help reduce symptoms of tiredness.

✓ Talking therapies

> › CBT – Consider this for mild/moderate depression.

> › Graded exercise therapies (GET) – Consider referring them for GET or activity-management programmes.

✓ Advise the patient to see a work-based occupational adviser or physician if they are having problems due to work.

*Medical*

✓ Anaemia – Consider ferrous supplements if there is evidence of them being low in iron.

✓ Dysmenorrhoea – *See Dysmenorrhoea section, page 335.*

✓ DM – *See Diabetes Mellitus section, page 201.*

✓ Hypothyroidism – *See Hypothyroidism section, page 210.*

✓ Myositis – Refer the patient to rheumatology to consider treatment with steroids or immunosuppressive agents (azathioprine).

✓ TB – Refer them to the respiratory team for therapy antibiotics (isoniazid and rifampicin for six months, with pyrazinamide and ethambutol for the first two months).

✓ Depression – Consider SSRIs (fluoxetine or sertraline) to treat depression. *See Depression section, page 541.*

## Referral

→ Refer them to speak to an OT about adaptations that can be made at home or regarding adaptations at work to maintain their ability to stay in employment.

→ Consider referring them to a pain clinic to maximise treatment if needed.

→ Refer them to a rheumatologist or CFS service if one is available locally.

→ Refer them according to the 2WW pathways if there are any red flags or cancer is suspected.

## Safety Netting

» Review them in four to six weeks for any response to the treatment or to check the diagnosis.

---

*References*

National Institute for Health and Care Excellence (2007). *CFS / myalgic encephalomyelitis: diagnosis and management.* https://www.nice.org.uk/guidance/cg53

# Vitamin D Deficiency

A vitamin D value (25-hydroxyvitamin D) of less than 25nmol/l indicates a vitamin D deficiency (note that an insufficiency is classed as 25–50nmol/l). Causes include sun avoidance, inadequate dietary intake, malabsorption syndromes and obesity.

There are many different forms of vitamin D and many different ways of obtaining it. Vitamin D3 is obtained from the skin, and vitamins D2 and D3 can be obtained from the diet. These forms are biologically inactive. In the liver, hydroxylation occurs and 25-hydroxyvitamin D is formed. However, this form is also inactive, and further hydroxylation occurs in the liver to activate this molecule to form 1,25-dihydroxyvitamin D.

## There are many causes of vitamin D deficiency:

➤ Nutritional – Dietary deficiency, lack of sunlight and altered/inefficient absorption.

➤ Drug-induced – Phenytoin and carbamazepine.

➤ CKD – Due to the reduced synthesis of 2,25-dihydroxyvitamin D.

➤ Hyperparathyroidism.

Insufficient vitamin D leads to the inadequate absorption of calcium and phosphate, which results in secondary hyperparathyroidism and a lack of new bone mineralisation, causing rickets in children and osteomalacia in adults.

## *History*

» Many patients are asymptomatic.

» They complain of muscle aches and sometimes have wasting of muscles (mainly the quadriceps).

» Patients may complain of generalised bone pain.

» They feel tired, and may complain that they 'feel off' or 'are not themselves'.

» Children may have poor growth or poor delay, and babies may be irritable.

» Ask about any history of lack of sunlight (poor mobility, lives in a residential home, wears covering clothing, etc.).

## Examination

» Commonly, a nil acute or unremarkable examination.

» In severe cases, bowed legs may be noted in children.

» In children, there may be skull softening with frontal bossing. There may be tender and swollen joints, mainly in the wrists.

## Differentials

➤   Iron-deficiency anaemia

➤   Depression

➤   Fibromyalgia

➤   Vitamin B12 deficiency

## Investigations

»   Bloods – Serum 25-hydroxyvitamin D, serum alkaline phosphatase (may be raised in rickets), serum calcium (normal), U&Es and LFTs.

»   Consider a dual energy x-ray absorptiometry (DEXA) scan in chronic vitamin D deficiency.

## Management

✓   Vitamin D insufficiency normally warrants conservative management. However, if any of the following are present, start treatment:

   ›   Increased risk of having a vitamin D deficiency.

   ›   Raised parathyroid hormones.

   ›   The patient takes anti-epileptic medications or steroids.

   ›   Malabsorption conditions are met.

   ›   CKD.

   ›   Liver disease.

✓   Vitamin D deficiency should be treated with loading doses: either daily split doses or weekly doses of up to a total of 300,000IU. This could be 50,000IU weekly for six weeks, 20,000IU twice weekly for seven weeks, or 4,000 IU daily for 10 weeks.

   ›   One month after commencing treatment, check the adjusted serum calcium levels.

   ›   Three to six months after commencing treatment, recheck the vitamin D levels (note that certain labs will not allow vitamin D to be retested more than once in 12 months).

   ›   If levels are still low after treatment, refer them to secondary care and consider causes (compliance, liver disease, etc.).

   ›   If treatment is successful, give a daily dose of 800IU per day.

   **Examples of vitamin D supplements include the following:**

   ›   Fultium-D3® (colecalciferol) capsules – These are available in 80mcg (3,200IU) and 500mcg (20,000IU) capsules for 15 days post diagnosis (note that these have gelatin, but are halal).

› InVita D3® (colecalciferol) oral solution – Available in 625mcg (25,000IU) per ml ampoules. Prescribe 50,000IU weekly for six weeks.

› Thorans

- Children of one to five months – 3,000IU (15 drops =0.3ml) daily.

- Children of six months to 11 years – 6,000IU (30 drops =0.6ml) daily.

- Children of 12–17 years – 10,000IU (50 drops =1ml) daily for 8–12 weeks.

## References

National Institute for Health and Care Excellence (2018). *Vitamin D deficiency in adults*. https://cks.nice.org.uk/topics/vitamin-d-deficiency-in-adults-treatment-prevention/

# 7

# Neurology

## Headache

Headaches are an extremely common symptom that patients present with in primary care. The vast majority of headaches are due to migraine and tension (also known as primary headaches). However, a small minority are due to a more sinister and serious cause, such as an intracranial bleed or a space-occupying lesion (SOL) (secondary headaches). The key to a good consultation is to take a comprehensive history about the headache, identify any associated features and to not miss any red flags.

### History

» Focused questions
  › Ask when the headache started and how long it has been going on for.
  › Ask about the site of the headache (unilateral, bilateral or always on the same side).
  › Ask about the onset, and if it was sudden (subarachnoid) or gradual.
  › Ask about the character (sharp, dull, throbbing or like a band).
  › Ask about the severity, including asking for a pain score.
  › Ask about timing (evening indicates tension).
  › Ask about the relieving and exacerbating factors (posture, stress, head movements, coughing, periods, sex and exercise).

» Associated history – Ask if they experience fever, nausea or vomiting, visual disturbances (zigzag lines, blurring or loss of vision) or photophobia; enquire about whether they wear glasses and when they last had their eyes tested.

» Past history – Ask if they have had migraines, a pregnancy, cancer, HTN or a stroke.

» Family history – Ask if there is a family history of migraines or cancer.

» Drug history – Ask if they have taken nitrates, CCBs, codeine or COCP. Ask if they have taken any painkillers, and if so, how often they are taking them (overuse for headaches is >14 days/month for three months or more).

» Social history – Ask what their occupation is; whether they have any stress or financial worries;, if they smoke, drink alcohol or take recreational drugs; and what their diet is like (cheese, chocolate and caffeine).

## RED FLAGS

» Sudden onset of severe pain that reaches its maximum intensity in five minutes (thunderclap indicates subarachnoid).

» A new headache or one that has changed in character in an >50-year-old (temporal arteritis).

» Persistent/progressive/changing headache (subdural).

» Dizziness.

» Features of meningitis.

» An atypical aura (lasting one hour or more or weakness) or while taking the COCP (CVA risk).

» Vomiting.

» A headache that is made worse by lying down (cerebral SOL).

» A headache that is made worse by coughing, sneezing or exertion.

» A head trauma within the last three months (subdural).

» Pregnancy (pre-eclampsia).

» A change in behaviour.

» Focal neurology.

## Differentials

*Sudden*

➤ Subarachnoid haemorrhage

➤ Minor viral headache

➤ Postcoital migraine

➤ Migraine

➤ Meningitis

*Periodic*

➤ Migraine

➤ Cluster headaches

➤ Sinusitis

➤ Glaucoma

➤ HTN

➤ Cervical spondylosis

*Continuous*

➤ Temporal arteritis

➤ Brain tumour

➤ Depression

## Differential Diagnosis

| | |
|---|---|
| Migraine | Unilateral throbbing/pulsating frontal or temporal headaches. Often lasting 4–72 hours. More common in women than men. It may present with or without an aura (flashing lights, loss of vision, zigzag lines, pins and needles, aphasia or motor weakness), but patients invariably suffer with nausea, vomiting and photophobia. Classically, patients sleep it off. It rarely presents with hemiplegia. Occasionally triggered by certain foods (caffeine or chocolate), drugs (OCP), stress and periods. |
| Tension headaches | Stress-induced headaches often lasting from 30 minutes to seven days. Often bilateral, of moderate intensity, and felt as a band (frontal/occipital) across the head that worsens throughout the day. It is not worsened by activity, nor associated with nausea and vomiting. An absence of neurological signs. |
| Cluster headaches | Common in 30–40-year-old males. These are recurrent attacks (five times or more) of unilateral pain (temporal/eye) lasting 15–180 minutes, which are often described as the most severe pain felt. It can awaken the patient from sleep, and it usually occurs same time every day (night). It can be triggered by alcohol. It is associated with rhinorrhoea, lacrimation, flushing, pupil constriction and a drooping eyelid. Attacks occur in clusters lasting several weeks, with periods of remission (one month or more). |
| Medication overuse | More common in women. Often affects people with migraines or tension headache who suffer from a chronic headache that is present for >14 days per month and that worsens with analgesia. This is likely if they have been taking analgesia for more than three months. Patients are at risk of this if they are taking triptans or opioids for >10 days per month, or are taking paracetamol, aspirin or NSAIDs for >15 days per month. |
| Temporal arteritis | Inflammation of the walls of medium/large arteries. Often found in the elderly (>50 years). Presents with a temporal headache, malaise, fever, scalp tenderness (combing hair) and jaw claudication (chewing). OE: temporal tenderness, decreased temporal pulse and cranial nerve (CN) palsy (III, IV and VI). Can cause sudden blindness. Associated with raised ESR (>50) and PMR. Confirmed with a biopsy. |

## Examination

» Vitals – BP, pulse and temperature.

» Rheumatology – Palpate the temporal arteries for tenderness if a >50-year-old has a headache and temporomandibular joint disorder (TMJ).

» MSK – Examine the neck, frontal, temporal, masseter, sternocleidomastoid and trapezius for muscle tenderness and stiffness (tension), as well as meningeal irritation.

» Neurological – Perform a focused CN examination (CNs 2,3,4 and 6) and a neurological assessment dependent on symptoms (Kernig's sign and Brudzinski's sign indicate meningitis; also assess their gait).

» Eyes – Inspect the pupils and examine the fundi (papilloedema); if indicated, press on the eyeballs (intraocular pressure [IOP]). Check for pupillary reflexes and asymmetry.

## Investigations

» Bloods – FBC, iron (anaemia), ESR and CRP.

» CT/MRI – Brain scan if suggestive of pathology.

» Specialist – Lumbar puncture (LP) (subarachnoid).

## Imaging in Headaches

» An urgent MRI scan (CT if contraindicated) is to be performed wthin two weeks for patients with progressive or sub-acute loss of central neurological function.

» An urgent referral (<48 hours) should be considered to assess for brain or central nervous system cancer in young people (<24 years) with newly abnormal cerebellar or other central neurological function.

## Management

*Treat the underlying cause*

*Conservative (general)*

✓ Diary – Offer the patient a headache diary to monitor their symptoms for at least eight weeks. Advise them to record the duration, frequency and severity of headaches, along with associated symptoms, any possible triggers and any medication that helps relieve it.

✓ General – Advise them to try to not miss meals, to avoid triggers (dietary and stress), to try to manage stress and to have good sleep.

*Migraine* – See Migraine section, page 239.

*Sinusitis* – See Trigeminal Neuralgia section, page 246.

### Tension headache

✓ Conservative – Reassure the patient, advise them to manage stress, offer CBT, advise them to use relaxation techniques, and recommend exercise. They should avoid missing or delaying meals, and maintaining poor sleep patterns. Recommend fluid hydration and advise them to avoid caffeine. Suggest that they consider acupuncture.

✓ Medical – Offer paracetamol or NSAIDs, and advise that they avoid opioids. If their headaches are frequent, consider amitriptyline (10–75mg) or nortriptyline if contraindicated.

### Cluster headache

✓ Conservative – Advise them to avoid triggers such as alcohol, fumes (solvents or oil products), smoking, some forms of exercise, and that they should maintain a good sleep routine (they should thus avoid caffeinated tea and coffee).

✓ Oxygen – Consider providing oxygen (100%) at home for 20 minutes.

✓ Medical – Consider sumatriptan by injection (6mg) or administered intranasally (10–20mg into one nostril and repeat two-hourly if it recurs, up to a maximum of 40mg/day). Try zolmitriptan intranasally (5mg into one nostril and repeat two-hourly if it recurs, up to a maximum of 10mg/day). Avoid NSAIDs, paracetamol, opioids and oral triptans during an acute cluster headache. For prophylaxis, consider verapamil 40mg bd (up to 960mg, with an ECG required to check for AV block), prednisolone (60–100mg od for two to five days, reduced by 10mg every three days), lithium, melatonin or sodium valproate.

### Medication overuse

✓ Attempt to stop the medication (triptans and simple non-opioids) completely for at least one month. Advise the patient that their headaches may worsen before improving (2–10 days). They may experience withdrawal symptoms for 7–21 days (nausea, vomiting, restlessness, anxiety or sleep problems). Consider topiramate for headache prophylaxis; opioids / benzodiazepines (BDZ) may require gradual reduction under specialist or inpatient care.

### Postcoital headache

✓ If it is the first presentation, consider excluding a subarachnoid haemorrhage. Recommend NSAIDs (indomethacin) or propranolol as prophylaxis. There is some evidence to support triptan use.

### Temporal arteritis

✓ Refer the patient urgently to hospital. Consider prednisolone 40–60mg daily if they are without visual symptoms (visual loss, double vision or field defects), or 60mg, as a one off (as it needs a same-day ophthalmology referral), if they are with visual symptoms, with a low dose of aspirin and PPI. May warrant bone biphosphonates if they are on long-term steroids.

### Acute Glaucoma – *See Red Eye section, page 319.*

## Referral

→ Cluster headaches – For the first episode, consider neuroimaging. If they are not responding to verapamil or require treatment during pregnancy, refer them for specialist advice.

→ Temporal arteritis – Refer them urgently to an ophthalmologist for a temporal biopsy.

→ Tension headache – Refer them to the headache clinic if they have a poor response to treatment.

## Safety Netting

» Review after two to four weeks if their symptoms are not improving.

---

*References*

British Association for the Study of Headache (2010). *Guidelines for all healthcare professionals in the diagnosis and management of migraine, tension-type headache, cluster headache, medication-overuse headache.* https://www.bash.org.uk/wp-content/uploads/2012/07/10102-BASH-Guidelines-update-2_v5-1-indd.pdf

National Institute for Health and Care Excellence (2012). *Headaches in over 12s: diagnosis and management.* https://www.nice.org.uk/guidance/cg150

National Institute for Health and Care Excellence (2015). *Suspected cancer: recognition and referral.* https://www.nice.org.uk/guidance/ng12

# Migraine

Migraine is a common condition that causes episodic headaches that can be debilitating at times. They are the commonest cause of headaches and often affect teenage women more than men. Most experience moderate to severe pain that can affect their ability to work or function. They often present with headaches that last from 4–72 hours, which are throbbing, unilateral and aggravated by performing daily physical activities. They can also cause nausea or vomiting, with sensitivity to light (photophobia) or sound (phonophobia). They may also occur with auras (visual, sensory or speech disturbance) that can last up to one hour. Migraines are usually classified into episodic (<15 days/month) and chronic (>15 days/month).

## Diagnosis of Migraine in Adults

| | |
|---|---|
| *Without aura* | More than five attacks with a headache lasting 4–72 hours. |
| *With one or more of* | Nausea/vomiting or photophobia/phonophobia. |
| *With two or more of* | Unilateral, moderate/severe pain, pulsating or aggravated by normal physical activity. |
| *With aura* | More than two attacks with visual aura (zigzag lines, flickering lights, spots, lines or loss of vision), sensory aura (pins and needles, or numbness) or dysphasic speech disturbance. Each symptom lasts less than an hour. |

## *History*

» Focused questions

› Ask when the headache started, how long it has been going on for and how long it lasts for.

› Ask about the site (unilateral).

› Ask about the onset (sudden or gradual).

› Ask about the character (throbbing) and how they would describe it.

› Ask about the frequency (how often they get the headaches).

› Ask if there are any exacerbating factors (food, lack of sleep, stress or anxiety).

› Ask if there are any relieving factors (medication).

› Ask about the severity (pain score).

» Associated history – Ask if they have any nausea and vomiting, limb weakness, dysphasia, vertigo, visual symptoms, photophobia or phonophobia.

» Prodromal symptoms – Ask if they have any prodromal symptoms (i.e. they get a warning before the headache starts), such as a change in mood, appetite, temperature, or sensitivity to light, sound or smell.

» Past history – Ask if they have previously had migraines.

» Family history – Ask if there is a family history of migraines.

» Drug history – Ask if they have taken COCP or HRT.

» Social history – Ask what their occupation is, if they are suffering from any stress, and if they smoke.

» Triggers

  › Diet (cheese, chocolate or caffeine)

  › Alcohol

  › Related to their menstrual period

  › A change in sleep pattern

  › Stress at home or work

  › Exercise

  › Certain smells or bright lights

## RED FLAGS

» A migraine with an aura while on COCP.

» Atypical features (weakness, diplopia, unilateral visual symptoms, ataxia or reduced level of consciousness).

» A worsening migraine.

## Examination

» Vitals – BP.

» Eyes – Inspect the pupils and examine the fundi.

» Neurological – If it is indicated clinically, perform a focused CN examination (e.g. CNs 2, 3, 4 and 6 if there are visual disturbances), and examine their gait (ataxia), sensation perceptions and the power of their limbs.

## Investigations

Investigations are not usually indicated unless there are red flags.

## Management

*Conservative*

✓ Diary – Advise the patient to keep a headache diary to monitor their symptoms for eight weeks.

✓ Occupation – Advise them to avoid work that can affect sleep patterns (shift work) or provide exposure to triggers.

✓ Avoid triggers – Advise them to have regular meals and avoid eating too quickly. They should avoid cheese, chocolate and red wine. They should avoid flickering lights, loud sounds and strong smells. They should stop smoking. Advise them to consider relaxation techniques to reduce stress or anxiety.

✓ Adjunct treatments – Advise them to consider massage and acupuncture (10 sessions over five to eight weeks) as adjunct treatments.

*Medical*

✓ Stop any COCP or HRT (increased risk of strokes). Avoid treating with opioids (overuse headache).

✓ For acute presentation

› Consider combined therapy or monotherapy (if preferred)

› Combined – Oral triptan and NSAID (ibuprofen), or triptan and paracetamol.

› Triptan – Consider sumatriptan (50 or 100mg) or other (zolmitriptan, naratriptan or frovatriptan). If there is excessive vomiting, consider subcutaneous (SC) or a nasal spray. Side effects are tingling sensations, heat, heaviness, pressure on body parts (vasoconstriction), flushing, dizziness, fatigue, and nausea and vomiting. It is contraindicated for patients with a previous stroke, TIA, PVD, severe HTN or cardiovascular disease.

› Monotherapy – Oral triptan, NSAID or paracetamol with an antiemetic (metoclopramide 10mg for five days or less, domperidone for seven days or less, or prochlorperazine 10mg).

✓ Preventative

› Consider if they have more than two attacks a month that cause disability lasting for three days or more, they are at risk of medication-overuse headaches, triptans are contraindicated/ineffective, or they have an uncommon migraine (prolonged aura or hemiplegic). Offer propranolol or topiramate as the first-line treatment.

› Propranolol – Start at 40mg bd titrating up to 240mg in divided doses, depending on symptom control. Consider if the patient suffers from anxiety or HTN. Contraindicated in asthma, COPD, PVD and uncontrolled HF.

› Topiramate – Start at 25mg od for one week, increasing in 25mg steps at weekly intervals to 50–100mg in two divided doses. There is an increased risk of foetal malformation and it reduces the effectiveness of the COCP.

✓ Other

› Acupuncture if the first-line treatment does not work after two months.

› Riboflavin (400mg od) can reduce the intensity and frequency.

› Amitriptyline daily can be considered if they have four or more migraine attacks a month.

› Gabapentin should not be used as prophylaxis.

### Pregnancy

✓ Recommend paracetamol. NSAIDs are to be avoided. Triptans are to be avoided, but if used, it should be sumatriptan.

### Menstrual migraine

✓ Offer NSAIDs (mefenamic acid) during their period (if they have dysmenorrhoea) or triptan (frovatriptan 2.5mg bd) starting two days before and until the end of the menstrual migraine. Consider COCP for migraines without an aura (take three cycles back to back, then have a seven-day hormone-free period). Offer progesterone (Cerazette) or Nexplanon implants.

## Referral

→ Refer the patient if there are any atypical features (weakness, diplopia, unilateral visual symptoms, ataxia or reduced level of consciousness) or it becomes chronic on maximal treatment.

→ Refer them urgently if the patient has severe, uncontrolled status migrainosus (>72 hours).

## Safety Netting

» Review after completing the first pack of triptans (six doses), if there is a change in symptoms (frequency or severity) or there is poor tolerance to medication.

### References

National Institute for Health and Care Excellence (2012). *Headaches in over 12s: diagnosis and management.* https://www.nice.org.uk/guidance/cg150

National Institute for Health and Care Excellence (2012). *Headaches: diagnosis and management of headaches in young people and adults.* https://www.nice.org.uk/guidance/cg150/update/CG150/documents/headaches-nice-guideline-for-consultation2

Scottish Intercollegiate Guidelines Network (2018). *SIGN 155 Pharmacological management of migraine.* https://www.sign.ac.uk/media/1091/sign155.pdf

# Temporal Arteritis

Temporal arteritis is an immune-mediated vasculitis that is characterised by granulomatous inflammation in the walls of medium- and large-sized arteries. It is more common in the elderly (>50 years), particularly women of northern European descent. There is a clear association with PMR (upper arm stiffness and tenderness, and pelvic girdle pain), where almost 40% of patients will have the underlying condition. It can present with the recent onset of temporally located pain, scalp tenderness, jaw claudication, and potentially transient or permanent visual symptoms, such as blindness (20%). There may be tenderness to the temporal artery and a reduced temporal artery pulse. Often, the ESR is raised, with the diagnosis confirmed by a temporal artery biopsy.

## Diagnosis Criteria of Temporal Arteritis

➤ Symptoms start when the patient is >50 years

➤ New onset or localised head pain

➤ Temporal tenderness and reduced pulse of the temporal artery

➤ ESR is raised (>50)

➤ Biopsy confirms vasculitis

## History

» Focused questions

  › Ask when the headache started, how long it has been going on for and how long the pain lasts for.

  › Ask about the site (temporal).

  › Ask about the severity (pain score).

  › Ask about the character (throbbing).

  › Ask if there are any triggers or alleviating factors (scalp tenderness when combing the hair, and for jaw claudication, ask if it is painful when chewing food or brushing their teeth).

  › Ask if there are any vision disturbances (amaurosis fugax).

  › Ask if there are any PMR symptoms (shoulder tenderness, joint stiffness in the neck or hips, which is worse in the morning).

» Associated history – Ask if they have experienced any fatigue, muscle pain, fever or night sweats, weight loss, oedema, or pins and needles (neurological symptoms).

» Past history – Ask if they have had PMR.

» Family history – Ask if there is a family history of temporal arteritis or PMR.

» Drug history – Ask if they have taken any steroids.

» Social history – Ask what their occupation is, and if they smoke or drink alcohol.

## RED FLAGS

Visual disturbances (diplopia or loss), stroke symptoms and neuropathy.

## Examination

- » Vitals – Temperature, BP and pulse.

- » Inspection – Inspect for ulceration of the scalp skin.

- » Palpation – Check for tenderness, prominence, thickening or pulsing of the temporal artery.

- » Auscultation – Listen for bruits over the carotids.

- » Ophthalmology – Check visual acuity, pupillary exam, visual fields and eye motility. Perform a fundoscopy, looking for ischaemic changes: optic disc pallor/oedema, small haemorrhages or cotton-wool spots.

- » If clinically indicated, also perform the following:

  - › MSK – Examine the shoulder for muscle tenderness or stiffness.

  - › Neurological – Perform a CN examination (CNs 3, 4 and 6). Check for power (hemiplegia) and sensation (mono/polyneuropathy).

## Differentials

- ➤ Migraine
- ➤ Tension headache
- ➤ Trigeminal neuralgia
- ➤ TIA

## Investigations

- » Bloods – ESR, CRP and Hb (anaemia).

- » Specialist – CT/MRI and a temporal artery biopsy to confirm the diagnosis.

## Management

*Medical*

- ✓ Steroids

  - › Visual symptoms – Start at 60mg prednisolone stat, for urgent same-day review by an ophthalmologist.

> ›   No visual symptoms – Start at 40–60mg prednisolone od. Initiate 75mg aspirin (with PPI).

✓   Aspirin – Start at 75mg od and PPI, unless contraindicated (PU).

✓   Ongoing recipe (Rx) – Continue high-dose steroids until the symptoms and ESR/CRP normalise (usually at four weeks), reduce the dose at two-weekly intervals by 10mg until 20mg od is reached. Reduce the dose in smaller quantities by 2.5mg every two to four weeks until it reaches 10mg od, then reduce by 1mg every one to two months.

✓   Monitor the inflammatory markers regularly. Check for DM, raised BP, weight gain, glaucoma and fractures (side effect of steroids).

✓   Bone protection – Offer bisphosphonate, calcium and vitamin D if they are >65 years, have a fragility fracture or have a DEXA scan T score (-1.5).

✓   Relapses – If there are new onset visual symptoms, increase the dose to 60mg od and refer them to ophthalmology urgently. Similarly, if they develop jaw claudication, increase to a higher dose and seek advice. If they develop headaches or PMR symptoms (stiffness/pain) but no jaw claudication, then increase the steroid dose to the previous higher regime and seek advice.

## Referral

→   Refer the patient urgently (within two weeks of starting steroids) to a specialist (follow the local pathway) if a diagnosis is suspected. This requires a temporal artery biopsy.

→   Refer them immediately to an ophthalmologist if there is a sudden loss of vision.

## Safety Netting

»   Advise the patient that if they develop visual symptoms, they should seek immediate advice. Review two days after initiating prednisolone, as the response is often rapid. If there is a poor response, review the diagnosis and refer them to a specialist.

*References*

Mackie, S.L., Dejaco, C., Appenzeller, S., Camellino, D., Duftner, C., Gonzalez-Chiappe, S., Mahr, A., Mukhtyar, C., Reynolds, G., de Souza, A.W.S., Brouwer, E., Bukhari, M., Buttgereit, F., Byrne, D., Cid, M.C., Cimmino, M., Direskeneli, H., Gilbert, K., Kermani, T.A. Dasgupta, B. (2020). *British Society for Rheumatology guidelines for the management of giant cell arteritis. Rheumatology,* 59(3), e1–e23. doi: https://doi.org/10.1093/rheumatology/kez672

Royal College of Physicians (2010). *Diagnosis and management of giant cell arteritis.* https://www.rcplondon.ac.uk/guidelines-policy/diagnosis-and-management-giant-cell-arteritis

# Trigeminal Neuralgia

Trigeminal neuralgia is a rare-but-chronic debilitating condition that gives rise to intense, excruciatingly painful, episodic facial pain. It is more common in women, and it increases with age. It is due to a neuropathy, or a disorder of one or more branches of the trigeminal nerve (fifth CN) causing unilateral discomfort (3% are bilateral). Episodes may occur infrequently up to >100 times a day, lasting anything from a few seconds to many minutes. Classically, there are trigger points and certain actions that bring on the attacks, such as shaving, eating or brushing teeth.

## Types of Trigeminal Neuralgia

➤ Classic (type 1) – Usually idiopathic with relapsing and remitting symptoms of piercing, stabbing pain

➤ Atypical (type 2) – Constant throbbing pain with a burning sensation or associated sensory loss

➤ Symptomatic – Symptoms are due to an underlying condition, such as MS

## *History*

» Focused questions

› Ask when the facial pain started and how long it has been going on for.

› Ask about the onset and the site (cheek, forehead or chin).

› Ask which side it is on (unilateral or both).

› Ask about the character (stabbing, burning or electric shock).

› Ask about the timing (if the episodes come and go, and how long they last for).

› Ask about the severity of the pain (pain score).

› Ask if there are any triggers (chewing, eating, talking, washing, shaving or brushing teeth).

» Associated history – Ask if they have any paraesthesia (tingling or burning in the face) or autonomic responses (eye redness or eye watering).

» Past history – Ask if they have had MS, HTN, a brain tumour or shingles.

» Family history – Ask if there is a family history of MS or similar headaches.

» Drug history – Ask if they have taken any analgesia.

» Social history – Ask what their occupation is, and if they smoke or drink alcohol.

## RED FLAGS

Optic symptoms (MS), herpetic lesions, <40 years old, deafness (mass) and optic neuritis.

## Diagnostic Criteria for Trigeminal Neuralgia

A.   Paroxysmal attacks of pain lasting from one second to two minutes, affecting one or more divisions of the trigeminal nerve, and fulfilling criteria B and C.

B.   The pain has at least one of the following characteristics:

›   Intense, sharp, superficial or stabbing.

›   Precipitated from trigger zones or by trigger factors.

C.   Attacks are stereotyped in the individual patient.

D.   There is no clinical evidence of a neurological deficit.

E.   The symptoms cannot be attributed to another disorder.

## Differential Diagnosis

| | |
|---|---|
| Trigeminal neuralgia | Affects more women than men. Usually found in patients >50 years old. Commonly involves short-lived, unilateral facial pain that comes and goes (which is lancinating in nature) after touching trigger spots, eating, talking or exposure to cold air. They are often pain free between attacks. May be associated with other conditions, such as MS. Often varying in frequency. Atypical features include pain between paroxysms. |
| Postherpetic neuralgia | Occurs following a shingles eruption. Burning, stabbing and gnawing pain that persists for three months once the rash has faded. |
| TMJ dysfunction | Causes pain and limited movement around the joint. May note crepitus. Multifactorial aetiology due to muscle overactivity, dental problems and underlying OA. |
| Temporal arteritis | Inflammation of the walls of medium/large arteries. Often in older (>50 years) women. Presents with temporal headache, malaise, fever, scalp tenderness (when combing hair) and jaw claudication (chewing). OE: temporal tenderness and decreased temporal pulse. Can cause sudden blindness (20%). Associated with a raised ESR (>50) and PMR. Confirmed with a biopsy. |

## Examination

»  Vitals – Temperature, BP and pulse.

»  Inspection – Inspect for vesicles of the scalp skin. Examine the face and oral cavity to exclude dental causes of pain.

»  Palpation – Check for tenderness, prominence, thickening or pulselessness of the temporal artery. Feel over the TMJ joint for crepitus. Request that the patient opens, closes and moves their jaw side to side, and look for restricted movements.

»  If clinically indicated, then do the following:

>  MSK – Examine their shoulder for muscle tenderness.

>  Neurological – Perform a CN examination, check for trigeminal sensory deficit and absent reflexes. Check for power (hemiplegia) and sensation (mono/polyneuropathy).

## Investigations

The following are done to exclude other causes:

»  Bloods – ESR (to exclude temporal arteritis) and CRP.

»  Specialist – MRI if a brain tumour / MS is suspected.

»  Advise them to see a dentist for a dental x-ray if appropriate.

## Management

### Conservative

✓  Lifestyle – Advise them to complete a pain diary and record their triggers.

✓  Reassure – Advise them it is not a life-threatening condition, but it can be debilitating.

✓  Support group – Advise them to contact the Trigeminal Neuralgia Association (TNA) UK for support.

✓  Depression – Treat and refer them if appropriate.

### Medical

✓  Carbamazepine – Start at 100mg bd and titrate according to their response. The usual maintenance dose is 200mg tds, but it can be increased to a maximum daily dose of 1,600mg.

>  When the pain is in remission, titrate down to the lowest possible dose.

>  Consider a modified release preparation for night pain.

>  Monitor FBC, LFTs and U&Es before commencement, and six monthly ongoing.

>  Advise them regarding the side effects, which include nausea, vomiting, dizziness, skin reactions and mood changes.

> › Warn them about the signs of agranulocytosis (fever, sore throat, rash, bruising and bleeding).

✓ Alternatives can be initiated by a specialist, such as oxcarbazepine.

## Referral

Refer the patient to neurology for any of the following:

→ Atypical presentations (a burning sensation between paroxysms, numbness or neurological signs).

→ If they are <40 years.

→ If you are unsure of the diagnosis; e.g. optic neuritis.

→ If there is a family history of MS.

→ If there is ophthalmic involvement.

→ If there are uncontrolled symptoms with carbamazepine.

## Safety Netting

» Review them in six to eight weeks for their response to treatment. If there is a poor response, review the diagnosis and refer them to a specialist.

*References*

National Institute for Health and Care Excellence (2013). *Neuropathic pain in adults: pharmacological management in non-specialist setting.* https://www.nice.org.uk/guidance/cg173

Zakrzewska, J.M. and Linskey, M.E. (2015). *Summaries of BMJ clinical evidence: trigeminal neuralgia.* https://new-learning.bmj.com/course/10052816

# Stroke and Transient Ischaemic Attacks

TIAs are focal transient neurological events that are caused by vascular ischaemia from microemboli or an occlusion affecting the brain, spinal cord or retina. By definition, the symptoms last <24 hours, with complete resolution and no ongoing deficit. Headaches are not typical features of a TIA. It is important to treat TIA, as there is a 20% risk of a stroke in the first month with the highest risk being in the first three days.

Strokes are sudden onset or rapidly developing focal or global neurological deficits that persist for >24 hours, and are usually ischaemic (85%) or haemorrhagic (15%) in origin. They often cause unilateral weakness, numbness, slurred speech, dysphagia and/or visual symptoms (hemianopia).

## Risk Factors

➤ Lifestyle – Smoking, drinking alcohol, poor diet or inactivity

➤ CVD – BP, AF, carotid artery disease, CCF, valvular disease, DM or high cholesterol

➤ Medical conditions – CKD, OSA, antiphospholipid syndrome or sickle cell disease

➤ Male

➤ >55 years

## History

» Focused questions

> Ask when the symptoms started, how long they have been going on for and if there has been any improvement.

> Ask about weakness and numbness (affecting arms, face or legs), and if so, which side.

> Ask if there is any dysphasia (slurred speech).

> Ask if there is any dysphagia.

> Ask about their vision and visual disturbances (loss of vision [when like a curtain falling down, it indicates amaurosis fugax] or diplopia).

> Ask about their coordination (feeling unbalanced).

> Also ask about confusion, severe headaches (subarachnoid haemorrhage [SAH]) or a change in sensation.

» Associated history – Ask if they have had any previous episodes, or any recent head injury or falls. Ask about their mood.

» Past history – Ask if they have had any IHD (TIA/CVA, AF, DM, HTN, CVD or high cholesterol), cardiac issues (endocarditis or valve disease) or haemorrhagic disorders.

» Family history – Ask if there is a family history of CVA, DM, HTN, CVD or high cholesterol.

» Drug history – Ask if they have taken NSAIDs, aspirin or warfarin.

» Social history – Ask what their occupation is; if they have any carers; if they smoke, drink alcohol or take recreational drugs; if they drive; and if they have any problems with looking after themselves.

## RED FLAGS

Symptoms prolonged for more than one week.

## Differential Diagnosis

| | |
|---|---|
| TIA/Stroke | TIA if <24 hours; stroke if >24 hours. Neurological symptoms of contralateral motor or sensory disturbance, ipsilateral visual signs or amaurosis fugax (a curtain coming down). Other symptoms include vertigo diplopia, dysarthria, weakness or numbness affecting the limbs. OE: hemiplegia, homonymous hemianopia, dysphagia, hemisensory loss, neglect and carotid bruit. |
| Hypoglycaemia | Often seen in diabetics on a new medication (gliclazide or insulin) or with concurrent illness. Presents with sweating, tremors, anxiety, confusion, slurred speech, a personality change or hunger. |
| Migraine | Unilateral throbbing headaches. May present with or without an aura (flashing lights or loss of vision), but patients invariably suffer with nausea, vomiting and photophobia. Classically, patients sleep it off. Can present with slowly evolving hemiplegia for several days in contrast to acute TIA symptoms. |
| Labyrinthitis | Inflammation of the vestibular nerve or labyrinth. Caused by recent onset URTI. Often affects 20–30-year-olds. Presents with severe acute-onset vertigo, nausea and vomiting, which recurs for several days. Head movements can precipitate symptoms. Hearing loss may be present. Nystagmus fast direction to the healthy side. Patients sway to the ipsilateral side during a Romberg test or on assessment of gait. |
| Subdural haemorrhage | Brain injury after trauma. More common in the elderly and alcoholics. Presents with fluctuating conscious levels with lucid periods, along with headaches, a personality change and confusion. Can present with ipsilateral hemiparesis (false localising sign). Can have a latent phase of weeks to months. |
| Bell's palsy | Facial paralysis caused by a latent viral infection. Presents with acute unilateral facial paralysis, often after a bout of postauricular pain. OE: the inability to frown or close an eye with loss of wrinkles of the brow. The corner of the mouth may drop and drool. |

## Examination

» Vitals – BP (for HTN), pulse (for AF) and BMI.

» Neurological (perform a focused exam based on the clinical findings)

› Gait – Hemiplegic gait or a broad-based gait (cerebellar).

› Inspection – Look for signs of CN 7 nerve palsy / drooping face.

› Tone – Check for hypertonia.

› Power – Check the power of their limbs compared to their normal side.

› Reflexes – Check the reflexes of their biceps, triceps, knee and ankle.

› Sensation – Check with a light touch compared to their normal side.

› CNs – Conduct a CN examination, including their visual fields.

› Cerebellar – Check for inattention, dysdiadokinesis and past-pointing.

» Cardiovascular – Listen for heart murmurs and carotid bruits. Check their peripheral pulses.

## Investigations

» Bloods – Hb (anaemia), HbA1c (DM), lipids and BM (hypoglycaemia).

› Other – Coagulation screen, thromophillia if haemorrhagic, ESR and U&Es.

» ECG – AF.

» Echo – Heart murmurs.

» Imaging – Urgent CT/MRI and carotid Doppler (endarterectomy).

## Management

### Suspected TIA

✓ Risk assessment – Assess the risk of stroke after a TIA using ABCD2:

› **A**ge >60 years (one point).

› **B**P >140/90 (one point).

› **C**linical – Unilateral weakness (two points) or speech disturbance without weakness (one point).

› **D**uration of symptoms – 10–60 minutes (one point) or >60 minutes (two points).

› **D**M (one point).

### Other risk – AF

✓ If they are high risk, refer them immediately to secondary care and do a CT scan within 24 hours. If they are low risk, refer them for review by a specialist and for a CT scan within one week.

> High risk – ABCD2 score of four or more, AF, more than one TIA in a week or a TIA while on an anticoagulant.

> Low risk – ABCD2 score of three or less, attended one week after symptoms or not in AF.

### Medical

✓ Antiplatelet – Offer aspirin 300mg stat (unless contraindicated). Give PPI if at risk of a GI bleed.

## Safety Netting

» If they are low risk and awaiting an appointment in the week, advise them to seek urgent medical attention if there is a further episode during that time or focal neurology persists.

» Follow up one month after the event.

# Suspected CVA

If CVA is suspected, refer them urgently (within one hour) to a specialist stroke unit. Check ABC (airways, breathing and circulation) and give oxygen if saturation is less than 95%. If diagnosed on the phone, advise them to call 999. Do not start antiplatelet treatment until they have had a brain scan to exclude haemorrhagic stroke. Patients should be NBM until reviewed using SALT.

### Secondary prevention for TIA/stroke

#### Conservative

✓ Offer smoking-cessation advice.

✓ Advise them to reduce their alcohol intake.

✓ Recommend a cardioprotective diet (low fat, low salt, and containing fruit and vegetables).

✓ Recommend that they take 30 minutes of aerobic exercise five times a week. Advise them to aim for a BMI <25.

✓ Advise them that, after a TIA they must not drive for one month. They must be free of further attacks for three months to be able to drive if there are multiple TIAs in a short period.

✓ Advise them that, after a stroke they cannot drive for one month. The DVLA must be notified if there is a residual deficit for more than one month (visual, cognitive or limb function).

✓ The patient may be entitled to sick pay, employment and support allowance (ESA), personal independence payment (PIP) or attendance allowance. Carers may be entitled to the carer's allowance. They should consider amended duties or altered hours if they are finding it difficult to carry out certain tasks or attend work. Advise them to attend the jobcentre/ Citizens Advice for advice around benefits, income support and disability.

✓ Perform a depression screen.

*Medical*

✓ Offer clopidogrel 75mg daily.

✓ Consider MR dipyridamole 200mg bd and aspirin 75mg if clopidogrel is not tolerated.

✓ If they have dyspepsia, give PPI.

✓ Ensure patients are on atorvastatin (80mg) for ischaemic CVA/TIA. Recheck lipids one to three months after initiating medication, and aim to reduce non-HDL by at least 40%. Consider ezetimibe if there is familial hypercholesterolaemia (avoid in instances of intracerebral haemorrhage).

✓ Offer the annual flu vaccination.

✓ Ensure optimal control of the following:

  › AF – Anticoagulation unless contraindicated.

  › DM.

  › HTN – Systolic <130.

  › Stop any COC, and use only progestogen-only pills (POP) / barrier methods.

  › Stop HRT.

## QOF

» Maintain a register of patients with TIA/CVA. Refer new patients within three months of presenting. Monitor BP (<150/90) yearly and offer the flu vaccination yearly. Ensure those without haemorrhagic stroke are on antiplatelet treatment.

## Long-term Stroke Complications

» Mobility – Hemiparesis/hemiplegia, ataxia, falls and spasticity.

» Sensory – Reduced sensation to temperature, touch and pain.

» Swallowing – Dysphagia, oral ulceration, dehydration and increased risk of aspiration.

» Vision – Blurred vision, double vision and reduced acuity.

» Continence – CKD, OSA, antiphospholipid syndrome and sickle cell disease.

» Pain – Neuritic pain and MSK pain due to immobility.

» Cognitive/communication – Poor concentration, poor attention, the inability to plan or carry out tasks, reduced cognition, dysphasia and dysarthria.

» Emotional – Depression, anxiety and anger.

## Referral

→ Physiotherapy – To assess mobility, and to treat weakness or poor balance.

→ OT – To assess, and to offer equipment and any adaptations.

→ SALT – To assess and treat communication or swallowing difficulties.

→ Dietician – To offer advice about a healthy diet.

→ Continence adviser – To assess and manage urinary or faecal incontinence.

→ CBT – Consider referring them for psychological intervention if they are depressed or anxious.

### References

National Institute for Health and Care Excellence (2019). *Stroke and transient attack in over 16s: diagnosis and initial management.* https://www.nice.org.uk/guidance/ng128

Scottish Intercollegiate Guidelines Network (2017). *SIGN 149 Risk estimation and the prevention of cardiovascular disease.* https://www.sign.ac.uk/assets/sign149.pdf

Tyrrell, P., Swain, S. and Rudd, A. (2010). *Diagnosis and initial management of transient ischaemic attack. Clinical Medical Journal, April 2010.* doi: https://doi.org/10.7861/clinmedicine.10-2-164

# Epilepsy

Epilepsy is a chronic brain disorder that causes seizures. Almost 500,000 people in the UK have been diagnosed with epilepsy, making it the second most common neurological condition in the UK. However, in most cases (66%), we do not know the cause; some people suffer from epilepsy due to a head injury, brain cancer, a stroke, or as a result of alcohol or drug abuse. It is diagnosed when a person has had at least two seizures occurring >24 hours apart and other causes are excluded. Seizures may be generalised or partial, with generalised ones giving rise to tonic-clonic, absence or myoclonic seizures. Status epilepticus is defined as a continuous seizure lasting for >30 minutes or recurrent seizures that occur without the patient regaining consciousness for a similar period.

## History

» Focused questions

  › Seizure – Ask what happened, when it occurred and how it started.

  › Before – Ask what they were doing before, and if they were feeling faint, suffering from stress or were exposed to flashing lights. Ask if there was any aura (warning symptoms before the fit, such as an odd taste in the mouth, a smell or déjà vu).

  › During – Ask if there were any witnesses. Ask about the fit itself; did their whole body shake (clonic), go firm (tonic) or cause muscle twitching (myoclonic); and did they have a blank stare (absence), jerks, or odd sensations in their arm(s) or leg(s) (partial). Ask about their symptoms (tongue biting, passing urine or limb weakness).

  › After – Ask if they were feeling drowsy or had a headache afterwards, if there was a postictal phase, and if they had any amnesia.

» Associated history – Ask if there have been any previous episodes; if so, when exactly; and if there has been any LOC, a head injury or a recent fall (subdural or haemorrhagic).

» Past history – Ask if they have had CVA, a brain tumour, epilepsy, tuberous sclerosis, neurofibromatosis, febrile seizures as a child, or a brain trauma or injury.

» Family history – Ask if there is a family history of epilepsy.

» Social history – Ask what their occupation is (bus or train driver, or a DJ); what support they have at home; if they smoke, drink alcohol or take recreational drugs; and if they drive.

## RED FLAGS

Sudden onset, recent head injury, focal neurology and a prolonged fit (>30 minutes).

## Differentials

➤ Brain tumour

➤ Meningitis

➤ Cardiac arrhythmia

➤ Panic attacks

## Examination

» Vitals – BP, pulse, Glasgow coma scale (GCS) and temperature.

» Inspection – Look at their general appearance (anxious or pale).

» Neurological – Perform a focused examination based on the clinical findings. The patient should be asymptomatic after the fit. Exclude features of a brain tumour using the following:

  › Tone – Check for hypertonia.

  › Power – Check the power of the limbs.

  › Reflexes – Consider the reflexes in the biceps, triceps, supinator, knee or ankle.

  › CNs – Conduce a CN examination (e.g. nystagmus, visual fields, and CNs 3, 4 and 7).

  › Cerebellar – Check for intentional tremors, dysdiadokinesis and past-pointing.

  › Fundoscopy – Perform this to exclude raised intracranial pressure.

## Investigations

» Bloods – Hb, ESR, HbA1c, U&Es, LFTs and calcium. Check epilepsy drug levels if there is poor compliance.

» Cardiac – ECG (arrhythmia, WPW, Long QT syndrome and bradycardia) and a 24-hour ECG if the ECG is normal.

» Specialist – CT/MRI (brain tumour) and electroencephalogram (EEG).

## Management

*Conservative*

✓ Emergency – Prevent injury by cushioning the head. Remove any harmful or sharp objects from their surroundings. When they recover, protect the airway and place them in a recovery position. Call 999 if the fit lasts for more than five minutes.

✓ Drugs – Buccal midazolam / PR diazepam.

✓ Safety netting

> Occupation – Advise them to avoid working at heights or with heavy machinery.

> Driving – Advise them to stop driving, and to inform their car insurance company and the DVLA. They must not drive for one year or for three years if they have fits during their sleep. If medication is being withdrawn, there should be no driving during the withdrawal period and for six months after. They should avoid cycling. If the patient is not keen to stop driving, tell them that you may have to inform the DVLA.

> Others – Advise them to avoid bathing a baby alone. It is better for them to have a shower; however, if they do use a bath, they should keep the bathroom door open. They should avoid swimming alone.

*Medical*

✓ A referral to a specialist should be initiated after the second seizure. Conduct a trial of one agent, but add a second drug if the seizures continue.

✓ Advise them that they are entitled to free prescriptions.

✓ Medication – Do FBC if there are mouth ulcers, bruising or an infection (sore throat). Check LFTs and U&E.

> Sodium valproate – Side effects are pancreatitis, liver toxicity, blood dyscrasias, tremors and weight gain. They must be on a pregnancy-prevention programme, including contraception.

> Carbamazepine – Side effects are blood dyscrasias, liver toxicity, a rash, drowsiness and fluid retention.

> Phenytoin – Side effects are blood dyscrasias, drowsiness, a rash, gum hyperplasia and cerebellar symptoms.

> Withdrawal – If they are fit-free for two to three years, consider withdrawing the medication.

> Osteoporosis – Advise them that the long-term use of carbamazepine, phenytoin and valproate can increase the risk of osteoporosis and bone fractures.

✓ COCP – Medication can affect the efficacy of the COCP (except sodium valproate). Barrier methods should be considered. Consider ethinylestradiol monophasic 50mcg (up to 100mcg if breakthrough bleeding), oestrogen or tricycling (taking three packs with no breaks).

✓ Before conception – These drugs are teratogenic. Carbamazepine has the least risk. Try to rationalise the patient to a single agent if they are on polypharmacy. They should take extra folic acid (5mg) until reaching 12 weeks of pregnancy.

✓ Pregnancy – Refer them early for shared care (obstetrician and neurologist). There is an increased risk of miscarriage if they are fitting, and the teratogenicity risk is increased without treatment. Give Vitamin K 20mg tablets after 36 weeks gestation.

✓ Breastfeeding – It is safe to breastfeed on these medications.

## Referral

→ Refer them urgently to a neurologist on the first seizure to exclude any underlying pathology (tumour) and to get advice.

---

*References*

National Institute for Health and Care Excellence (2012). *Epilepsy: diagnosis and management.* https://www. nice.org.uk/guidance/cg137

# Multiple Sclerosis

MS is an immune-mediated disease affecting the insulating covers of the central nervous system (brain and spinal cord). Its trigger is not clear, but the body's immune system is directed against itself, attacking the white matter (demyelination), and continued destruction leads to the disruption of the conduction pathways of the nerves, causing signs and symptoms in the areas it affects. It is usually suspected when a person suffers from distinct neurological symptoms that are disseminated in space and time. It largely affects young people (women are two to three times more likely to have this than men) from 20–40 years old, and it presents in four distinct patterns.

## Types of MS

> Relapsing/remitting – The symptoms come and go with periods of remission interspersed with relapses. This is the most common.

> Primary progressive – The symptoms begin and gradually worsen over time.

> Secondary progressive – The patient is initially relapsing/remitting, but goes on to have fewer remissive periods, and more, longer relapses.

> Benign – The symptoms present less frequently and cause no permanent damage.

## *History*

» Start by asking the patient what symptoms they have been experiencing and what has been troubling them.

» Focused questions

  › Ask about eye symptoms (which eye is affected, or both), optic neuritis (pain in the eye that is worse with movement), visual loss (loss of the colour red, blurred vision, losing sight in one eye, or losing a small part of vision [scotoma]) and diplopia (double vision).

  › Sensory – Ask if they have had any odd sensations in the body, if it spreads slowly anywhere else, or if there has been any numbness, pain (burning or shooting), or Lhermitte's sign (shooting pain down the spine when bending the neck forwards).

  › Motor – Ask if there are any symptoms affecting the muscles. Ask about tremors (hands, arms, face or legs), muscle spasms, ataxia (clumsy movements) and any issues with walking.

  › Bowel/bladder – Ask if they are passing urine more often or experiencing leaking, or if they have any constipation or bad diarrhoea.

  › Ask about slurred speech and erectile dysfunction.

  › Timing – Ask about the onset, how long the symptoms have gone on for and if there was a period when there were no symptoms.

» Associated history – Ask if they have any cognition issues (memory or concentration), fatigue, dizziness or low mood, and how they are managing everyday activities (cooking, feeding themselves, washing, dressing and mobility).

» Past history – Ask if they have had any autoimmune disorders (thyroid, type 1 DM or IBD), low vitamin D levels or a slipped disc.

» Drug history – Ask if they have taken TCAs or infliximab for rheumatoid arthritis (RA).

» Family history – Ask if there is a family history of MS.

» Social history – Ask what their diet (vitamin B12) is like, what their occupation is, if they smoke or drink alcohol, and if they drive.

## Differential Diagnosis

| MS | Affects women three times more than men. Usually young (20–40 years). Neurological symptoms disseminated in time and space. Common symptoms include visual (optic neuritis, which is often unilateral; hemianopia; diplopia; and nystagmus), muscle spasticity (legs), neuropathic pain, paraesthesia (trigeminal neuralgia), cerebellar damage (ataxia, dysarthria and nystagmus), and bladder (incontinence) and bowel dysfunction (faecal incontinence, though this is rare). |
|---|---|
| Transverse myelitis | A rare disorder that comes on acutely and affects the lower spine. Believed to be caused by a viral illness that instigates progressive sensory loss and weakness. Patients present with sharp, shooting pain, and numbness and tingling over the legs or abdomen. May also be associated with limb weakness (reduced tone and lower motor-neurone signs) and urinary incontinence, along with reduced sensory level (typically mid-thoracic). |

## Examination

» Vitals – BP, pulse and BMI.

» Inspection – Look at their general appearance and identify any tremors.

» Eyes – Inspect the pupils; check for nystagmus, diplopia, scotoma and colour plates (red colour); and assess visual acuity.

> Fundoscopy – Examine the fundi (pale discs).

» Neurological – Perform a focused examination based on the clinical findings:

> Tone – Check for hypertonia.

> Power – Check the power of the limbs compared to the normal side.

> Reflexes – Consider increased reflexes in the biceps, triceps, supinator, knee or ankle.

> › Sensory – Check for reduced sensation (pain, light touch and vibration) in affected areas.

> › CNs – Conduct a CN examination (e.g. CNs 3, 4 and 6).

## Investigations

» Bloods – Hb (anaemia), ESR (sarcoid), vitamin B12, HbA1c, U&Es (dehydration), TFT, HIV, calcium and LFTs.

» Specialist – MRI (sclerotic lesion in brain or spine) and CT (to exclude other causes).

## Management

*Conservative*

✓ Driving – Advise them that they must inform the DVLA, but there are usually no restrictions. They should consider driving adaptations (hand controls, so no pedals, and wheelchair access).

✓ Support group – Suggest that they join the Multiple Sclerosis Society (www.mssociety.org.uk) or the MS Trust (www.mstrust.org.uk).

✓ Lifestyle

> › Exercise – Advise them that regular exercise – such as jogging, swimming and cycling – helps to reduce stress and release tension. It also helps to build muscle strength, tone and balance.

> › Smoking – Advise the patient to stop smoking.

> › Reduce stress – Recommend relaxation techniques, and advise that they should try to reduce stress.

> › Keep cool – Advise them that MS symptoms are worse when they are feeling hot. They should use air conditioning, swimming and cold water to cool down.

> › Rest – Advise them to ensure they have plenty of rest when fatigued.

> › Diet – Advise them to eat a healthy, balanced diet. They should eat foods that have a high vitamin D content (dairy, fish and mushrooms).

*Medical*

✓ Refer them to a neurologist to confirm the diagnosis. A specialist would consider IV/oral methylprednisolone in a relapse and interferon beta as disease-modifying therapy (to reduce the frequency of relapses).

✓ Consider referring them to physiotherapy, a continence nurse, OT, SALT and for CBT.

✓ Spasticity – Consider baclofen (side effects are drowsiness and weakness) or gabapentin. Refer them to physiotherapy.

✓ Incontinence – Offer oxybutynin. If they have nocturia, consider desmopressin.

✓     Erectile dysfunction – Offer sildenafil 25–100mg PRN.

✓     Pain – Simple analgesia (paracetamol or codeine) or NSAIDs can be prescribed as topical creams or oral medications. Add PPI if prescribing NSAIDs to the elderly. For neuropathic pain, treat this with gabapentin, carbamazepine or amitriptyline.

✓     Emotional lability – Consider amitriptyline and refer them for CBT.

✓     Vitamin D – Some studies advise giving vitamin D supplements to reduce relapse rates.

✓     Immunisation – Offer an annual flu vaccination.

## Relapse

If a patient has a relapse, exclude infection (UTI/URTI) before considering treatment with a steroid (oral methylprednisolone 0.5g od for five days) if appropriate. This may help reduce the severity and duration of relapse. Consider admission.

## Acute Symptoms

»     Optic neuritis – Refer them to an ophthalmologist for corticosteroids as an emergency.

»     Transverse myelitis – Refer them to a neurologist to consider corticosteroids as an emergency.

---

*References*

National Institute for Health and Care Excellence (2003). *Multiple sclerosis: management of multiple sclerosis in primary and secondary care.* https://www.nice.org.uk/guidance/cg8

# Loss of Consciousness

Transient LOC or a blackout episode refers to a rapid onset LOC with complete recovery. Most commonly it is due to low cerebral oxygenation as a result of the impairment of cerebral perfusion because of postural hypotension, cardiac causes or hypoglycaemia. In such cases, the symptoms are acute and short lived, and the patients will eventually return to full consciousness without any loss of function. Other causes of LOC include epilepsy or, less commonly, a TIA. These may recur if the patient is not diagnosed or managed correctly.

## Causes of LOC

➤ Syncope – Diagnosis of exclusion: vasovagal, situational, carotid sinus, orthostatic or neurogenic

➤ Metabolic – Hypoglycaemia (common), hypocapnia (hyperventilation) or hypoxia

➤ Epileptic – Primary/secondary seizures or temporal lobe epilepsy (memory lost).

➤ Psychiatric – Panic attacks (young, no injury and coordinated movements during attack)

➤ Cardiac – Bradycardia, tachycardia or structural disease

➤ Other – Narcolepsy, Lewy body dementia or transient global amnesia

## History

» Focused questions

› LOC – Clarify what they mean by LOC or a blackout. Ask when it happened.

**Before**

- Ask if there was there any warning or any odd taste in the mouth.

- Posture – Ask if they had been lying down then suddenly stood up, or if they had been standing for a long period of time before it occurred.

- Circumstances – Ask what they were doing and before they felt faint (passing urine, defecating, coughing or exercising). Ask if they were suffering any stress or pain, were looking at flashing lights, had a tight collar or were shaving (carotid sinus).

- Prodromal – Ask if there was any chest pain or palpitations (arrhythmia), if they were feeling sweaty and hot (panic or hypoglycaemia), or their speech was slurring (TIA).

**During**

- If the patient is unsure what happened, then try to obtain a witness statement.

- Ask about the duration of the unconsciousness.

- Ask about the onset, and if it came on slowly or suddenly (cardiac).

- Ask if there was any fitting.

- Ask if their eyes were open (seizure or syncope) or closed (pseudoseizure or psychogenic).

- Ask if they bit their tongue, passed urine, their face went pale, or there was any weakness of limbs.

### After

- Ask how they felt after recovering (confused or had a headache), if they recovered quickly (syncope), and how long it took to come around.

- Amnesia – Ask if they are able to remember everything that happened.

» Associated history

  › Ask if there have been any previous episodes; if it has happened before, ask when exactly it happened and how many times.

  › Ask if they have had a head injury or fall recently (subdural or haemorrhagic).

» Past history – Ask if they have had any AF, DM, HTN, CVD, epilepsy, panic attacks or anxiety.

» Drug history – Ask if they have taken any antihypertensives, diuretics, nitrates (postural hypotension or hypoglycaemia) or antiarrhythmics.

» Family history – Ask if there is a family history of epilepsy or early death.

» Social history – Ask what their occupation is, how things are at home, if they smoke or drink alcohol, if they drive, and what their diet is like.

## RED FLAGS

Sudden onset, recent head injury, exercise-induced LOC and focal neurology.

## Differential Diagnosis

| Vasovagal syncope | A simple faint. Precipitated by prolonged standing, stress, emotion, pain, strenuous exercise, micturition, coughing, dehydration, a warm environment or a heavy meal and alcohol. Often experiences prodromal symptoms; e.g. sweating or feeling hot prior to the LOC. During the episode, they can appear pale and clammy, and they may experience a headache and nausea after an attack. |
|---|---|

| | |
|---|---|
| Carotid sinus syncope | History of cardiac condition (heart murmur or hypertrophic obstructive cardiomyopathy [HOCM]). Can have a family history of sudden death. Chest pain or palpitations may precede the syncope. |
| Cardiac syncope | History of cardiac condition (heart murmur or HOCM). Can have a family history of sudden death. Chest pain or palpitations may precede the syncope. |
| Generalised seizures | Requires more than one seizure for a diagnosis of epilepsy. The episodes can last for anything from seconds to minutes. May present with clonic, myoclonic, tonic or tonic-clonic seizures or absences. Can get warning auras (smell, tastes, déjà vu or jamais vu). Patients may bite their tongue, develop pallor or turn their head to one side during the LOC, they may sweat before the episode, and be confused post event. |
| Postural hypotension | Dizziness or blackouts due to impaired cerebral perfusion, precipitated by a postural change, prolonged standing (in hot places) and improved by lying flat. Often caused by medication (antihypertensives or diuretics), a big meal, dehydration, anaemia or autonomic-affecting conditions (PD). OE: drop in BP >20/10 within three minutes of standing. |
| TIA/stroke | Neurological symptoms of contralateral motor or sensory disturbance, ipsilateral visual signs, amaurosis fugax (a curtain coming down in the vision), vertigo, diplopia or dysarthria. |
| Hypoglycaemia | Rare in non-diabetics (except Addison's disease, severe liver disease and alcohol excess), often seen in diabetics on new medication (gliclazide or insulin) or those with concurrent illness. Presents with sweating, tremors, anxiety, confusion, slurred speech, personality change or hunger. |
| Panic attack | Unpredictable, recurrent panic attacks with severe anxiety, palpitations, tremors, SOB, chest pain or paraesthesia. Often lasts 5–10 minutes, but can last for a few hours. |

## Examination

» Vitals – Lying and standing BP (hypotension), pulse (AF and bradycardia), and BMI.

» Inspection – Look at their general appearance (anxious or pale).

» Neurological

**Perform a focused examination based on the clinical findings:**

› Tone – Check for hypertonia.

› Power – Check the power of the limbs compared to the normal side.

› Reflexes – Consider the reflexes in the biceps, triceps, supinator, knee or ankle.

> › CNs – Conduct a CN examination (e.g. visual fields, and CNs 5 and 7).

» Cardiovascular – Listen for heart murmurs (AS).

## Investigations

» Bloods – Hb (anaemia), glucose (DM), U&Es (dehydration) and LFTs (liver damage).

» CXR – Enlarged heart.

» Cardiac – ECG (arrhythmia, WPW, Long QT, bradycardia or ST-T abnormality), 24-hour ECG if the ECG is normal and cardiac sounding, and an echo (heart murmurs or HOCM).

» Specialist – CT/MRI (subdural or subarachnoid), carotid Doppler (TIA), tilt-table, carotid sinus massage and EEG (epilepsy).

## Management

*Treat the underlying cause*

### Driving

✓ Vasovagal – No restrictions and the DVLA does not need to be informed.

✓ Cardiac cause – Driving licence is revoked for six months if there is no cause, or for one month if there is an identifiable cause.

✓ Seizure markers – If there is a strong suspicion of epilepsy (but not diagnosed), they must not drive for six months; if they have a past medical history of this, they must not drive for 12 months.

✓ No markers – If there has been LOC, but it has been investigated and no abnormality was detected, the driving licence is revoked for six months.

### Postural hypotension

#### Lifestyle

✓ Fluids – Advise them to drink plenty of fluids and reduce their alcohol intake. They should avoid drinking caffeine at night.

✓ Diet – Advise them to not miss meals. They should add salt to their meals (low BP), and eat small amounts with little carbohydrate.

#### Prevention

✓ Advise them to sit up for a short period before standing.

✓ Standing – Advise them to avoid standing for long periods. They should not go out if it is very hot. They should get up slowly from sitting.

✓ Bending – Advise them to squat down, bending their knees not their waist, to pick things up.

✓ Bed – Advise them to raise the head of their bed by 15cm with books or bricks.

✓ Stockings – Advise them to wear leg-compression stockings to stop the pooling of blood in the legs.

✓ Polypharmacy – Rationalise their medications if they are on multiple medications for BP.

✓ Medications – Consider fludrocortisone to increase salt and water retention (specialist initiated).

✓ Referral – Refer them to an endocrinologist if you suspect autonomic neuropathy.

## Carotid sinus syncope

✓ If this is suspected, refer them for a carotid sinus massage (five seconds in the supine and upright position). They may be symptomatic / show bradycardia during the massage. If there are more than two syncope episodes, consider a dual-chamber pacemaker.

## Cardiac

✓ Bradycardia – Consider changing medications if they are on b-blockers.

✓ AF – Find the cause if relevant (hyperthyroidism, pneumonia, HF or alcohol). Consider a b-blocker or antiarrhythmic drug (specialist initiated).

✓ Referral – Refer the patients for a cardiovascular assessment, except if they have had an uncomplicated faint, situational syncope, orthostatic hypotension or history suggestive of epilepsy. Also refer them if there has been LOC with an abnormal ECG or HF, LOC with exertion, a family history of sudden death <40 years, unexplained SOB, a heart murmur, or LOC in someone of >65 years without prodromal symptoms.

## Epilepsy

✓ Referral – Refer them urgently to a neurologist if it is their first seizure with LOC (bitten tongue, prolonged limb jerking, confusion after event and déjà vu / jamais vu).

*Panic Attacks* – *See Shortness of Breath section, page 100*

*TIA* – *See Stroke and Transient Ischaemic Attack section, page 250.*

### References

National Institute for Health and Care Excellence (2010). *Transient loss of consciousness: management in adults and young people.* http://guidance.nice.org.uk/CG109/NICEGuidance/pdf/English

National Institute for Health and Care Excellence (2013). *Postural hypotension in adults: fludrocortisone.* https://www.nice.org.uk/advice/esuom20/chapter/intervention-and-alternatives

# Bell's Palsy

Bell's palsy is an acute, unilateral facial nerve (CN 7) weakness or paralysis of rapid onset (<72 hours) with an unknown cause. Herpes simplex virus (HSV), varicella zoster virus (VZV) and autoimmune disorders may contribute to the development of it, but their significance remains unclear.

## Risk Factors

➤   Ages 15–45 (median is 40)

➤   Previous stroke

➤   Brain tumour

## *History*

»   A diagnosis of Bell's palsy can be made when no other medical condition is found to be causing facial weakness or paralysis.

»   Ask about the following symptoms:

›   Rapid onset (<72 hours).

›   Facial muscle weakness (almost always unilateral) involving the upper and lower parts of the face. This causes a reduction in movement on the affected side, often with the drooping of the eyebrow and corner of the mouth, and the loss of the nasolabial fold.

›   Pain in the ear and postauricular region on the affected side.

›   Difficulty chewing, dry mouth and changes in taste.

›   Incomplete eye closure, dry eye, eye pain or excessive tearing.

›   Numbness or tingling of the cheek and/or mouth.

›   Speech articulation problems or drooling.

›   Hyperacusis.

›   A recent rash (a vesicular rash over the ear or pharynx indicates Ramsay Hunt syndrome).

›   A recent viral infection.

## Differential Diagnosis

| Stroke | The forehead is spared, but with extremities often affected. |
|---|---|
| Brain tumour | Mental state changes, with gradual onset. |
| MS | *See Multiple Sclerosis section, page 260.* |

## Examination

» Take a focused examination of the scalp, ears, mastoid region, parotid glands, eyes and CNs.

› There is ipsilateral paralysis of the upper and lower facial muscles (lower motor-neurone lesion).

› The eyebrow droops, and the wrinkles of the brow are smoothed out; frowning and raising the eyebrows are impossible (whereas, in a stroke, the forehead is not affected).

› The eye cannot be closed. When asked to close the eyes and show the teeth, the eyeball rotates upwards and outwards (Bell's phenomenon)

› The eye may appear to tear excessively due to loss of lid control.

› The patient is unable to blow out their cheeks. The lips cannot be pursed, and whistling is impossible. The effects tend to be more pronounced in the elderly.

› The sensory component of the corneal reflex is intact (trigeminal nerve), but the motor component is lost.

› An ipsilateral rash or vesicles in the ear.

› Exclude parotid gland tumours.

## Investigations

» Routine tests and diagnostic imaging are not required for new onset Bell's palsy.

## Management

*Conservative*

✓ Pure Bell's palsy should resolve within two weeks.

✓ Advise the patient to keep the affected eye lubricated by using lubricating eye drops during the day and ointment at night.

✓ If the ability to close the eye at night is impaired, the eye should be taped closed at bedtime, using microporous tape, or an eye patch should be used.

*Medical*

✓ For patients presenting within 72 hours of the onset of symptoms, consider Prednisolone as follows:

› 50mg daily for 10 days; or

› 60mg daily for five days, followed by a daily reduction in dose of 10mg (for a total treatment time of 10 days) if a reducing dose is preferred.

## Referral

→ Refer the patient urgently under certain circumstances, including the following:

> A worsening of existing neurologic findings or new neurologic findings.

> Features suggestive of an upper motor neuron cause.

> Features suggestive of cancer.

> A systemic or severe local infection.

> Trauma.

→ Refer them to a facial-nerve specialist if there is doubt about the diagnosis or there is one of the following:

> No improvement after three weeks of treatment.

> An incomplete recovery three months after the initial onset of symptoms.

> Any atypical features.

→ Refer them to an ophthalmologist if the patient has eye symptoms (e.g. pain, irritation or an itch).

---

*References*

National Institute for Health and Care Excellence (2019). *Bell's palsy: scenario: management of Bell's palsy.* https://cks.nice.org.uk/topics/bells-palsy/management/management/

# Parkinson's Disease

PD is a progressive neurodegenerative disorder caused by a reduction in dopamine. This is due to the degeneration of the dopamine pathways in the substantia nigra. The cause of this is idiopathic. Specific drugs – such as tranquilisers and antiemetics such as metoclopramide – can cause either a reduction in the storage of dopamine or block receptors, giving rise to similar symptoms.

## Risk Factors

- More common in men
- Old age (peaks at 60–70 years)
- It has been reported that there is an increased risk with pesticide use

## *History*

- » Focused questions
    - › Ask about the initial symptoms experienced, including the impairment of dexterity, the dragging of one foot, a blank expression on the face, infrequent blinking, drooling (due to impaired swallowing) and a quiet voice.
    - › Ask if any other symptoms have been experienced, including a resting tremor (may initially only be apparent unilaterally on one limb before becoming generalised), rigidity and bradykinesia.
    - › Ask if any late symptoms have been experienced, including having difficulty standing from a sitting position, and gait-related symptoms such as shuffling steps, difficulty turning around and difficulty stopping.

## Differentials

- Gait apraxia caused by small vessel cerebrovascular disease
- Benign essential tremor
- Huntington's disease
- Wilson's disease
- Lewy body dementia
- Psychogenic tremor

# Examination

» Inspection

> Look for a tremor. If there is no clear tremor on observation, it can be induced by asking the patient to concentrate on a task.

> Check for a rigidity increase in resistance to passive movement (cogwheel rigidity).

> Check for bradykinesia, which is most noticeable when observing the arm swing on walking.

# Investigation

» A clinical diagnosis is usually required, based on the Parkinson's Disease Society Brain Bank criteria for diagnosis, as follows:

| Step 1: Diagnosis | Bradykinesia and one of the following:<br><br>> Muscular rigidity<br>> 4–6Hz resting tremor<br>> Postural instability not caused by primary, visual, vestibular, cerebella or proprioceptive dysfunction |
|---|---|
| Step 2:<br>Exclusion criteria | • History of repeated stroke<br>• History of repeated head injury<br>• History of definite encephalitis<br>• Oculogyric crises<br>• Neuroleptic treatment at onset of symptoms<br>• More than one affected relative<br>• Sustained remission<br>• Strictly unilateral features after three years<br>• Supranuclear gaze palsy<br>• Cerebella signs<br>• Early severe autonomic involvement<br>• Early severe dementia with disturbances of memory, language and praxis<br>• Babinski's sign<br>• Presence of a cerebral tumour or communicating hydrocephalus<br>• Negative response to large doses of levodopa (L-dopa) |

| Step 3: Definitive diagnosis | Three or more of the following are required for a definitive diagnosis of PD: |
|---|---|
| | › Unilateral onset<br>› Rest tremor present<br>› Progressive disorder<br>› Persisting asymmetry affecting the side of onset most<br>› An excellent response to L-dopa<br>› Severe L-dopa-induced chorea<br>› An L-dopa response for five years or more<br>› A clinical course of 10 years or more<br>› Hyposmia<br>› Visual hallucinations |

» CT or MRI brain scan may be done to exclude other causes for presentation in one of the following:

› A patient who has not responded to L-dopa (at least 600mg/day) after 12 weeks.

› A patient with atypical symptoms.

## Management

*Conservative*

✓ After diagnosis, do the following:

› Arrange a nursing assessment.

› Arrange a health and social care assessment.

› Refer them to physiotherapy.

› Refer them to speech therapy.

› Advise them to inform the DVLA.

› Arrange a specialist review every 6–12 months.

*Medical*

✓ Consider the following drug treatments (this is initiated by a specialist):

› Monoamine-oxidase-B inhibitors – Selegiline or rasagiline.

› Oral or transdermal dopamine agonist – Pramipexole, ropinirole or rotigotine.

› L-dopa.

› Amantadine or an anticholinergic.

*Surgical*

✓    Rarely required.

*Other*

✓    Deep brain stimulation (rare).

## Referral

→    Refer the patient immediately to a specialist (treatment is not to be initiated by anyone other than a specialist neurologist or geriatrician):

    ›    A two-week referral for those with late disease and/or complex issues.

    ›    A six-week referral for those with mild suspected PD.

---

*References?*

National Institute for Health and Care Excellence (2018). *Parkinson's disease.* https://cks.nice.org.uk/topics/parkinsons-disease/

# 8

# Ear, Nose and Throat

## Ear Pain

Ear pain or otalgia is a fairly common presentation in primary care. It is usually caused by local aural disease processes (primary otalgia), it or can be referred from other head and neck sites radiating into the ear. While it is a common symptom, it is often transient in nature, particularly affecting children when presenting with URTIs or ear infections.

### History

» Focused questions

> Otalgia – Ask when it started, and which side is affected or if it affects both ears.

> Ask about the character (sharp, fullness, dull or aching), severity, radiation or referred pain (tooth, throat or jaw).

> Ask what makes it worse (chewing, a change in pressure or swallowing).

> Ask about any recent trauma (cotton bud, loud noise or injury).

» Associated history – Ask about any dizziness, tinnitus, hearing issues or discharge (purulent, blood or waxy).

» Past history – Ask if they have had eczema, psoriasis, dental work or ear trauma.

» Drug history – Ask if they have taken SSRIs, lamotrigine or zolpidem.

» Social history – Ask what their occupation is.

» Travel history – Ask if they have travelled on a plane recently, and if they went diving or scuba diving while away.

### RED FLAGS

» Persistent, unilateral ear pain with a normal examination (referred otalgia).

» Painless, persistent, cheesy-smelling discharge or bloody discharge (cholesteatoma).

## Examination

» Vitals – Temperature and pulse.

» Face – Look for any facial rash (herpetic blisters).

» Ear exam

> Hold an otoscope like a pen, stabilising the hand against the cheekbone; use the right hand for the right ear and the left hand for left ear. With the other hand, pull the ear upwards and backwards in adults, and downwards and backwards in children. This is to straighten the external canal.

> Inspect the pinna (and behind) for sinuses, abscesses or furuncles. Look inside the ear canal for inflammation, impacted wax, foreign bodies, grommets or debris. Note any discharge. Before inserting the otoscope, check that the pinna is not painful (otitis externa).

> Observe the tympanic membrane (TM) (intact or perforated), its colour (red, yellow or cloudy), its shape (bulging or retracted), and whether an anterior-inferior light reflex is present. Check for an air-fluid level (effusion) appearing as bubbles.

> Palpate the mastoid process for any tenderness (mastoiditis).

» TMJ – If indicated, palpate the TMJs while at rest and with the jaw opened, noting crepitus or restricted movement.

» If there is referred pain or associated dizziness, consider a CN assessment.

## Different Types of Discharge from the Ear

➤ Cheesy smell – Cholesteatoma

➤ Sanguineous – Trauma

➤ Purulent – Otitis media or externa

➤ Watery – Possible cerebrospinal fluid (CSF) fluid

## Differential Diagnosis

| Otitis externa | Itchy ear with smelly discharge; caused by use of cotton buds, often after going swimming or visiting humid countries. Inflammation and/or infection of the outer ear canal. May be associated with eczema or psoriasis of the ear canal. OE: ear canal harbours debris or discharge. |
|---|---|
| Acute otitis media | High fever, sweats, URTI and discharge from the ear; pain improves after the discharge (perforation). Infection of the middle ear. Often unilateral ear pain with fever, typically after a URTI. OE: bulging red or cloudy eardrum. |

| Otitis media with effusion (glue ear | Causes the collection of fluid within the middle ear in the absence of acute infection. Most common cause of mild childhood hearing impairment. Common in two- to five-year-olds in winter. |
|---|---|
| Dental | Pain when eating or drinking cold fluids. |
| Eustachian tube dysfunction | A feeling of the ears popping or crackling, or muffled hearing; it feels better after swallowing. |
| TMJ dysfunction | Causes pain (full or uni/bilateral), typically in front of the tragus of the ear and limited movement around the joint. Described as the joint 'catches', 'gets stuck' or 'locks'. May note crepitus as well. Multifactorial aetiology due to muscle overactivity, bruxism, dental problems and underlying OA. |
| TM perforation | Sudden pain on one side, bloody discharge and reduced hearing. |
| Mastoiditis | Rare. Can occur from an otitis media infection spreading to the mastoid bone. Causes throbbing ear pain, profuse whitish (creamy) discharge with hearing loss. OE: mastoid process is tender with the ear sticking out. |
| Cholesteatoma | Skin that is trapped within the middle ear. Presents with persistent/recurrent, foul-smelling discharge and hearing loss. Local invasion can result in vertigo, facial nerve palsy or brain abscess. OE: crusting marginal eardrum perforation or retraction, and conductive hearing loss. |
| Impacted wax | Can cause irritation, ear pain, hearing loss and tinnitus. |
| Barotrauma | Linked to poor eustachian tube dysfunction. Seen in air travel or diving. Presents with pain or pressure in the ears with hearing loss. OE: haemorrhagic areas on the TM and fluid behind the eardrum. |

## Investigations

> » Bloods – FBC (raised WCC), ESR (temporal arteritis) and TFTs (thyroiditis).

> » MC&S – Swab any discharge.

## Management

*Conservative (general)*

✓ Dewaxing – Advise the patient to not use cotton buds to clear out the ears, as they can cause impaction. They should use a pipette to place a few drops of olive oil into the affected ear, then place cotton wool in the ear to prevent the oil from leaking out. They should do this two to three times a day for 10 days.

✓ Flying – Ear pain can be made worse by flying. Advise them to suck a sweet and swallow when the plane is taking off or descending.

✓ Analgesia – Paracetamol or NSAIDs. Ensure there is no contraindication for NSAIDs (ulcers or gastritis). Add a PPI in the elderly. Consider a weak opioid (co-dydramol or co-codamol) if others fail, and consider laxatives for constipation.

## Otitis media

✓ Most cases are viral and resolve within three days without antibiotics. They are self-limiting up to seven days. Recommend fluids and analgesia, and give a delayed prescription for antibiotics if it persists for more than three days. Consider a referral to ENT in children if they are under two, have an ear discharge, are systemically unwell or have a recurrent infection. Admit them if they are severely unwell (e.g. if you suspect mastoiditis).

## Glue ear

✓ Conduct active monitoring over 12 weeks. Reassure the patient that the vast majority improve without complication. Consider a referral to ENT for hearing tests, and possibly hearing aids or grommets. If a child suffers from Down's syndrome or a cleft palate, refer them immediately.

## Otitis externa

### Conservative

✓ Advise them to not use cotton buds or any kind of object within the ear canals. Use a warm flannel.

✓ If they are swimming, advise them to keep their ears dry; to do so, they should consider using a swimming cap covering the ears, or special ear plugs.

### Medical

✓ Offer analgesia for the pain.

✓ Offer steroid and antibiotic ear drops (neomycin or clioquinol). In mild cases, 2% acetic acid can be used.

✓ Consider oral antibiotics if it is a spreading preauricular infection. Send a swab for MC&S to guide sensitivities if there is resistance or it is recurring.

## Perforated ear drum

✓ These often heal spontaneously (usually within four weeks). If it persists for more than six weeks, refer them to ENT for surgical repair.

## Cholesteatoma

✓ Refer them to a specialist if cholesteatoma is suspected. Admit them if it is associated with facial nerve palsy or vertigo.

## Furunculosis

✓ Consider antibiotics (flucloxacillin), incision and drainage if there is severe pain and swelling.

## Impacted wax

✓ Advise them to use ear drops (olive oil, Otex or sodium bicarbonate). They should avoid using cotton buds. If it persists, refer them for microsuction or ear irrigation.

## TMJ dysfunction

✓ Advise them to avoid eating anything that will involve a lot of chewing, such as chewing gum. They should try a soft diet to relax the jaw. They should try placing ice packs over the joints. They should use relaxation techniques if they are stressed (as they may clench their teeth or suffer nocturnal bruxism). They should gently stretch the ligaments in the joint by opening and closing the jaw slowly, and by doing relaxing exercises.

✓ Offer analgesia (NSAIDs), muscle relaxants or TCAs. Refer them to maxillofacial (max fax) if there is no improvement.

# Referral

→ Refer the patient to ENT for any of the following:

› Any evidence of mastoiditis (this needs IV antibiotics and possible surgery).

› Any suspicion of cholesteatoma.

› A persistent, unexplained, unilateral pain for more than four weeks in the head or neck with otalgia but a normal otoscopic examination warrants an urgent referral.

→ Recommend that the patient sees a dentist to discuss TMJ or dental caries.

## Safety Netting

» If the pain in the ear persists for four weeks, the patient should attend for a review.

---

## References

National Institute for Health and Care Excellence (2018). *Otitis media (acute): antimicrobial prescribing.* https://www.nice.org.uk/guidance/ng91

National Institute for Health and Care Excellence (2018). *Hearing loss in adults: assessment and management.* https://www.nice.org.uk/guidance/ng98

# Hearing Loss and Tinnitus

Hearing loss is a subjective reduction in the ability to hear things. It is often assessed objectively using an audiogram (pure tone audiogram). Hearing loss can be due to damage anywhere along the hearing pathway from the outer ear (auricle) through the middle and on to the inner ear. Broadly speaking, it is classified into conductive or sensorineural loss, with the Weber and Rinne tests being useful to distinguish between the two types. Tinnitus relates to the unwanted hearing of a ringing, buzzing, humming or clicking sound from within the ear. It is not audible to others and denotes a symptom rather than a diagnosis. It affects around 10% of the population, but only 1% has a severe form that is debilitating.

## Causes of Hearing Loss

### Conductive

➤ Ear canal impaction with wax or a foreign body

➤ Eardrum perforation

➤ Ear infection

➤ Collection of middle-ear fluid

➤ Otosclerosis

➤ Cholesteatoma

### Sensorineural

➤ Congenital

➤ Presbycusis

➤ Ototoxic drugs

➤ Previous meningitis

➤ Mumps or measles

➤ Acoustic neuroma

➤ Noise exposure

### History

» Focused questions

› Hearing loss – Ask when it started, which side ear it is, if the hearing is muffled, about the onset (sudden or gradual), about the types of sounds that cannot be heard (e.g. high or low pitched), and about any exposure to prolonged loud noises at work or during recreation (concerts, etc.).

› Tinnitus – Ask when it started, what it sounds like (ringing, clicking, hissing or buzzing), if it is pulsatile, if it comes and goes, if it affects sleep and/or social/work activities, which side ear it is or if it is both, and if there are any relieving or worsening factors.

» Associated history – Ask about dizziness, fever, recent cough or colds, and if there is any ear pain or any discharge.

» Past history – Ask if they have used hearing aids, or have had any recurrent ear infections, neurofibromatosis or craniofacial syndromes.

» Surgical history – Ask if they have had any previous operations (grommet, tympanoplasty or mastoidectomy).

» Drug history – Ask if they take gentamicin, chloroquine, methotrexate, diazepam (withdrawal), erythromycin or valproate.

» Travel – Ask if they have recently travelled abroad or been diving.

» Social history – Ask what their occupation is, or if they have had any recent exposure to loud sounds on a daily basis.

» Family history – Ask if there is a family history of hearing problems (otosclerosis or osteogenesis imperfecta).

## Occupational Causes for Hearing loss

➤ Noise levels of >80 decibels can lead to damage

➤ UK law states that persons who are regularly exposed to 85 decibels daily must be offered ear protection; e.g. construction workers, aeroplane workers, those using firearms or DJs.

## RED FLAGS

» Unilateral or sudden deafness (less than three days) that is fluctuant with no signs of a URTI.

» Unilateral tinnitus that is sudden and pulsatile, neurological signs such as facial weakness and/or paraesthesia, or severe vertigo.

» Persistent cheesy-smelling discharge or bloody discharge.

» Depression or suicidal ideation.

## Differential Diagnosis

| Otitis media | Ear pain, fever, sweats, and a recent cough or cold. Infection of the middle ear. Often unilateral. Ear discharge (perforation) often resolves the pain. OE: bulging, red or cloudy ear drum. |
|---|---|

| Ménière's disease | Dizziness or vertigo pressure with fullness in the ear. Condition affects the middle-aged. Patients complain of periodic episodes of tinnitus, intense rotary vertigo (requiring them to sit down) and a progressive, fluctuating hearing loss. The fullness in the ear lasts from minutes to hours. The patient may feel nauseous after an attack. OE: normal otoscopy, but decreased hearing and nystagmus during episode. |
|---|---|
| Earwax | Muffled hearing and the gradual onset of reduced hearing. Can cause irritation, ear pain and tinnitus. |
| Head injury | A recent blow or knock to the head. |
| Cholesteatoma | Cheesy-smelling discharge. Skin that is trapped within the middle ear. Presents with persistent/recurrent foul-smelling discharge and hearing loss. Local invasion can result in vertigo, facial-nerve palsy or a brain abscess. OE: discharging or crusty marginal eardrum perforation or retraction, and conductive hearing loss. |
| Perforation | Sudden onset, trauma and bloody discharge. |
| Otosclerosis | An inherited condition that may have a strong family history. Usually seen in 20–40-year-old females, and presents with tinnitus and deafness. Worsens in pregnancy. OE: conductive deafness, typically bilateral with gradual onset. |
| Presbycusis | Usually bilateral, with gradual onset, reduced hearing of high-pitched sounds and difficulty hearing background noise. Most common in the elderly (>75 years). Causes progressive, sensorineural hearing loss. Patients may complain of not being able to hear people in noisy environments. May be associated with tinnitus. OE: nil to find (high-pitched-sounds hearing loss on audiology). |
| Acoustic neuroma | Rare condition causing unilateral symptoms. May have a family history of this, and bilateral symptoms found in neurofibromatosis type 2. Patients complain of deafness, tinnitus and/or vertigo. They may have a headache or report occipital pain. If it is large, it can cause facial-nerve palsy. OE: unilateral sensorineural deafness with or without tinnitus (CN 8), absent corneal reflex (CN 5) and facial palsy (CN 7). |
| Glue ear | Sequel to recurrent otitis media, which leaves behind an effusion. It normally affects children, and hearing loss is the main complaint. If it is not treated early, children may develop a speech and language delay, or problems with balance. OE: usually a dull and retracted eardrum, behind which you may see air bubbles or fluid levels. |

| Otitis externa | Inflammation and /or infection of the outer ear canal. May be associated with eczema or psoriasis of the ear canal. Described as 'Mediterranean ear', as it is often seen in visitors to humid countries, swimmers or regular cotton bud users. Often causes an itch, ear pain and discharge (offensive smelling). OE: the pinna can be painful to touch or move, and the ear canal harbours debris or discharge. |
| --- | --- |

# Examination

» Hearing tests

> Whisper test – At a 1m distance from the test ear, with the patient's eyes closed to prevent lip-reading, mask the contralateral ear, whisper three letters or numbers into the patient's other ear, and ask them to repeat them back.

> Weber test – Strike a tuning fork (512Hz), place it on the middle of the forehead, and ask if the sound is equal in both ears or if it is louder to one side. If it is lateralised to one ear, then suspect conductive hearing loss on that side or a sensorineural hearing loss in the other ear.

> Rinne test – Strike a tuning fork and hold the stem against the mastoid process for three seconds. Ask when they can no longer hear it vibrate. Next, hold it 2.5cm away from their ear and check if the vibrations can still be heard.

**Interpreting the Rinne Test:**

- Positive – If vibrations are heard through the ear canal, air conduction is greater than bone conduction. This represents a normal finding (i.e. there is no conductive hearing loss), although sensorineural hearing loss cannot be excluded.

- Negative – If vibrations cannot be heard through the ear canal, bone conduction is greater than air conduction. This suggests a conductive hearing loss in that ear or possibly a dead ear on that side (false negative), whereby bone conduction is being detected by the contralateral side.

» Otoscope

> Hold the otoscope like a pen, stabilising the hand against the cheekbone, using the right hand for the right ear and the left hand for the left ear. With the other hand, pull the ear upwards and backwards in adults, or downwards and backwards in children, to straighten the external canal.

> Inspection – Inspect the pinna (and behind) for scars, sinuses, tags, abscesses and furuncles. Look inside the ear canal for inflammation, impacted wax, foreign bodies or debris (otitis externa). Note any discharge. Before inserting the otoscope, check that the pinna is not painful (otitis externa).

> › Observe the TM (intact or perforated), its colour (flamingo tinge, red or dull), its shape and whether a light reflex is present. Inspect for a fluid level behind the TM (glue ear) or the presence of any grommets. Look for cholesteatoma on the attic just in front of the TM.

» Neurology – Do a focused CN exam (CNs 5, 6 and 7) if acoustic neuroma is being considered.

» Objective tinnitus – Listen out for any clicking or pulsatile noises. Examine the jaw for any snapping or clicking (TMJ). Auscultate the periauricular area. Listen for a carotid bruits jugular venous hum and arteriovenous malformation (AVM) thrills.

## Investigations

» Bloods – FBC (anaemia), TFT and glucose.

» MC&S – Swab any discharge.

» Specialist – Audiogram and brain MRI (acoustic neuroma).

## Management

### Hearing loss

#### Conservative

✓ Suggest that the patient sits in closer proximity to the person speaking.

✓ Advise them to ask people to speak more slowly, and to consider learning to lip read.

✓ Suggest using phone amplifiers.

✓ Advise the patient of the benefits available such as the Disability Living Allowance (DLA), ESA or Industrial Injuries Disablement Benefit (IIDB).

#### Treatment

✓ Hearing aids – Refer them to an audiology department for consideration and fitting.

✓ Cochlear implants – These may be considered in cases of severe hearing loss in both ears, or for those who have had little or no benefit from a hearing aid.

### Tinnitus

#### Conservative

✓ Reassure the patient that if red flags are not present, tinnitus may not have a serious underlying cause and can be self-limiting.

✓ Refer them for counselling if it is intrusive, as such tinnitus can have a large negative impact on life.

✓ Put the patient in contact with support groups (such as the Tinnitus Association).

✓ Advise the use of background music, a white-noise device from the ENT department or wearable devices similar to earphones/hearing aids.

✓ Refer them for audiological assessment, particularly if it has persisted for more than six months.

*Treat the underlying cause*

### Glue ear

✓ Reassure them, as up to 80% of cases resolve within three months. Otherwise, it may require grommets, although hearing aids would be an option. Consider speech therapy, particularly in the young. There is no evidence for the use of antibiotics, antihistamines, decongestants or steroids.

### Ménière's disease

✓ In an acute attack (if severe), admit them for IV sedatives and fluids. The patient should remain still, and if their eyes are open, they should fix them on a single spot. Advise them to avoid fluids, as this may induce vomiting. They should remain in a stationary position until the peak of the vertigo attack is over. Advise them that most attacks resolve within 24 hours. Treat this with buccal or intramuscular (IM) prochlorperazine 5–10mg tds or cinnarizine 15–30mg tds if they are vomiting a lot.

✓ In between episodes, suggest that they stop smoking, and restrict salt and fluid intake. Advise them to reduce the amount of coffee and alcohol they consume. This can be treated with betahistine 16mg tds to prevent episodes. Direct them to support groups, and refer them to ENT if it is not settling and to confirm the diagnosis.

### Barotrauma

✓ Reassure the patient that it often heals within three weeks. Recommend that they yawn or suck on boiled sweets during take-off or descent when flying. Consider nasal decongestants.

### Impacted wax

✓ Advise them to use ear drops (olive oil, Otex or sodium bicarbonate). They should not use cotton buds. If it persists, consider ear irrigation or microsuction.

## NICE Referral Guidance for Hearing Loss (National Institute for Health and Care Excellence, 2018)

→ Rapid onset – Refer the patient to ENT immediately if this developed suddenly (under three days) within the last 30 days.

→ Refer them to ENT if their hearing was lost suddenly >30 days ago, or has worsened rapidly over 90 days.

→ Refer them to ENT immediately if they have unilateral hearing loss with a facial drop (same side) or altered sensation.

→    Refer them to ENT urgently if they are Chinese or of Southeast Asian descent with hearing loss and middle-ear effusion that is not associated with a URTI.

→    A routine referral is appropriate if their hearing loss is unilateral/asymmetric, fluctuates and is not associated with URTI, or for persistent tinnitus or unresolved, recurrent vertigo.

## References

Baguley, D. and McFerran, D. (n.d.). *Tinnitus guidance for GPs*. British Tinnitus Association https://www.tinnitus.org.uk/guidance-for-gps

National Institute for Health and Care Excellence (2018). *Hearing loss in adults: assessment and management*. https://www.nice.org.uk/guidance/ng98

Meehan, T. and Nogueira, C. (2014). Tinnitus. *The BMJ, 348*. doi: https://doi.org/10.1136/bmj.g216

# Vertigo

Vertigo is a debilitating symptom that is a subset of dizziness. A patient feels an abnormal sensation that everything around them or they themselves are moving or spinning, but in the absence of any actual movement. It is usually accompanied with symptoms such as nausea or vomiting. Dizziness as a symptom is extremely common; however, effort should be made to confirm what the patient means by their dizziness, and to ensure that a patient is suffering from true vertigo, and not generalised unsteadiness or presyncope. The majority of patients presenting in primary care with balance problems suffer from generalised unsteadiness, and only 20–30% have true vertigo. Vertigo is classified as peripheral or central, depending on the location of the dysfunction on the vestibular pathway.

## Causes of Vertigo

*Central*

➤ Migraine

➤ Acoustic neuroma

➤ CVA

➤ TIA

➤ MS

➤ Cerebellar tumour

➤ Epilepsy

## Peripheral

➤ Benign paroxysmal positional vertigo (BPPV)

➤ Vestibular neuronitis

➤ Ménière's disease

➤ Labyrinthitis

➤ Eustachian tube dysfunction

## *History*

» Focused questions

› Vertigo – Ask whether, when they feel dizzy, they feel light-headed or they feel everything spinning: *'Does it feel like you just got off a playground roundabout?'*

› Ask about the onset, and if they have recently had a cold.

› Ask about the duration of the episodes, and if they come and go.

› Ask if there are any periods where they have no symptoms at all.

› Ask about any triggers, the severity and if they have had any falls as a result.

» Associated history – Ask if they have had any nausea or vomiting, hearing loss, otorrhoea, tinnitus, or any visual symptoms such as double vision or flashing lights.

» Past history – Ask if they have had any migraines, strokes, epilepsy, MS, BP issues, a brain tumour, DM or meningitis. Also ask if they have had anxiety, depression or panic attacks.

» Family history – Ask if there is a family history of Ménière's disease or migraines.

» Drug history – Ask if they have taken gentamicin, furosemide, carbamazepine, benzodiazepines, aspirin or anti-hypertensives.

» Social history – Ask if they live alone, what their occupation is and if the symptoms have affected them at work.

» Travel history – Ask if they have recently travelled on a plane.

## RED FLAGS

» Acute onset of severe and persistent vertigo.

» Headache.

» Acute deafness in the absence of ear symptoms.

» Focal neurology.

## Differential Diagnosis

| BPPV | The sudden onset of vertigo that lasts for a few seconds (<30 seconds) and is precipitated by head movement related to gravity (e.g. lying down, looking upwards or bending over). Often worse in the mornings or when turning over in bed. Affects those of any age, but is common those in their 50s. Can be precipitated by a virus (labyrinthitis) or a head injury. Associated with nausea, but with no hearing loss or tinnitus. |
|---|---|
| Ménière's disease | Sudden onset of severe rotatory vertigo (needing them to sit down) that is unaffected by the posture, which is associated with reduced hearing, fullness and tinnitus of the affected ear. Episodes last anything from 30 minutes to two to three hours, with severe nausea and vomiting. Can experience the clustering of episodes (6–11 per year). Ear symptoms are often unilateral, but develop bilaterally later. Typically affects those of middle age. |

| Vestibular neuritis / labyrinthitis | Inflammation of the vestibular nerve or labyrinth. Caused by the recent onset of a URTI. Often affects 20–30-year-olds. Presents with the acute onset of vertigo, nausea and vomiting that recurs for several days. Head movements can precipitate symptoms. There may be hearing loss. Resolves within two to six weeks. |
| --- | --- |
| Migraine | Throbbing headache, visual symptoms (flickering lights, spots and zigzag lines), and nausea or vomiting. |
| Postural hypotension | Dizziness starts first thing in the morning when getting up or when standing. |
| TIA/CVA | Slurred speech and weakness in the limbs. |
| Epilepsy | Warning signs (prodromal – taste or smell), a stiff body, seizure, tongue biting and urinary incontinence. |
| MS | Eye symptoms, and urine or bowel problems. |

## Examination

»   Vitals – Temperature, sitting and standing BP, and pulse.

»   Gait – Assess their gait to look for waddling. Consider a Romberg's test (ask the patient to stand up straight with their feet together then shut their eyes – they will sway to ipsilateral side in neuronitis).

»   Inspection – Inspect for facial asymmetry or a resting tremor.

»   Neurological – Inspect the eyes for nystagmus. Perform a CN examination (CNs 5, 7, 9 and 10 if acoustic neuroma is suspected). Check power and sensation. Check for dysdiadochokinesia (finger–nose test) to exclude cerebellar causes.

»   ENT – Check the ears for infection (vesicles indicate Ramsay Hunt syndrome), discharge and cholesteatoma. If there is hearing loss, consider performing the Weber and Rinne tuning-fork tests.

   **Specialist**

   ›   Dix-Hallpike manoeuvre (for BPPV) – Ask the patient to keep their eyes open, sit upright on a couch at a 45° angle with their head facing to one side, then lie down rapidly with their head extended (30°). This test is positive if you see nystagmus. Repeat on the other side.

   ›   Unterberger's test (for labyrinthitis) – Ask the patient to close their eyes and march on the spot for 30 seconds. With labyrinthine dysfunction, the patient may rotate laterally to the side of the lesion.

## Investigations

»   Bloods – (Not usually performed in primary care.) CRP and FBC for infection or anaemia (ferritin).

»   ECG – To exclude cardiac causes for dizziness.

» Specialist – MRI (brain tumour or MS), audiometry (sensorineural hearing loss) and vestibular testing.

## Management

### Conservative (general)

✓ Recommend that during episodes they do not drive and do not operate any machinery.

✓ Advise that they reduce their salt and fluid intake, stop smoking, and reduce their coffee and alcohol intake.

### BPPV

✓ Reassure them that recovery is usually over a few weeks. Advise that they get out of bed slowly, and avoid activities/tasks that require them to look up.

✓ Epley manoeuvre – If they have a positive Dix-Hallpike manoeuvre, get them to rotate their head 90° to the other side. Roll the patient to that side, with their head fixed and looking to the ground. Sit the patient up.

✓ Brandt-Daroff exercise – The patient should start in upright seated position on a bed, then lie down to one side, turning their head 45° to look up at the ceiling. They should hold position for 30 seconds. Then they sit upright and hold that position for 30 seconds. Repeat on the other side. They should repeat this two-minute cycle five times (for 10 minutes in total), three times a day for two weeks.

### Labyrinthitis

✓ Recovery is usually over a few weeks. Advise them to avoid alcohol, and advise bed rest during the acute phase.

✓ Offer buccal/IM prochlorperazine, or oral prochlorperazine if it is less severe. They should take this regularly for three days, then PRN. Advise them regarding the side effects of a dystonic reaction. Consider antihistamines (cinnarizine or cyclizine).

### Ménière's disease

✓ Suggest they follow a low-salt diet, avoid caffeine and alcohol, and stop smoking. Recommend support groups (Ménière's Society) to them. Advise them to inform the DVLA regarding driving. Advise them to avoid loud sounds. Inform them that most attacks last <24 hours.

### Other

✓ For tinnitus, consider masking devices or sound therapy.

✓ If they have hearing loss, refer them to audiology for hearing aids.

✓ Offer buccal/oral prochlorperazine for 7–14 days or IM prochlorperazine if it is severe. Consider antihistamines (cinnarizine or cyclizine).

✓ Trial betahistine 16mg tds (with food) as a preventative measure, which will reduce the severity and frequency of attacks.

## Referral

→ Admit the patient if there is severe vomiting and they are unable to keep fluids down.

→ Refer them for education on the Epley manoeuvre if BPPV symptoms last longer than four weeks.

→ Refer them if labyrinthitis symptoms persist for longer than six weeks, or if they are not improving despite treatment of more than one week.

→ Refer them to ENT for a formal diagnosis of Ménière's. Admit them if it is severe, as they may need an IV sedative and fluids.

## Safety Netting

» Typically review them one week after the onset of symptoms to ensure they are improving.

### References

Al-Malky, G., Cane, D., Morgan, K. Radomskij, P., Rutkowskij, R., West, P. and Wilkinson, A. (2016). *Recommended procedure – Positioning tests. British Society of Audiology.* https://www.thebsa.org.uk/wp-content/uploads/2015/12/Positioning-Tests-September-2016.pdf

Parnes, L.S. and Nabi, S. (2019). *Benign paroxysmal positional vertigo.* BMJ Best Practice. https://bestpractice.bmj.com/topics/en-gb/73

# Rhinitis

Rhinitis refers to a feeling of congestion or blockage of the nasal passage, which is often associated with a watery discharge, and is caused by inflammation. Although an allergenic cause is typically found, this might not always be the case. Common allergens include grass and tree pollen, cat dander, or house dust mites. Non-allergic causes include a hormonal imbalance, air pollution, emotion or a side effect of medication. Symptoms are often severe enough to affect the quality of life – particularly in the young, who may miss school – or it may affect performance at work. It affects around 26% of adults, with the peak prevalence in those in their 30s and 40s.

## *History*

» Focused questions

  › Ask when the symptoms started and how long they have been going on for.

  › Ask which side is affected and if it alternates.

  › Ask if it is there all the time (perennial), it comes and goes, or it occurs during particular months (seasonal).

  › Ask if there is any discharge, and if so what colour it is (clear, yellow or bloody).

  › Ask about postnasal drip (i.e. if they have a feeling of liquid dripping down the back of the throat).

  › Ask about nasal itching, if they have a blocked nose, or if there is any snoring.

  › Ask if there are any triggers (stress, food, fumes, trees/grass, work or exercise).

  › Ask if the symptoms get better when they are on holiday or off work.

» Associated history – Ask if they have a change in their sense of smell or reduced taste.

» Past history – Ask if they have had asthma, hay fever, eczema or hypothyroid. Ask if there has been any past trauma or injury to the face (TMJ).

» Drug history – Ask if they have taken ACEis, b-blockers, chlorpromazine, aspirin or NSAIDs, which may worsen the condition. Ask if they have taken OTC nasal decongestants.

» Family history – Ask if they have a family history of asthma, eczema or hay fever.

» Social history – Ask if they smoke, drink alcohol or take recreational drugs (cocaine). Ask what their occupation is (a cook [using flour], or a painter, hairdresser or carpenter [all using chemicals]). Ask if they have any pets (cat or dog dander).

## RED FLAGS

Unexplained bloody or unilateral nasal discharge, nasal pain or non-traumatic deformity.

## Differential Diagnosis

| | |
|---|---|
| Allergic rhinitis | Seasonal or perennial itchiness, sneezing, bilateral nasal obstruction or nasal discharge (clear), with postnasal drip or nasal pruritus. Can be triggered by chemicals (tar, perfume, drugs or allergens, including cats/dogs, dust mites, pollen, etc.). Severe cases can affect sleep and daily activities. A family history of atopy may be present. OE: mucosal pallor, inflamed and congested turbinates, and red conjunctiva. |
| Sinusitis | Symptoms must include the cardinal features of nasal blockage and discharge. Facial pain without these cardinal sinonasal symptoms does not indicate sinusitis. OE: mucosal inflammation, mucosal oedema or discharge; tenderness over the cheeks, between eyes or across the forehead; and pain that is worse on stooping forwards. |
| Nasal polyps | Common in those with atopy, cystic fibrosis (CF) or asthma. Patients may complain of a disfigured nose, rhinitis, problems smelling or mouth breathing at night. OE: fleshy-, yellow- or grey-coloured, tear-drop-shaped mass in the nasal antrum. |
| Nasal carcinoma | More common in males from Africa and Southeast Asia (Chinese). Occupational exposure to fumes, dust and nickel have been implicated. Most patients are asymptomatic. However, they may notice enlarged cervical LNs, facial pain and drooping. Consider unilateral symptoms with bloody nasal discharge, especially if there are cervical LNs or facial pain. |

## Examination

» Nose exam – Perform a focused nose examination.

**Inspection**

› External – Note any obvious deviation (stand behind the patient on examination) or discharge. Inspect the vestibule (raise the tip of the nose with the thumb), looking for cartilaginous collapse (cocaine use or repeated operations). Check the patency of the nostrils. Look under the eyes for 'allergic shiners' and over the nasal tip for a horizontal crease ('allergic salute'). Observe for mouth breathing.

› Internal – Inspect the nasal septum, inferior, middle turbinates and mucosa, noting any collapse, ulceration, active bleeding, perforation, foreign body or nasal polyps.

> › Palpation – Palpate the frontal and maxillary sinuses (sinusitis). Press over the supra and infraorbital areas, and percuss gently to elicit any tenderness. Feel for the LN in the cervical chain, and head and neck chain.

## Investigations

» Bloods – FBC (eosinophilia), TFT, immunoglobulin levels, radioallergosorbent tests (RASTs) (grass pollen, tree pollen, cat/dog dander, house dust mites and dust), CRP and sputum culture.

» Specialist – CT sinuses/nasal passages (polyps), skin-prick tests and nasal endoscopy.

## Management

*Treat the underlying cause*

### Allergic rhinitis

#### Conservative

✓ Advise them to reduce allergen exposure by regularly cleaning the house, vacuuming carpets and curtains, changing bed linen, avoiding pets (keep them off the bed), keep windows shut and avoid cut grass. They should remain aware of pollen charts on the news. They should avoid walking in grassland in the morning or evening. They should avoid going out in thunderstorms.

✓ Occupation – Advise them to wear a mask or use latex-free gloves. They should ensure that there is an adequate air and ventilation in the workplace.

#### Medical

✓ Consider an intranasal saltwater spray (Sterimar). Offer an intranasal solution (sodium cromoglycate) or antihistamines (azelastine) as first-line treatment. Consider intranasal steroid spray/drops (this takes up to two weeks to work), such as Beconase (OTC), Flixonase and mometasone. If it persists, try oral steroids. Try a short course of nasal decongestants (ephedrine) or anticholinergics (ipratropium bromide if the discharge is the most problematic).

### Non-allergic rhinitis

#### Conservative

✓ This may resolve spontaneously if it is due to a virus. Advise the patient to avoid triggers such as smoky or polluted environments. They should reduce their intake of spicy food and alcohol. They should stop any OTC nasal decongestant use.

*Medical*

✓ Consider changing any medication that may be implicated. Offer an intranasal salt water spray (Sterimar) or solution to use as a nasal douche first thing in the morning. Consider an intranasal steroid spray, or a short course of nasal decongestants (ephedrine) or anticholinergics (ipratropium bromide if the discharge is the most problematic).

## Sinusitis

✓ Most are self-limiting (<10 days). Advise the patient to try simple analgesia, increase their fluid intake and try steam inhalation. Consider a short course of decongestants (7–10 days), steroid nasal sprays or oral antibiotics (though there is poor evidence for this being efficacious).

## Polyps

✓ Consider steroid nasal drops (Flixonase drops) until they shrink (one month), then maintain with steroid nasal sprays. If they persist, consider oral steroids before referring for a polypectomy. They may recur post surgery.

# Referral

→ Allergy clinic – Consider referring the patient for skin-prick tests in allergic rhinitis.

→ ENT – Refer them if they have unilateral polyps with an irregular shape, or if the polyps are ulcerated and bleeding.

→ Admission – Admit the patient if clear fluid is dripping from the nose post trauma (CSF rhinorrhoea).

## Safety Netting

» Review the patient in two to four weeks if their symptoms are not improving.

*References*

Scadding, G.K, Kariyawasam, H.H., Scadding, G., Mirakian, R., Buckley, R.J., Dixon, T., Durham, S.R., Farooque, S., Jones, N., Leech, S., Nasser, S.M., Powell, R., Roberts, G. Rotiroti, G., Simpson, A., Smith, H. and Clark, A.T. (2017). BSACI guideline for the diagnosis and management of allergic and non-allergic rhinitis (Revised edition). *Clinical & Experimental Allergy, 47*(7), 856–889. https://doi.org/10.1111/cea.12953

# Mouth Ulcers

Most mouth ulcers are painful lesions located within the oral cavity. They are a great nuisance for patients, as they can interfere with essential everyday tasks, such as eating, drinking or brushing teeth. They are a very common problem, but, thankfully, are usually self-limiting, lasting up to two weeks. However, persistent mouth ulcers may be indicative of a significant underlying illness.

## *History*

» Focused questions

  › Ask when the ulcers started and how long they have been there.

  › Ask about the site (inner cheek, lip, tongue or palate), and if there are any anywhere else in the body (anus or groin).

  › Ask if they come and go, or are there all the time.

  › Ask about pain and bleeding.

» Associated history – Ask if they have had any recent stress or anxiety, trauma (have bitten the tongue or lip, or toothbrush abrasion), wear dentures. Ask what their diet is like (lack of fruit and vegetables), and if they chew anything other than food (tobacco or paan leaves). Ask if they have had any weight loss.

» Past history – Ask if they have had Crohn's disease, coeliac disease or malabsorption. Ask if they have worn dentures or braces.

» Drug history – Ask if they have taken steroids, nicotine, aspirin, NSAIDs, methotrexate or bisphosphonates, which can worsen mouth ulcers.

» Social history – Ask if they smoke, drink alcohol or take recreational drugs. Ask what their occupation is.

» Family history – Ask if there is a family history of bowel issues (coeliac disease) or aphthous ulcers (canker sores).

## Differentials

➤ Trauma – Ask if they have had any recent injuries to the mouth, such as having bitten their tongue or inner cheek. Ask if they have loose dentures.

➤ Crohn's disease – Ask if they have any blood or mucus in the stools, any ulcers in the back passage, abdominal pain or bloody diarrhoea.

➤ Coeliac disease – Ask if they have had any pale stools that were difficult to flush away, rashes on their legs, or symptoms linked to particular foods (wheat, rye or barley).

➤ Hand, foot and mouth – Ask if they had a fever a few days before the ulcers started, or any spots on the hands or feet.

➤ Kawasaki disease – Ask if they have had a persistent fever, any eye infections in both eyes, or any rashes.

## Differential Diagnosis

| Minor ulcers | Aphthous ulcers are more common in young adults. These affect the buccal, floor of the mouth, soft palate and lingual mucosa more commonly. They are yellowish-grey in appearance and <10mm in size. They resolve spontaneously within 10 days. |
|---|---|
| Herpetiform | More frequently affects women. Numerous very painful, <3mm lesions in clusters. May last many months. |
| Cancer | More common in males >45 years old. Usually heavy smokers or alcoholics. Red, painful ulcers that bleed and are friable. Persists for over four weeks. |
| Behcet's disease | Common in those of Middle Eastern and Central Asian decent. Presents with recurrent mouth ulcers (at least three times a year), genital ulcers and visual problems, including uveitis and iritis. |

## Examination

» Mouth exam

> Inspection – Inspect the ulcer regarding its site, size, colour, shape (irregular margins) and bleeding.

> Palpation – Palpate the lesion with a gloved finger (if it is hard this may indicate cancer). Palpate the neck for LNs.

## Investigations

» Bloods – FBC (anaemia), ferritin, vitamin B12, folate, ESR, CRP and coeliac screen.

» Specialist – Biopsy for persistent mouth ulcers.

## Management

*Treat the underlying cause*

*Aphthous ulcers*

*Conservative*

✓ Reassure the patient that there is no underlying disease and they will spontaneously resolve in <10 days.

✓ Mouthwash – Offer chlorhexidine 0.2% or difflam to reduce the pain and encourage healing.

✓ Barrier creams – Consider carmellose sodium (Orabase).

✓ Analgesics – Advise them to use analgesia such as Bonjela or benzydamine spray (difflam).

✓    Steroid lozenges – Consider this for ulcers that are difficult to treat.

✓    Food – Advise them to avoid spicy food, peanuts, chocolate and coffee.

### Herpes simplex

✓    Try acyclovir cream (five times a day for up to five days), or oral acyclovir if symptoms are severe or the patient is immunocompromised.

### Coeliac disease

✓    Suggest a lifelong gluten-free diet. Advise them to check the labels on foods. *See Diarrhoea section, page 114.*

### Crohn's

✓    Offer an elemental diet. *See Per Rectum Bleeding section, page 154.*

### Malabsorption

✓    Treat the cause. Consider vitamin B12, folate or iron replacement if they are deficient.

### Behcet's disease

✓    Offer high-dose corticosteroid therapy. Refer them to a specialist for assessment.

## Referral

→    Refer the patient to a specialist if ulcers persist.

→    Refer them to a dentist for wax treatment if their braces are causing ulcers.

→    Persistent ulcers in patients who are alcoholic or smokers should be referred under the 2WW pathway.

→    Refer the patient urgently for mouth ulcers if they have any of the following:

>    Ulceration of the oral mucosa persisting for more than three weeks.

>    A persistent and unexplained lump in the neck.

>    A lump on the lip or in the oral cavity.

>    Red or red-and-white patches in the oral cavity that are consistent with erythroplakia or erythroleukoplakia.

## Safety Netting

»    Review the patient if their symptoms worsen or persist for more than three weeks.

## References

National Institute for Health and Care Excellence (2015). *Suspected cancer: recognition and referral.* https://www.nice.org.uk/guidance/ng12

# Facial Pain

Facial pain describes any pain that may be experienced within the confines of the face. This can include pain originating from structures underlying the skin (e.g. the nose, sinuses, teeth, muscle or bone) or from deeper neurological and vascular structures. Do not overlook the fact that the pain may be referred into the facial area from an external site, such as the ear or throat. Although most cases of facial pain are benign, it is important to exclude serious causes such as malignant tumours and temporal arteritis (also known as giant cell arteritis).

## Causes of Facial Pain

➤ Local – Sinusitis, dental, ear pathology, TMJ dysfunction, cervical spine or salivary glands

➤ Vascular – Migraine, temporal arteritis or cluster headache

➤ Neuralgia – Trigeminal neuralgia

➤ Other – Atypical facial pain

## *History*

» Focused questions

   › Ask when the facial pain started, how long it has been going on for and how often it happens.

   › Ask about the site (jaw, eye, teeth or temporal area), radiation and character (sharp, dull ache, throbbing or lancinating).

   › Ask if anything makes it worse (touch, washing, shaving, periods, eating, yawning or a change in head posture).

   › Ask if anything makes it better (the avoidance of light or analgesia).

» Past history – Ask if they have had polymyalgia rheumatica or TMJ.

» Drug history – Ask if they are taking any medications.

» Social history – Ask if they smoke or drink alcohol, and what their occupation is.

## RED FLAGS

» Trigeminal neuralgia (atypical facial pain in those <50 years) or a failure to respond to treatment.

» Temporal arteritis – Blurred vision or a sudden loss of vision.

» Periorbital oedema – Signs of infection, periorbital swelling or cellulitis.

# Examination

» Skin – Inspect for shingles (a rash that does not cross the midline) and cold sores. Feel over the maxillofacial sinuses for any localised tenderness.

» Nose – Inspect for polyps, mucosal inflammation, mucosal oedema or discharge.

» Neurology

› CN 5 – Check the sensation over the face with your finger / cotton wool.

› CN 7 – Inspect the facial symmetry and for evidence of weakness. Ask the patient to raise their eyebrow, screw their eyes tight shut and blow out their cheeks. Ask them to bite their teeth together and to move their jaw from side to side. Palpate for crepitus.

» Ear exam – Inspect the skin near the ear for a rash (Ramsey Hunt syndrome). Touch the pinna for any pain (otitis externa). Look inside the ear for any debris or infection.

» Vascular – Palpate the temporal artery for any tenderness or rigidity.

# Investigations

» Bloods – FBC, ESR (temporal arteritis) and CRP (infection).

» Specialist – CT/MRI (nasopharyngeal cancer) and USS (salivary gland stones).

# Management

*Treat the underlying cause*

## Trigeminal neuralgia

✓ Offer carbamazepine, which reduces the frequency and intensity of attacks. For severe cases, consider surgery. *See Trigeminal Neuralgia section, page 246.*

✓ Post-herpetic neuralgia.

✓ Advise the patient to have cool baths or use ice packs for the pain, to wear loose cotton clothing (to reduce irritation), and to apply cling film / plastic dressing over the sensitive area. Start with paracetamol/codeine then consider amitriptyline, gabapentin or pregabalin.

› Amitriptyline – Initiate 10mg at night, which can be increased to 75mg od if necessary.

## TMJ dysfunction

### Conservative

✓ The majority of cases improve. Advise the patient to avoid chewing gum. They should eat a soft diet to relax the jaw. They should avoid opening the jaw widely, such as in singing or yawning. They should try placing ice packs over the joints. They may use relaxation techniques if stressed (as they may clench their teeth). They should gently stretch the ligaments in the joint by opening the jaw slowly and doing relaxing exercises. They should use ice, a warm flannel or a heat pad.

### Medical

✓   Consider offering bite guards for use at night. Offer physiotherapy or simple jaw exercises. They may require a low dose of BDZ (diazepam 2mg), amitriptyline or gabapentin. Consider intra-articular joint injections.

## Temporal arteritis

✓   Initiate a high dose of prednisolone, with the dose dependent on the presence of visual symptoms. If suspected, refer the patient urgently for ESR and/or temporal artery biopsy. *See Temporal Arteritis section, page 243.*

## Sinusitis

### Conservative

✓   Most cases are self-limiting (<10 days). Advise them to increase their fluid intake and try steam inhalation.

### Medical

✓   Try simple analgesia (paracetamol/NSAIDs), OTC nasal saline or decongestants. If it has persisted for >10 days, consider a high-dose corticosteroid nasal spray (mometasone 200mcg bd for 14 days). Consider a back-up antibiotics prescription of penicillin V, or doxycycline/clarithromycin if the patient is allergic to penicillin.

# Referral

→   Neurologist – Refer the patient to a neurologist if they have atypical features of trigeminal neuralgia, <50 years old, treatment fails or there is a neurological deficit between attacks.

→   Ophthalmologist – Refer them urgently to an ophthalmologist if a shingles-like rash is noted on the tip of nose (nasociliary branch of the trigeminal nerve), which may indicate eye involvement.

→   Dentist – If there is a dental abscess or pain, refer them to a dentist for further treatment.

→   ENT – Refer them to ENT if the cardinal sinonasal symptoms of nasal blockage and discharge are associated with facial pain.

→   Max fax – Refer a patient with TMJ if there is a history of trauma to TMJ, or a marked limitation to the mouth opening.

## Safety Netting

» Follow-up – Review the patient in two to four weeks if the symptoms are not improving.

---

## References

National Institute for Health and Care Excellence (2016). *NICE guidance on Sepsis: recognition, diagnosis and early management.* https://www.nice.org.uk/guidance/ng51

National Institute for Health and Care Excellence (2017). *Sinusitis (acute): antimicrobial prescribing.* https://www.nice.org.uk/guidance/ng79

# Sleep Apnoea

Snoring refers to the noise made during sleep due to upper airway relaxation. This results in turbulent airflow and the vibration of floppy, soft tissues. Although most cases of snoring are mild, with little impact on life, it can occasionally be so severe that it affects both the patient and their partner, causing undue strain on the relationship. Snoring is part of a spectrum of sleep-disordered breathing, which includes OSA, where the patient suffers from periods of absent breathing in their sleep. OSA affects people as they age, mainly those >60 years, with men being affected three times more than women. Although these episodes may only last for a few seconds a time, they may have profound effects on the patient's life and health, with research showing an increased incidence of HTN, MI and strokes.

Patients suffering with OSA may not realise they have a problem, making the diagnosis a tricky affair. Classically, they may attend with a partner who is at the end of their tether due to poor sleep as a result of their partner's snoring. The relationship may even be close to termination, with both partners sleeping in separate rooms. In other cases, patients may attend complaining of a headache, poor sleep, lack of libido, and symptoms that may suggest depression or stress.

## History

» Focused questions

**Sleep apnoea**

> Ask when it started, how long it has been going on for and how often it happens.

> Ask if they have had any disturbed sleep, and if they snore at night.

> Ask if they are in a relationship, if it affects their partner's sleep as well and if they have to sleep in a separate room.

> Ask if there are any triggers (lying on their back, drinking alcohol or caffeine, or taking sedatives).

**OSA**

> With respect to stopping breathing occasionally during sleep, ask how often it occurs in a single night, and how long the episodes of pauses in breathing are (5–10 seconds).

> Ask if they feel refreshed when they wake up, if they ever feel sleepy first thing in the morning, and if they have had trouble concentrating during the day.

» Associated history

> Perform a depression screen, and ask if they have had any change in personality.

> Ask if they feel tired all the time.

> Ask if they have a headache first thing in the morning.

> Ask if they have any nocturia.

» Past history – Ask if they have had hypothyroidism, IHD, CVA, HTN or CKD (water retention).

» Drug history – Ask if they have taken any b-blockers (tiredness) or SSRIs. Ask if they have taken any sedatives, such as diazepam, zopiclone or TCAs.

» Family history – Ask if they have a family history of IHD or OSA.

» Social history – Ask if they smoke or drink alcohol, what their occupation is (if they do shift work / work nights), and if they drive.

## Differential Diagnosis

| OSA | Typically affects 30–60 year olds. Snoring and daytime somnolence are the most common symptoms. Witnessed apnoeas or choking noises while asleep. Patients often report poor concentration, mood swings and being unrefreshed after sleep, with mood swings. Patients may be obese and have associated IHD risk factors. OE: raised BMI and a large neck circumference. |
|---|---|
| Tonsillitis | Common illness mainly seen in children. May present with sore throat, painful swallowing, headache and loss of voice. Pain may radiate to the ears. OE: red tonsils with exudate, and tender anterior cervical LNs. |
| Hypothyroidism | Patients complain of tiredness, weight gain, cold intolerance, constipation and menstrual irregularities. OE: dry skin, thinning hair, reduced reflexes, and a goitre may be present. |

## Examination

» Vitals – BP and BMI.

» Collar size – Use a tape measure to determine the neck/collar size. A size >43cm is associated with OSA.

» ENT exam – Inspect the nasal passages for any nasal polyps, and inspect the throat for enlarged tonsils or tonsillitis, and a floppy, elongated uvula. Look for a small jaw.

» Thyroid exam – If indicated, examine the thyroid gland for the presence of a goitre.

## Investigations

» Bloods – FBC, TFT, cholesterol and DM.

» Other – Use the Epworth Sleepiness Scale (ESS) to measure the level of sleepiness. Refer them for sleep studies if they have five or more episodes of apnoea per hour.

## Management

### *Conservative*

✓ Lose weight – If they have a raised BMI, encourage them to lose weight until their BMI is <25. Consider referring them to a dietician or an exercise programme.

✓ Smoking cessation – If they are a smoker, advise them to stop. Refer them for smoking-cessation advice/clinic.

✓ Alcohol – Suggest they cut down on alcohol and avoid evening consumption.

✓ Caffeine – Advise them to avoid or cut down on caffeine consumption.

✓ Sleep position – Advise them to avoid sleeping on their back. They should elevate the head of the bed with bricks to at least a 30° angle. Have one thick or two thin pillows for ideal pharyngeal opening.

✓ Ear plugs – Suggest that their partner wears ear plugs.

✓ Sedatives – Advise that they avoid medications that induce sedation, such as sleeping tablets.

✓ Occupation – Advise them to avoid working with machinery.

✓ DVLA – Those diagnosed with moderate or severe OSA and sleepiness affecting driving must not drive, and they must notify the DVLA. Grade 1 requires the three-yearly confirmation of control of symptoms, and grade 2 requires this annually. Those with mild OSA can drive once the symptoms are controlled. If they have had symptoms for more than three months, they must inform the DVLA.

### *Medical*

✓ Nasal congestion – Offer beclomethasone nasal spray (two puffs bd) or ipratropium bromide nasal spray (two puffs once per night [on]) to treat symptomatic nasal congestion.

✓ Retrognathia – Consider a mandibular-advancement device.

## Referral

→ Respiratory – Refer the patient for sleep studies to confirm the diagnosis and for continuous positive airway pressure (CPAP) therapy.

→ ENT – Refer them if there is an ENT-related problem (e.g. enlarged tonsils, nasal polyps or an obstructive septal deviation).

→ When to refer patients with OSA – If the ESS >10, the patient is experiencing sleepiness in dangerous situations, or the ESS is normal in combination with symptoms associated with obstructive sleep apnoea-hypopnoea syndrome (OSAHS), then this should prompt referring the patient to a sleep service.

## Safety Netting

» Follow-up – If the symptoms persist or the patient feels drowsy in the morning, review in two to four weeks.

## References

British Thoracic Society (2018). *BTS position statement driving and obstructive sleep apnoea (OSA)*. https://sleep-apnoea-trust.org/wp-content/uploads/2020/08/BTS-Position-Statement-on-Driving-Obstructive-Sleep-Apnoea-OSA-2018.pdf

National Institute for Health and Care Excellence (2015). *Obstructive sleep apnoea syndrome*. https://cks.nice.org.uk/topics/obstructive-sleep-apnoea-syndrome/

Scottish Intercollegiate Guidelines Network (2003). *Management of obstructive sleep apnoea/hypopnoea syndrome (OSAHS) in adults.*

# Halitosis

Halitosis is the medical term for bad breath, which is a common problem experienced by patients (it is estimated up to 50% of people suffer with this). Although it is not usually a sign of a sinister disease, the symptom may have a significant impact on the patient's work life and relationships. Usually, the source is located in the oral cavity and is due to poor oral hygiene, food impaction, tongue coating or periodontal disease. It is of note that, while it is common, it should be distinguished from halitophobia (the fear of bad breath in the absence of any). Family members or a partner's opinion should be sought to confirm the presence of the problem.

## History

» Focused questions

› Ask when it started and how long it has been going on for.

› Timing – Ask if it is worse first thing in morning after waking or worse between meals.

› Smell – Ask what the smell is like (fish or sweet).

› Triggers – Ask what makes it better (mouthwash) or worse (foods).

› Diet – Ask what types of foods they eat.

› Lifestyle – Ask if they smoke or drink alcohol.

› Dental hygiene – Ask how often they brush their teeth, and if they floss regularly.

» Differentials questions

› Gingivitis – Ask if their gums bleed after brushing their teeth.

› Tonsillitis – Ask if they have a sore throat, fever or swollen cervical LNs.

› Sinusitis – Ask if there is a nasal blockage and/or nasal discharge, a reduced sense of smell, or facial pain.

› GORD – Ask if there is burning after eating foods or when hungry, a bitter taste, or excess saliva in the mouth.

› Pharyngeal pouch – Ask if there is a bulge in the side of the neck, and if they bring up undigested food.

» Past history – Ask if they have had DM, liver disease or a hiatus hernia. Ask if they have seen a dentist (gum disease).

» Drug history – Ask if they have taken any disulfiram, melatonin, phenothiazines, mycophenolate or isosorbide dinitrate.

» Social history – Ask if they smoke, drink alcohol or take recreational drugs; ask what their occupation is; and ask what their diet is like.

## Examination

» ENT

› Assess for halitosis subjectively by smelling the patient's breath. Advise the patient to pinch their nose and then breathe out (if halitosis is present, then it is likely oral). Then advise them to breathe through the nose only (if halitosis is present, then it has a sinus/nasal origin).

› Inspection – Check for ill-fitting dentures, poor dental hygiene (gum hypertrophy or bleeding gums), tonsillitis and sinusitis. Check the tongue, buccal mucosa, palate and floor of the mouth.

› Palpation – Palpate the sinuses for any tenderness (sinusitis). Palpate the floor of mouth and buccal sulci (salivary problems).

## Investigations

*Not routinely needed*

» Bloods – HbA1c (DM) and LFTs.

» Urine – Dipstick for ketones.

» Stools – Check for H. pylori.

» Specialist – OGD if no cause is found, barium swallow (pharyngeal pouch) and nasal endoscopy.

## Management

*Conservative*

✓ Advise the patient to avoid certain foods that may perpetuate the problem, including onions, garlic, curry/spices, radishes, cheese, fizzy drinks, Brussels sprouts and cauliflower.

✓ Advise them to stop chewing betel or tobacco.

✓ Recommend smoking-cessation. Refer them to a smoking-cessation clinic if necessary.

✓ Advise them to stop drinking alcohol.

✓ Oral hygiene – Advise them to do the following:

› Brush their teeth at least twice a day and floss between their teeth.

› Clean the back of their tongue with a scraper or toothbrush.

› Gargle regularly using mouthwash (two to three times daily).

› Ensure their dentures are left out at night.

› Chew gum regularly to increase the amount of saliva in the mouth.

*Medical*

✓ Offer chlorhexidine 0.2% to reduce the formation of dental plaque.

✓ Dry mouth – Offer artificial salivary substitutes (mucin spray or lozenge) for xerostomia.

✓ H. pylori – Treat if present. *See Dyspepsia section, page 124.*

## Referral

→ Advise the patient to see a dentist if there is evidence of gum disease.

→ Refer them to ENT for recurrent tonsillitis, sinonasal disease or a pharyngeal pouch.

→ Refer them to a psychologist if halitophobia is suspected.

*References*

National Institute for Health and Care Excellence (2019). *Halitosis.* https://cks.nice.org.uk/topics/halitosis/

Singh, V.P., Malhotra, N., Apratim, A. and Verma, M. (2017). *Assessment and Management of Halitosis. Dental Update, 42(4).* https://doi.org/10.12968/denu.2015.42.4.346

# Epistaxis

The nasal mucosa is highly vascularised, making it prone to bleeding. Epistaxis can be anterior or posterior. Anterior epistaxis is more common. The anterior part of the nasal septum is made up of the Kiesselbach plexus / Little's area (arteries). The arteries that make up the Kiesselbach plexus / Little's area include the anterior ethmoidal, sphenopalatine, greater palatine and superior labial arteries.

## Risk Factors

- Haematological disorders; e.g. thrombocytopaenia
- Drugs; e.g. anticoagulants/antiplatelets
- Vasculitis
- Upper respiratory infection
- Trauma
- Oro-facial malignancy
- HTN

## History

» Simple epistaxis is usually transient/acute/bilateral and small in volume.

» The patient might complain of a preceding URTI with a cough precipitating epistaxis.

» Benign/malignant epistaxis would be subacute/chronic, and the patient might complain of facial pain, anosmia, night sweats, weight loss, headaches, rhinorrhoea or double vision.

» Focused questions

  › Ask if it is unilateral or bilateral.

  › Ask if there is any other source of bleeding.

» Past history – Ask if there has been any facial trauma, or if there has been a recent infection/fever.

» Associated history – Ask if there have been changes to smell/vision, or any facial pain.

» Drug history – Ask if they are taking any blood-thinning medication e.g. warfarin.

» Family history – Ask if there is a family history of bleeding.

## Examination

» Vitals – Pulse (tachycardia/atrial fibrillation, which might point to anticoagulation as cause of epistaxis) and BP (hypotension).

» Inspection – Examine both nostrils with a light source to visualise the source of bleeding if it is an anterior bleed.

» Perform a mouth examination to check for any obvious mass.

» CN – Examine the CNs to check for visual changes.

» Other – Perform an otoscopy to check for signs of infection, and a chest examination if an infection is suspected.

## Differentials

➤ Sinusitis

➤ Allergic rhinitis

## Investigations

» Bloods – FBC (anaemia) and coagulation (clotting disorders).

» Orifice test – OGD/colonoscopy if there is haematemesis or PR bleed.

» ECG – Might see tachycardia if there is haemodynamic instability.

» Specialist – CT facial bones/sinus and nasal endoscopy.

## Management

✓ Acute/small, resolved epistaxis can usually be managed in primary care.

✓ Ensure the patient is haemodynamically stable. If not, admit them to hospital.

✓ If the source of the bleeding cannot be visualised in primary care, it means there may be posterior epistaxis, and the patient should be admitted to hospital.

### Conservative

✓ Advise the patient to lean forwards, pinch their nose and open their mouth for about 15 minutes.

✓ On discharge, advise the patient to avoid lifting heavy objects, strenuous exercise and blowing their nose.

### Medical

✓ If the bleeding stops with first aid, the patient can be discharged with topical antiseptics to prevent crusting. First-line treatment is naseptin (chlorhexidine and neomycin) qds for 10 days. Mupirocin (bd/tds for five days) can be used if they are allergic to naseptin.

### Surgical

✓ If bleeding can't be stopped after 15 minutes and the source can be seen, the next step is nasal cautery if it can be tolerated. Otherwise, nasal packing can be used instead.

## Referral

→    Refer the patient to ENT if they have/are any of the following:

  ›    Recurrent epistaxis

  ›    Aged >50 years

  ›    Chinese nationals

  ›    History of telangiectasia

  ›    Signs of cancer, such as lymphadenopathy

  ›    Facial pain or proptosis

---

*References*

National Institute for Health and Care Excellence (2019). *Epistaxis (nosebleeds)*. https://cks.nice.org.uk/topics/epistaxis-nosebleeds/

# Quinsy

Quinsy is also known as a peritonsillar abscess and, in most cases, it occurs as a complication of acute tonsillitis. Cultures normally reveal a mixed culture containing Streptococcus pyogenes, Staphylococcus aureus or Haemophilus influenza. The majority of cases begin as acute tonsillitis, which then leads to peritonsillitis, and this, in turn, leads to the formation of a peritonsillar abscess.

## Risk Factors

➤ Aged 5–25 years

➤ A history of infectious mononucleosis or acute tonsillitis.

## *History*

» Associated history – Ask if there is any dysphagia or trismus, earache (referred pain), headache and general malaise, any drooling or any fever.

» Past history – Ask if they have a recent or current history of tonsillitis or infective mononucleosis.

## Examination

» Examination may be difficult due to trismus; there may be a strong odour noted from the mouth.

» LNs – Check for tender, enlarged ipsilateral cervical LNs.

» Inspection – Check the throat for the unilateral bulging of the tonsils. Look for pus/exudate inside the cheeks (buccal mucosa). Inspect for an oedematous uvula, which is displaced downwards by the infected tonsillitis; this may look like a white grape.

» Other – There may be signs of dehydration in severe cases.

## Differentials

➤ Acute tonsillitis

➤ Epiglottitis

## Investigation

» Usually requires a clinical diagnosis.

» Bloods – FBC, U&E, CRP and LFTs (may be done to assess the inflammatory markers and severity of dehydration).

» Swab culture – May also be obtained from the abscess itself once drained.

## Management

### Medical

✓    IV antibiotics – Amoxicillin/clarithromycin.

✓    The patient may also have IV fluids, depending on their dehydration status.

### Surgical

✓    Abscess drainage – Aspiration with a wide-bore needle under LA. GA may be used in children.

✓    Tonsillectomy – An immediate tonsillectomy is occasionally advised as part of urgent treatment, although this can be done at a later date (six weeks later).

Referral

→    If quinsy is suspected, refer the patient immediately / on the same day to ENT.

---

### References

Knott, L. (2014). *Peritonsillar abscess.* https://patient.info/doctor/peritonsillar-abscess

National Institute for Health and Care Excellence (2018). *Sore throat – acute.* https://cks.nice.org.uk/topics/sore-throat-acute/

# 9

# Ophthalmology

## Red Eye

The term 'red eye' refers to the reddish appearance of the eye that may be caused by infection, inflammation or allergy. It is an extremely common problem that presents regularly in both the primary- and emergency-care settings. It is usually non-life threatening, but may represent underlying systemic disease and illness. Any of the structures of the eye may be implicated, such as the conjunctiva, sclera, episclera or uvea, and a clear history of symptoms and onset must be taken to make a discernible diagnosis.

### Differentials of Red Eye

➤ Unilateral – Acute angle-closure glaucoma, corneal ulceration, subconjunctival haemorrhage, foreign body and arc-welder's eye

➤ Bilateral – Conjunctivitis, episcleritis, scleritis, blepharitis, anterior uveitis and foreign body

### *History*

» Focused questions

> Ask when they first noticed the red eye and how long it has been going on for (hours/days).

> Ask which eye (one or both) is affected, and if the eyelids or eyelashes are affected (blepharitis).

> Ask about the onset (sudden indicates glaucoma or subconjunctival haemorrhage, and gradual indicates uveitis or conjunctivitis).

> Ask what the relieving factors (sleep, washing eyes or a dark room) and aggravating factors (watching TV, reading, pollen, dust and coughing) are.

» Associated history

> Ask if it is painful (uveitis, glaucoma, corneal ulcer or conjunctivitis), if it keeps them up at night (scleritis), and if there is any pain around the eyebrow (glaucoma).

> Ask if there is any fever, sweats or shakes.

›　　Ask if there is a rash (herpes).

›　　Ask if there is any nausea or vomiting (glaucoma).

›　　Ask if there are any visual disturbances (photophobia indicates uveitis, glaucoma or an ulcer, and blurred vision indicates uveitis, glaucoma or scleritis).

›　　Ask if there has been any trauma or injuries to the eye.

»　Past history

›　　Medical – Ask if they have had AS, RA, IBD, sarcoidosis, SLE or polyarteritis nodosa, or if they have had a chronic disease such as DM or HTN (subconjunctival haemorrhage).

›　　Ophthalmological – Ask if they have had any eye operations or a history of uveitis.

›　　Contact lenses – Ask if they sleep with contact lenses in (ulcer), how often they wash the contact lenses and if they routinely follow lens hygiene recommendations.

›　　Glasses – Ask when their last eye test was.

»　Family history – Ask if there is a family history of glaucoma.

»　Drug history – Ask if they have taken any eye drops, anti-coagulants (haemorrhage), high-dose steroids (glaucoma), amiodarone or anti-TB drugs (optic neuropathy).

»　Social history – Ask what their occupation is, who lives with them at home, and if they smoke or drink alcohol.

## RED FLAGS

Sudden onset of severe pain, photophobia, a fixed mid-sized pupil, loss of vision, zoster skin rash or high-velocity injuries.

## Differentials Diagnosis

| Acute closed-angle glaucoma | Occlusion to the angle of the eye resulting in a sudden increased intraocular pressure. Often seen in those >50 years, those with hypermetropia (long-sightedness) and females of a Southeast Asian descent. Associated with a family history of the condition. Presents with acute, severe pain in the orbit, reduced acuity with halos around lights, nausea, vomiting and a headache. OE: fixed, unreactive, semi-dilated pupil that is hard on palpation, and a hazy cornea. |
| --- | --- |

| Conjunctivitis | Inflammation of the conjunctiva. The commonest cause of red eye. A gritty feeling or itchy (allergic) sensation in the eye. Infective cause often presents with purulent, mucoid discharge and with the sticking together of the eyelids. Allergic reaction caused by pollen, dust, cats, etc. |
|---|---|
| Uveitis | Inflammation of the iris and ciliary body. Mainly affects the young or middle-aged patients, and is more common in human leukocyte antigen (HLA) B27 positive patients (RA or AS). Presents with pain that is worse on reading, photophobia and reduced acuity. Often seen as a patient who is unresponsive to treatment for conjunctivitis. OE: pupil may be small and irregular, with redness around the corneal edge (ciliary injection). |
| Subconjunctival haemorrhage | Due to the rupture of a conjunctival vessel between the sclera and conjunctiva. May be due to trauma, such as sneezing, coughing or scratching. Often associated with raised BP and warfarin use. OE: painless, unilateral red eye that does not cover the cornea. |
| Corneal ulceration | Causes an acutely painful red eye with reduced acuity. Often feels as if a foreign body is in the eye. Can experience blurred vision and photophobia. Seen with contact lens use, trauma or injection. OE: often has circumcorneal injection, but the conjunctiva can be inflamed (keratoconjunctivitis). Keratitis of white/grey patches on the cornea. Fluorescein reveals an ulcer. |
| Scleritis | Inflammation of the sclera. Presents with a severe, painful eye, which is worse at night and with the eventual loss of vision. Can be bilateral or unilateral with diffuse redness. Associated with autoimmune conditions (RA, AS, SLE and IBD) or infections (herpes zoster virus [HZV], TB or syphilis). More common in >40-year-olds and women. |
| Episcleritis | Inflammation of the episclera. Often unilateral and self-limiting. Patients can have only mild irritation of the eye with redness and normal acuity. |

## Examination

»   Vitals – BP, pulse and temperature.

»   Inspection – Inspect the conjunctiva, cornea, sclera and lids. Inspect the pupil size and shape. Inspect the reflexes (fixed, semi-dilated and not reactive to light indicates glaucoma; small and irregular indicates anterior uveitis; and chemosis indicates conjunctivitis).

»   Palpation – If indicated, press on the eyeballs (rock hard indicates glaucoma).

»   Neurological – Consider visual fields and acuity, and perform a CN examination (CNs 3, 4 and 6).

## Investigations

» Bloods – Not routinely required; ESR and CRP with the Rh factor if a systemic cause is suspected.

» Swabs – MC&S (viral, bacterial and chlamydia).

» Specialist – Slit-lamp fluorescein staining (FB or corneal ulcer) and IOP measurements.

## Management

*Treat the underlying cause*

### Allergic conjunctivitis

#### Conservative

✓ Advise the patient to avoid allergens.

#### Medical

✓ Offer topical antihistamines (xylometazoline, azelastine, olopatadine, etc.). Other treatments include sodium cromoglycate and nedocromil. Avoid steroid drops (risk of glaucoma or cataracts).

### Infective conjunctivitis

#### Conservative

✓ Often self-limiting (three to five days). Suggest bathing the eyes with clear water or OTC eye drops (hypromellose). Advise that they can wash the eye with wet cotton wool. They should avoid wearing contact lenses during the illness. The infection can be contagious, so advise them to wash their hands, not to share towels and to avoid contact with children.

#### Medical

✓ If it is bacterial, offer chloramphenicol or fusidic acid eye drops for 7–10 days.

### Acute glaucoma

#### Conservative

✓ Advise them to avoid using a computer or watching the TV in dim or low-lit rooms.

#### Medical

✓ Refer the patient urgently to an ophthalmologist and advise that they avoid wearing an eye patch (a dilated pupil worsens the symptoms).

✓ Pilocarpine for pupillary constriction and acetazolamide to reduce IOP are usually given by the hospital.

## Uveitis/Scleritis

### Medical

✓ Refer them urgently to an ophthalmologist for consideration of steroid or antibiotic drops. They are not to be treated in primary care.

## Corneal injury

✓ Foreign body – Remove the foreign body if possible. Irrigate the eye with water or 0.9% saline. Offer pain relief and topical antibiotics to prevent infection. All patients with high-velocity injuries (e.g. hammering, glass or darts) should be referred as an emergency.

✓ Chemical – Remove the contact lens. Irrigate the eye immediately with water or 0.9% saline for 15 minutes. Refer them for an emergency assessment.

## Corneal ulceration

✓ Refer the patient urgently to an ophthalmologist to establish the type and treatment.

## Subconjunctival haemorrhage

### Conservative

✓ Usually self-limiting. Consider artificial tears to reduce mild irritation.

## Blepharitis

### Conservative

✓ Advise them on good lid hygiene. They should use a cloth warmed in hot water that is applied to the closed eyelid for 10 minutes. They should clean the eyelids every morning with a cleanser / cooled boiled water and a cotton bud.

### Medical

✓ Consider topical antibiotics if there are signs of infection.

## Safety Netting

» Review after two to four weeks if symptoms are not improving. If there is any deterioration or loss of vision, advise them to attend eye casualty / emergency department.

### References

National Institute for Health and Care Excellence (2017). *Glaucoma: diagnosis and management*. https://www.nice.org.uk/guidance/ng81

# Loss of Vision

Loss of vision describes the alarming symptom of the complete or partial loss of sight. It may occur acutely or progress gradually over time, affecting one eye or both. It is an extremely distressing and debilitating symptom, as vision is an integral part of our sensory perception. Visual disorders may affect the sharpness or clarity of a patient's vision, restrict their visual fields, or reduce their ability to perceive colour.

Blindness is defined as a person having a visual acuity of less than 3/60, while partial sightedness is an acuity between 3/60 and 6/60.

## Differentials of Loss of Vision

> Sudden onset – Retinal artery (central or branch) or retinal vein occlusion, retinal detachment, optic neuritis, acute closed-angle glaucoma, vitreous haemorrhage, anterior ischaemic optic neuropathy (AION) (secondary to temporal arteritis) and wet macular degeneration

> Gradual onset – Cataract, diabetic retinopathy, chronic (open-angle) glaucoma and dry macular degeneration

## *History*

» Focused questions

› Loss of vision – Ask when they first noticed it, how long it has been going on for, and whether they cannot see anything at all or if it is just blurred.

› Site – Ask if it is unilateral/bilateral, in the central part of vision (macular degeneration or optic neuritis) or in the peripheral vision.

› Size – Ask if there are problems with colour vision (red desaturation). Ask if they have lost sight in a small part of their vision (optic neuritis, age-related macular degeneration [AMD] or migraine), half of it (CVA) or all of it (vessel occlusion, haemorrhage or migraine). Ask if they can see around the periphery of both eyes (retinitis pigmentosa, glaucoma or pituitary tumour). Ask if they see any zigzag lines or have a headache (aura with migraine).

› Onset – Ask if it was sudden (glaucoma, haemorrhage or TIA) or came on gradually (AMD or cataract).

› Timing – Ask if it is persistent (vessel occlusion or CVA), or if it comes and goes (migraine or TIA).

» Associated history

› Pain – Ask if there is any pain (glaucoma or optic neuritis), what the pain is like (gritty, boring or an ache), and if there is pain when looking at lights (migraine or closed-angle glaucoma).

› Visual disturbances – Ask if they have had any visual disturbances (including photophobia), flashing lights or floaters; if so, ask if they have happened suddenly with no pain.

> › Other – Ask if they have any fever, rash (herpatic keratitis), nausea, vomiting (glaucoma) or trauma.

» Past history

> › Medical – Ask if they have had DM, BP, AF or migraines.

> › Ophthalmological operations – Ask if they have had a cataract removal or AMD.

> › Corrective lenses – Ask if they wear contact lenses, and if so, ask how often they clean them. Ask if they wear glasses, when their last eye test was, and if they short-sighted (open-angle glaucoma or retinal detachment) or long-sighted (closed-angle glaucoma).

» Family history – Ask if they have a family history of glaucoma, retinitis pigmentosa or migraines.

» Drug history – Ask if they have taken any eye drops (high-dose steroids may cause glaucoma; amiodarone and anti-TB drugs may cause optic neuropathy) or COCP (migraine).

» Social history – Ask what their occupation is, who is at home, what their hobbies are, if they smoke or drink alcohol, and if they drive.

## RED FLAGS

Sudden onset of severe pain or acute loss of vision.

## Differential Diagnosis

| | |
|---|---|
| Acute closed-angle glaucoma | Occlusion to the angle of the eye resulting in sudden increased intraocular pressure. Often seen in those >50 years, hypermetropic females of Southeast Asian descent. Associated with a family history of the condition. Presents with acute, severe pain in the orbit, reduced acuity with halos around lights, nausea, vomiting and a headache. OE: fixed, unreactive semi-dilated pupil that is hard on the palpation of the pupil, and a hazy cornea. |
| AMD | The most common cause of loss of vision in those >50 years. There are two types: 'wet' and 'dry'. It is due to the degeneration of the cells of the macula, which affects the centre of vision. Dry is more common and is slowly progressive, giving rise to problems recognising faces or written text. Wet is more acute and is due to a haemorrhage from choroidal neovascularisation, which can lead to rapid loss of vision. OE: drusen (yellow deposits) and increased pigment. |

| Cataract | This is the clouding of the lens in the eye, which causes a gradual reduction in the clarity of vision. Age is the most common cause, but it may be accelerated due to trauma, medications and DM. OE: lack of red reflex in the affected eye. |
| --- | --- |
| Vessel occlusion | Retinal vein occlusions are usually due to thrombus formation, and are associated with DM, BP, raised cholesterol and obesity. Patients present with more gradual, painless, unilateral deterioration of their vision. OE: dilated vessels and increased tortuosity with dot-and-blot haemorrhages.<br><br>Retinal artery occlusions are associated with the same conditions and also present with more acute, painless loss of vision. OE: disc pallor, silver wiring, cherry-red spot and optic disc oedema on fundoscopy. Note that temporal arteritis is a rare cause of retinal artery occlusion that must be considered. |
| Retinal detachment | Caused by the detachment if the inner neurosensory retina from the retinal pigment. Causes a progressive and sudden loss of vision, which is often preceded with floaters and flashing lights. If not treated, it can lead to permanent vision loss. May be associated with a very high BP. OE: loss of red reflex, with pale, detached retinal folds on fundoscopy. |

## Examination

» Vitals – BP (raised indicates retinal detachment), pulse and temperature.

» Inspection

› Cornea – Inspect the cornea (ciliary injection indicates acute glaucoma). Consider using a fluorescein stain (corneal ulcer).

› Pupils – Inspect the pupil size and shape (fixed, semi-dilated and not reactive to light indicates glaucoma; small and irregular indicates anterior uveitis). Check the red reflex (cataract) and pupillary reflexes (MS). Check for scotoma and red desaturation (colour plates).

› Fundoscopy – Examine the fundi for pale discs and the cup-disc ratio (DM and BP may cause retinopathy, AMD and retinal detachment).

» Palpation – If indicated, press on the eyeballs (glaucoma).

» Neurological – Consider the visual fields (CVA or glaucoma) and acuity, and do a CN examination (CNs 3, 4 and 6).

» Systemic – Consider a systemic examination if suggested by their past medical history.

› Thyroid – Get the patient to outstretch their hands to check for a tremor. Inspect the eyes for signs of exophthalmos, and check for loss of hair in the outer one-third of the eyebrow, lid lag/retraction and ophthalmoplegia. Inspect and palpate the neck for the presence of a goitre.

> Temporal artery – Check for tenderness, thickening or pulselessness of the temporal artery.

## Investigations

» Bloods – Not routinely required. FBC, TFTs, ESR and CRP.

» MRI – To check for optic neuritis.

» Specialist – Slit-lamp fluorescein staining and IOP measurements.

## Management

✓ Visual aids

> Reading – Advise the patient to use a magnifying glass or large-print books for reading. Brighter lamps may also improve readability. They should also consider learning Braille.

> Gadgets – Advise them to purchase large-button telephones or remote controls to help.

> Talking – Advise them to consider using talking alarms, talking newspaper, audiobooks, and phone apps to read messages and text.

> Walking – Advise them to consider using a long cane or a guide dog for mobilisation.

✓ Driving – If they are registered as partially sighted or blind, they are ineligible to drive. They can only drive if visual acuity is 6/12 (i.e. they can read a number plate at distance of 20m).

✓ Support group – Suggest that they contact the Royal National Institute of Blind People (RNIB) for support.

✓ Registering as blind – A consultant ophthalmologist can register a patient blind or partially sighted by completing a certificate of visual impairment (CVI).

✓ AMD – Advise them to stop smoking, reduce their alcohol intake, increase omega-3 fatty acids via increasing their oily fish and oral antioxidant intake (vitamins A, C and E and zinc), control their BP and avoid direct sunlight by wearing sunglasses.

### Acute glaucoma (See Red Eye section, page 319.)

✓ Vessel occlusion – Advise them to control the risk factors, such as lowering BP, keeping DM controlled, losing weight, reducing cholesterol through diet and exercise, stopping smoking and reducing alcohol intake.

> Arterial – There is no proven treatment to improve vision. Consider commencing aspirin prophylaxis.

✓ Cataract – Advise them to keep DM under tight control. If they have mild cataracts, then advise simple reading aids and brighter lights. Patients may need a stronger prescription for glasses.

## Referral

→ AMD – Refer them to a low-vision clinic in the hospital for vision rehabilitation. For wet AMD, refer them to an ophthalmologist to consider laser treatment, anti vascular endothelial growth factor (VEGF) injections or surgery.

→ Retinal detachment – Refer them urgently to an ophthalmologist. Advise them to keep their BP well controlled.

→ Vessel occlusion

  › Arterial – If it presents early, refer them to the ophthalmologist an as emergency for immediate management.

  › Venous – Refer them to an ophthalmologist to consider laser treatment, steroid injections or anti-VEGF injections to the macular area.

  › Cataract – Once the cataract is mature, refer them for cataract surgery. They may need to wear glasses lifelong after the operation.

## Safety Netting

» Review in two to four weeks if the symptoms are not improving. If there is any deterioration or loss of vision, advise them to attend the emergency department.

### *References*

Driver & Vehicle Licensing Agency (2016). *Visual disorders: assessing fitness to drive.* Gov.uk. https://www.gov.uk/guidance/visual-disorders-assessing-fitness-to-drive

# Chalazion

A chalazion (also known as a meibomian cyst) is a common condition that affects the eyelid (usually the upper one). The meibomian glands are a set of glands that run along the eyelid margin. They produce meibum to help lubricate the eye. The obstruction of the gland means that the meibum cannot escape into tears, and may expand into a cyst and leak into the eyelid tissue. This triggers an inflammatory reaction against the meibum, which subsides with time. Consequently, the meibomian cyst often becomes painless and non-tender. Clinically, it is difficult to distinguish between a chalazion and a hordeolum (stye). However, the chalazion tends to be less painful and may be a larger swelling.

## Symptoms of a Chalazion

➤ They are most commonly found on the upper eyelid due to the increased number and length of meibomian glands present in the upper lid

➤ Usually 2–8mm in diameter

➤ Can affect one or both eyes

➤ They may rupture through the skin

➤ Vision is normal unless the cyst is especially large and causes obstructive visual changes

## Risk Factors

➤ Chronic blepharitis

➤ Seborrhoeic dermatitis

➤ Rosacea

➤ Pregnancy

➤ DM

➤ Elevated serum cholesterol

➤ Chronic hordeola (styes)

## *History*

» Focused questions

› Ask if there have been any changes in visual acuity.

› Ask if they have been exposed to any chemicals or toxins.

» Past history – Ask if they have had any recent viral infections, frequent skin infections, any lid trauma, significant allergies or recent antibiotic use.

## Examination

» Palpation – A chalazion will feel firm, non-erythematous, non-fluctuant and non-tender. However, a large or acute chalazion may be tender as a consequence of the size.

» Chalazia are more common on the upper lid.

## RED FLAGS

» Recurrent chalazia on the same site can be suggestive of meibomian gland carcinoma.

» A firm, warm, tender, erythematous, oedematous eyelid can be suggestive of associated periorbital or orbital cellulitis.

» An infection anterior to the orbital septum is periorbital cellulitis. Periorbital cellulitis does not affect eye movements, or cause visual impairment, protrusion of the eyeball or any oedema of the conjunctiva. The patient may complain of general malaise and a fever.

» An infection posterior to the orbital septum is orbital cellulitis. This infection involves the deep, soft tissue around the eyeball. Patients will complain of severe pain, eyeball protrusion, visual impairment, and painful or limited eye movements. The patient will also have general malaise, headache and a fever.

## Differentials

➤ Stye
➤ Blepharitis
➤ Dacryocystitis
➤ Malignant eyelid tumours

## Management

*Conservative*

✓ Chalazions are usually self-limiting, so it is important to reassure the patient.

✓ Advise patients to do the following:

› Apply a warm compress to the affected eye for 15 minutes up to five times a day. This will help with draining of the contents of the cyst.

› Gently massage the chalazion after the application of the warm compress (to aid with expression of the cyst's contents). This should be done in the direction of the eyelashes using clean fingers or a cotton bud.

## Referral

→    If the chalazion persists for more than four to six weeks, refer them to an
     ophthalmologist.

→    Arrange an urgent hospital admission if there are signs and symptoms of
     orbital cellulitis or symptoms to suggest malignancy.

*References*

Lowth, M. (2016). *Chalazion. Patient Info.* https://patient.info/eye-care/swollen-eyelid/chalazion

# Pterygium

A pterygium is a benign, raised, triangular or wedge-shaped growth of conjunctiva tissue. It usually occurs on the side of the eye nearest to the nose. In addition, if left, it may grow over the cornea in a triangular manner and grow large enough to affect vision (rare). A pterygium usually develops in individuals who have been living in a hot, dry climate, and it may be the eyes' response to long-term exposure to sunlight, and/or chronic eye irritation from a dry climate.

## Risk Factors

➤ Chronic/long-term exposure to ultraviolet (UV) light (always ask patients about their occupation), which is the highest known risk factor

➤ Age (highest prevalence in patients >40 years)

➤ Male

➤ Human papilloma and Epstein-Barr virus infection

## History

» It is usually asymptomatic; patients may just have cosmetic concerns.

» The patient may present with a red eye after suddenly noticing something on their eye.

» The patients may present with visual disturbances, such as blurred vision resulting from encroachment on the pupillary area.

» Associated history – Ask if they have had any irritation or tearing (eyes watering).

» Social history – Ask what their occupation is; if their job involves / has involved outdoor work for long hours, particularly in a hot/dry climate; and if they have lived for long periods in other countries.

## Examination

» Inspection – The diagnosis is usually made by just looking at the eye; look for a wing-shaped conjunctival overgrowth onto the corneal surface. It is usually bilateral and often asymmetrical. It is more commonly located on the side nearest to the nose.

» CN examination (CNs 1, 3, 4 and 6) – It may be found that the patient has loss of vision in the affected eye(s), and astigmatism may also be found.

## Differentials

➤ Pinguecula (no corneal involvement)

➤ Pannus

➤ Pseudopterygium

## Investigations

» Slit-lamp examination – This allows the accurate measurement of the nature and extent of the pterygium.

» Fluorescein staining – This may reveal an epithelial breakdown over the surface of the pterygium.

## Management

### Conservative

✓ Advise the patient on UV protection: they should wear a brimmed hat and tinted lenses. This reduces the risk of progression.

### Medical

✓ Consider applying topical ocular lubricants or steroids depending on the findings:

› Ocular lubricants for symptomatic relief – Hypromellose ophthalmic (two drops into the affected eye(s) every hour when required) or carmellose ophthalmic (two drops into affected eye(s) every four hours when required).

› Prescribe topical steroids alongside ocular lubricants if there is associated inflammation: fluorometholone ophthalmic (0.1%), one to two drops in the affected eye(s) two to four times a day.

### Surgical

✓ If they have any visual changes, refer for surgery as first-line treatment.

✓ If there is recurrent and significant irritation, despite first-line medical treatment, then surgical intervention is indicated.

✓ Simple excision is the most straightforward and common technique used. However, it should be noted that recurrence rates over 33% have been reported.

## Referral

» Refer them to an ophthalmologist if they are still symptomatic after medical treatment, or have cosmetic concerns or vision changes.

### References

College of Optometrists (2017). *Pterygium.* https://www.college-optometrists.org/guidance/clinical-management-guidelines/pterygium.html

# Female Health

## Menorrhagia and Dysmenorrhoea

Menorrhagia is the medical term for heavy periods. It is usually defined as the loss of more than 80mls of blood during the menstrual cycle. On average, a woman's period lasts for between two and five days. Periods that last for more than seven days are considered abnormal. In 60% of cases, no abnormality can be found, and this is termed dysfunctional uterine bleeding (DUB). Patients often complain of the increased use of sanitary towels and tampons, flooding or the passing of clots. Bleeding associated with secondary dysmenorrhoea (painful cramping) that occurs several days before the onset of menstruation may be indicative of fibroids, endometriosis, adenomyosis or ovarian tumours.

### Risk Factors for Endometrial Cancer

➤ Increased age – The average age of those with this cancer is 61.

➤ Hereditary nonpolyposis colorectal cancer (HNPCC) or Lynch syndrome. Lifetime risk of 40%

➤ Obesity

➤ Nulliparity

➤ DM

➤ PCOS

### *History*

» Focused questions

›   Menorrhagia – Ask when the heavy periods started, how long they last for and on which days they are the heaviest. Ask how many tampons / sanitary towels are being used each day, and if they are using more than normal. Ask if there is any flooding or soiling of the underwear with blood, including any clots.

›   Cycle – Ask how regular the periods are, how many days they last for, when their last menstrual period (LMP) was and how old they were when their periods began.

» Associated history

› Pain – Ask about pain during the period, when it occurs in the cycle, if the pain moves anywhere and how long it lasts for. Ask about dyspareunia.

› Anaemia – Ask if they have been feeling tired recently, and if they have had any SOB.

› Also enquire about thyroid-related symptoms, bloating, bowel symptoms and fever.

» Sexual – Ask if they have had any recent UPSI or vaginal discharge.

» Contraception – Ask if they have a coil in place, have an implant or take the POP.

» Smear history – Ask if they are up to date and what the last result was.

» Past history – Ask if they have had any fibroids, thyroid issues or clotting disorders.

» Surgical history – Ask if they have had a hysterectomy or hysteroscopy.

» Drug history – Ask if they have taken tamoxifen, HRT, warfarin or risperidone.

» Social history – Ask if they smoke.

» Family history – Ask if they have a family history of any bleeding disorders, ovarian cancer, endometriosis or HNPCC.

## RED FLAGS

Postcoital bleeding (PCB), intermenstrual bleeding (IMB), post-menapausal bleeding (PMB) or weight loss.

## Examination

» Vitals – BP (hypotension), pulse (tachycardia), temperature and BMI.

» Abdomen – Inspect the hands for signs of koilonychia (iron deficiency). Palpate the abdomen, particularly the lower segment, for any tenderness or guarding. Consider a PR examination if it is not clear where the blood is coming from. Examine for ascites (ovarian cancer).

» Pelvic exam – Visualise the cervix with a speculum. Look for any polyps. Inspect the vulva for irritation, ulceration, swelling or Bartholin's cyst. Attempt to palpate the uterus as well as the adnexa for masses or pain (salpingitis). Palpate the cervix for masses or tenderness (excitation). Ballot the uterus between the opposing fingers of your two hands to feel for fibroids or endometrial carcinoma.

» Thyroid exam – Perform a thyroid exam if clinically indicated.

## Investigations

» Bloods – FBC and ferritin (anaemia); TFTs; coagulation screen if there is a family history of bleeding disorders, etc.; CA125 (ovarian cancer); hormone profile; CRP (PID); and a pregnancy test.

» High vaginal swab (HVS) – Swab for STIs.

» USS – Pelvic / transvaginal (TV) USS for endometrial or ovarian cancer, fibroids, or structural abnormality.

## Differential Diagnosis

| Condition | Characteristic features |
|---|---|
| DUB | Represents 50% of complaints. No pathology found. |
| Fibroids | Benign uterine tumours. Often seen in Afro-Caribbean women in their 40s. Presents with menorrhagia, painful colicky periods, and they can press on the bladder causing urinary frequency or retention. Occasionally causes infertility. There may be a uterine mass on examination. |
| Endometrial polyps | Endometrial hyperplasia forming a mass of the inner lining of the uterus that often is pedunculated into the uterine cavity. Presents with menorrhagia, IMB or postmenopausal bleeding (PMB). |
| PID | Caused by an ascending STI (chlamydia or gonorrhoea) from the cervix. Risk factors include a contraceptive intrauterine device (IUD), multiple partners, a lack of barrier contraception and termination of pregnancy (TOP). Presents with lower abdominal pain, deep dyspareunia, purulent discharge and abnormal bleeding (PCB or IMB). OE: low abdominal tenderness with cervical excitation and fever. Complications include infertility and ectopic pregnancy. |
| Endometriosis | Endometrial lining found outside the endometrial cavity. Regresses during pregnancy or menopause. It presents with menorrhagia and dysmenorrhoea, deep dyspareunia, pelvic pain or infertility. |
| Endometrial carcinoma | Often an adenocarcinoma arising from the endometrium. Risk factors include nulliparity, obesity, late menopause (>52 years), HNPCC, tamoxifen and HRT. Presents with PMB. |

## Management

*Conservative*

✓ Advise the patient to keep a detailed menstrual diary regarding symptoms, and the number of pads or tampons used.

*Medical*

✓ Mirena intrauterine system (IUS) – This is the first-line treatment if long-term contraception is also sought. It is most effective in reducing heavy periods. It can cause amenorrhoea.

✓ Tranexamic acid – Take 1g tds for three to five days during heavy periods. Trial for three cycles.

✓ NSAIDs – Naproxen or mefenamic acid (500mg tds). This should be started the day before each period and continue for three to five days. Trial for three cycles. Tranexamic acid and an NSAID can be used concurrently.

✓ COCP – This offers contraception and period control.

✓ Norethisterone – Take 5 mg tds for 10 days. This will stop the bleeding. There is an increased risk of venous thromboembolism (VTE) on taking high doses of norethisterone for a long period of time. This should be avoided in those with obesity, a history of VTE, a family history of VTE and immobile patients. Consider using medroxyprogesterone.

## Referral

→ Refer the patient to gynaecology for any of the following:

› Heavy bleeding affecting the quality of life of the patient.

› If surgery (endometrial ablation or myomectomy) is being considered.

› Persistent iron-deficiency anaemia despite treatment.

→ Refer the patient urgently if they have PCB, IMB, a vulval mass/ulceration or an abdominal mass (not fibroid-like), or if ovarian cancer is suspected.

*References*

National Institute for Health and Care Excellence (2018). *Heavy menstrual bleeding: assessment and management*. https://www.nice.org.uk/guidance/ng88

Pitkin, J. (2007). Dysfunctional uterine bleeding. *The BMJ, 334, 1110*. doi: https://doi.org/10.1136/bmj.39203.399502. BE

# Endometriosis

In women of childbearing age, endometriosis is one of the most common gynaecological conditions. About one in 10 women of reproductive age in the UK have endometriosis. It is characterised by the growth of endometrium-like tissue outside the uterus. Deposits of the endometrium can be found in different areas of the pelvis. This includes the pouch of Douglas, ovaries, peritoneum and the uterosacral ligaments. The condition is associated with menstruation; the hormonal changes in the menstrual cycle induce bleeding, chronic inflammation and scar-tissue formation.

## *History*

- » Focused questions
  - › Ask how long they have had the pelvic pain (for endometriosis, chronic is defined as a minimum of six months of cyclical or continuous pain).
  - › Ask if the pain is it related to their period (dysmenorrhoea), and if it affects daily activities and their quality of life.
  - › Ask if there is any pain during or after sexual intercourse.

- » Associated history – Ask about any period-related or cyclical gastrointestinal symptoms; in particular, painful bowel movements. Ask if there are any cyclical urinary symptoms, including haematuria or dysuria.

## Differentials

- ➤ IBS
- ➤ PID
- ➤ Ovarian cyst torsion
- ➤ Uterine fibroids

## Examination

- » Examination is often normal. However, there may be one of the following:
  - › Posterior fornix or adnexal tenderness.
  - › Palpable nodules in the posterior fornix, or adnexal masses.
  - › Bluish haemorrhagic nodules that are visible in the posterior fornix.

## Investigations

- » The gold standard for a definitive diagnosis is the laparoscopic visualisation of the pelvis.

» However, other less-invasive methods (including USS) may be useful in assisting diagnosis. A pelvic/TV USS helps to exclude the diagnosis of an ovarian endometrioma.

## Management

### Conservative

✓ The management of endometriosis depends on the nature and severity of symptoms, and the need for any future fertility, and it is usually individually based.

✓ Managing pain with analgesia – Advise them to take paracetamol, an NSAID and/or hormonal treatment (COCP or POP) as appropriate.

### Medical

✓ An IUS (levonorgestrel) is quite effective at addressing the symptoms, once it has been used for at least three years.

### Surgical

✓ Surgical management includes ovarian cystectomies (for endometriomas), the removal of infiltrating lesions (which may help to reduce pain linked to endometriosis), adhesiolysis and bilateral oophorectomy (there is often a hysterectomy).

## Referral

→ Refer the patient to secondary care for any of the following:

› Severe, persistent or recurrent symptoms.

› Pelvic signs of endometriosis.

› If the initial management is not helping, not tolerated well or contraindicated.

### References

National Institute for Health and Care Excellence (2020). *Endometriosis.* https://cks.nice.org.uk/topics/endometriosis/

Tidy, C. (2020). *Endometriosis.* https://patient.info/womens-health/pelvic-pain-in-women/endometriosis

# Secondary Amenorrhoea

Amenorrhoea is the absence of a menstrual period in a woman of reproductive age. There are two types of amenorrhoea: primary and secondary. Primary refers to the complete absence of any menstrual flow in a girl >14 years old, along with the absence of secondary sexual characteristics; or the absence of menstruation in a >16-year-old girl. Secondary amenorrhoea refers to women who have had no periods for three to six months, despite previously having normal cycles, in the presence of a negative pregnancy test. It is worth remembering that amenorrhoea is a normal finding in prepubescent girls, during pregnancy and lactation, as well as for postmenopausal women.

## History

» Focused questions

› Ask about their LMP.

› Ask how long they have not had a period for.

› Ask whether or not their periods were regular.

› Ask what the length of their periods was.

› Ask when they had their menarche.

» Sexual history – Ask when they last had UPSI, if they use any contraception and if there is any chance they may be being pregnant.

» Associated history

› Ask if they have any symptoms related to thyroid disease.

› Ask if they have any symptoms related to PCOS: acne, hirsutism, or hair growth on the chest or abdomen.

› Ask if they have any symptoms related to prolactinoma: galactorrhoea, headaches or visual problems.

› Ask if they have any symptoms related to ovarian cancer: weight loss, bloating, constipation or diarrhoea, or urinary symptoms.

› Ask if they have any symptoms related to early menopause, such as hot flushes or vaginal dryness.

› Ask if they have any symptoms related to Asherman's syndrome.

› Ask if they have had any TOPs, including any surgical TOPs.

› Ask if they have any symptoms related to anorexia: appetite or weight loss.

› Ask about their mood.

» Past history – Ask if they have had any radiotherapy or chemotherapy.

» Surgical history – Ask if they have had a dilation and curettage (D&C), endometrial curettage, oophorectomy, endometrial ablation or hysterectomy.

» Drug history – Ask if they have taken methyldopa, cimetidine, opiates, metoclopramide, oral steroids (Cushing's disease), or any forms of contraception, and if so, what type.

» Social history – Ask if they smoke or if they have experienced any stress recently.

## RED FLAGS

Visual changes, galactorrhoea in the absence of a recent delivery, or amenorrhoea (Sheehan's syndrome).

## Differential Diagnosis

| | |
|---|---|
| Anorexia | Affects young girls >16 years old. Low BMI <17.5. Missing meals, vomiting or using laxatives. Obsessed with body image and looking in the mirror. OE: thin, yellow skin, pale conjunctiva, calluses on the knuckles, pallor, low BP and bradycardia. |
| PCOS | Hirsutism, obesity and acne. Irregular periods and fertility problems. |
| Premature menopause | Amenorrhoea in women <40 years old with raised FSH and a family history of premature menopause. Periods that are heavier or lighter than usual, hot flushes, vaginal dryness, irritability, mood swings and decreased libido. |
| Prolactinoma | Headaches, double vision, poor peripheral vision, galactorrhoea and infertility. |
| Ovarian cancer | The fifth most common cause of female cancer. Usually affects those >50 years old. Pelvic pain, bloating, decreased appetite and weight loss. |
| Hypothyroidism | Increased BMI, dry skin, thin hair, feeling cold, reduced reflexes, low BP, bradycardia, low mood, constipation and tiredness. |
| Cushing's disease | Central obesity, skin bruises easily, depression, decreased libido, puffy and red face, and purple striae. |

## Examination

» Vitals – BP and BMI.

» Inspection – Check for secondary sexual characteristics. Also check for the following:

› Turner's syndrome – Webbed neck and wide nipples.

CHAPTER 10 – FEMALE HEALTH

> › PCOS – Look at their fat distribution, for increased hair growth (hirsutism) and for acne.

> › Cushing's disease – Look for central fat obesity, striae, a buffalo hump and bruising.

> › Thyroid – Look for dry skin, midline neck swelling, tremors and sweating. Perform a focused thyroid exam if this is suspected.

» Perform a fundoscopy and check visual fields if a pituitary cause is suspected.

» Complete a breast exam if there is galactorrhoea.

## Investigations

» Urine – Pregnancy test.

» Bloods – TSH, thyroxine (T4) and CA125 (ovarian cancer). Also check for hormones LH, FSH, free testosterone, SHBG and prolactin.

» Imaging – Pelvic/TV USS (PCOS and ovarian cancer) and MRI head/pituitary (adenoma).

### Interpreting hormone levels

| Ovarian failure | Raised FSH and raised LH. |
|---|---|
| PCOS | Normal FSH, mildly raised LH and testosterone (<2.5 nmol). |
| Hypothalamic cause | Normal or low FSH, and normal or low LH. |
| Prolactinoma | If prolactin >1,000mIU/l, suspect a pituitary adenoma or hypothyroidism. |
| Testosterone | If <5nmol/l, investigate for Cushing's disease, congenital adrenal hyperplasia and an androgen-secreting tumour. |

## Management

### Conservative

✓ Anorexia – Advise them to try to increase their weight by eating a balanced diet. Aim for a BMI of 25. They should decrease the amount of exercise they do. Consider referring them to a dietician.

### Medical

✓ Medication – Stop the offending drug if appropriate. Change the POP or remove the Mirena/implant. Consider bone protection if they have low oestrogen levels.

✓ Hypothyroidism – Start thyroxine and monitor their response. It may take six months before their periods are corrected.

✓ Pregnant – *See Antenatal Care section, page 349.*

✓ PCOS – *See Polycystic Ovarian Syndrome section, page 345.*

✓ Premature menopause – *See Menopause section, page 381.*

✓ Infertility – Treat the underlying disorder. *See Infertility section, page 363.*

*Complications*

✓ There is an increased risk of CVD, similar to that found in postmenopausal women.

✓ Low oestrogen levels lead to osteoporosis.

✓ Infertility.

---

## References

National Institute for Health and Care Excellence (2013). *Fertility problems: assessment and treatment.* https://www.nice.org.uk/guidance/cg156

# Polycystic Ovarian Syndrome

PCOS is a common condition in the UK, which affects one in 10 women. It is an endocrine disorder that presents with multiple cysts in the ovaries, along with irregular periods (oligomenorrhoea or amenorrhoea), acne and hirsutism. It is more prevalent in the Southeast Asian population, who usually present earlier and with more prominent symptoms. PCOS has been identified as a significant cause of infertility in women. Patients with PCOS produce excess androgens (hyperinsulinaemia) and have raised LH relative to their FSH.

## Diagnosing PCOS

Patients must have two out of three of these symptoms:

➤ Clinical hyperandrogenism (e.g. hirsutism, acne, male-pattern baldness or alopecia) or elevated levels of total/free testosterone.

➤ Infrequent (less than six to nine menstrual bleeds per year) or no ovulation.

➤ Polycystic ovaries on pelvic/TV USS (>=12 follicles in one ovary, measuring 2–9mm or an ovarian volume 10cm$^3$ or more).

## *History*

» Focused questions

  › Ask when their LMP was; if their periods are irregular, light or absent; how many days they last; and how long these problems have been going on for.

  › Ask if they suffer from acne, and if so, where the spots are.

  › Ask if they have noticed any unusual hair growth on their face or body.

  › Ask if they have found that the hair on their head is thinning.

» Associated history

  › Ask if they are trying to get pregnant, and if so, how long they have been trying. Ask if they have ever been pregnant, and if they have had any terminations or miscarriages.

  › Ask if they have had any problems with their weight.

  › Ask if they have suffered from problems with their mood.

» Past history – Ask if they have ever suffered from raised BP, raised cholesterol or type 2 DM.

» Family history – Ask if there is a family history of PCOS or similar problems.

*When To Suspect PCOS*

Consider PCOS in women <18 who have had two years of irregular periods after menarche. Investigate after one year of irregular cycles. PCOS may cause evidence of insulin resistance (central obesity or acanthosis nigricans around the axilla).

## Examination

» Vitals – BP and BMI.

» Urine – Pregnancy test.

» Inspection – Observe the general habits of the patient and look at their fat distribution. Check for increased hair growth (hirsutism) on the face, chest and lower abdomen. Inspect them for acne (face, back and chest). Inspect the scalp for thinning hair.

## Differential Diagnosis

| Simple obesity | Androgen with or without other symptoms; usually a diagnosis of exclusion. |
|---|---|
| Prolactinoma | Oligo/amenorrhoea, galactorrhoea and increased prolactin levels. |
| Androgen-secreting tumour | High androgen levels, oligo/amenorrhoea, clitoromegaly, extreme hirsutism, male alopecia and striae. |
| Cushing's disease | Oligo/amenorrhoea, HTN, striae, bruising, increased 24-hour urine cortisol. |
| Acromegaly | Often oligo/amenorrhoea, enlarged extremities, coarse features, and raised GH and insulin-like growth factor (IGF). |
| Hypothyroidism | May have oligo/amenorrhoea, a goitre, raised TSH and reduced T4. |
| Premature ovarian failure | Oligo/amenorrhoea, associated autoimmune disorder, raised FSH and reduces oestrodiol. |

## Investigations

» Bloods – Hormonal blood test performed in the first week of the cycle to test for the following:

› LH (<10IU/l).

› FSH (LH:FSH ratio of 3:1).

› SHBG (normal or low).

› Testosterone (<2.5–5nmol/l) – Consider adrenal hyperplasia, Cushing's disease or an androgen-secreting tumour.

> › Prolactin (mildly elevated in PCOS; i.e. <500mU).
>
> › TSH and T4.
>
> › HbA1c and cholesterol.
>
> › Also determine the free androgen index = 100 x (total testosterone / SHBG)

» USS – Polycystic appearance to ovaries (one-third have polycystic ovaries on pelvic/TV USS).

## PCOS and DM

PCOS patients who are obese (BMI >30), have a strong family history of type 2 DM and are >40 years should be recommended to have a diabetic screening due to having an increased risk.

## Management

### Conservative

✓ Lifestyle – Advise them to try to lose weight by eating a balanced diet and increasing exercise. Aim for a BMI <25, consider referring them to a dietician and advise them to stop smoking.

✓ Hirsutism – Advise them to try to lose weight loss, and that they can try cosmetic solutions such as shaving, plucking, bleaching and waxing.

### Medical

✓ Fertility – Offer clomiphene and refer them to secondary care.

✓ Periods – Offer COCP, POP or Mirena if they are not wanting to become pregnant.

✓ Acne

> › Topical – Consider benzoic acid or retinoids, as advised by a dermatologist.
>
> › Oral – Consider COCP or antibiotics (e.g. lymecycline).

✓ Hirsutism – Offer Vaniqa cream (eflornithine). Refer them to secondary care for anti-androgens, spironolactone or finasteride.

✓ Insulin resistance – Offer metformin to help increase insulin sensitivity, improve the frequency of menstruation and improve ovulation rates.

✓ Weight – Consider orlistat.

### Surgical

✓ Laparoscopic ovarian drilling – A simple surgical procedure used as a treatment for fertility symptoms. It lowers testosterone levels and increases FSH, helping to balance the hormones and release an egg.

## Referral

→   Refer the patient to ENT if they show symptoms of sleep apnoea.

## Safety Netting

»   Always review the patient in three months to check their response to treatments. Consider referring them to a gynaecologist if there no response to the first-line treatment.

---

### References

Goodarzi, M. (2020). *Polycystic ovarian syndrome*. https://bestpractice.bmj.com/topics/en-gb/141

Royal College of Obstetricians & Gynaecologists (2014). *Long-term consequences of polycystic ovary syndrome*. https://www.rcog.org.uk/globalassets/documents/guidelines/gtg_33.pdf

# Antenatal Care

Once a woman has fallen pregnant, it is important that they have an early appointment (<10 weeks), as this will provide them with greater chances to participate in screening programmes and help develop a planned package of care. Women who are thought to have an uncomplicated and low-risk pregnancy can be managed using shared-care protocols between midwives and the GP. Those who have complex needs (mental health, multiple miscarriages or a previous stillbirth) or are high risk (HTN, DM or epilepsy) should be overseen by a consultant obstetrician and have access to relevant specialist input as needed.

## History

» Focused questions

› Ask how they feel about their pregnancy.

› Ask when their LMP was. From this, calculate the gestation and estimated date of delivery (EDD) using an obstetric wheel.

EDD = LMP – 3 months + 1 year + 7 days + (cycle length – 28)

Pregnancy

› Ask if they have felt the baby move or kick recently (>=18 weeks).

› Ask if they have noticed any leg swelling or breast tenderness (oedema).

› Ask if they have felt nauseous or vomited. If so, ask if it is worse in the morning (morning sickness).

› Ask if they suffer from burning or a feeling of indigestion in their stomach.

› Abdominal pain – Ask if they have experienced any abdominal pain.

› Mood – Ask how their mood is; if they have been bothered by feeling down, depressed or hopeless; and if they feel nervous, anxious or on edge.

› PV bleeding – Ask if they have had any PV bleeding. If so, ask when it began and how long it was for. Ask if there has been any spotting on their clothes, if they have had to use any sanitary products and if there have been any clots.

» Past history

› Obstetric – Ask if they have had any previous pregnancies, what type of deliveries (spontaneous/induced, Caesarean section, or ventouse/forceps) they have had, if they have had any miscarriages (if so, how many), if they have had any stillbirths, and if they have any history of preeclampsia or preterm babies.

› Medical – Ask if they have had HTN, DM, epilepsy, VTEs, anaemia or thyroid issues.

› Psychiatric – Ask if they have had depression, bipolar disorder or schizophrenia. Ask if they have had any postnatal depression or puerperal psychosis during any previous pregnancies.

» Family history – Ask if there is a family history of DM or HTN, twins, blood disorders or inherited disorders.

» Drug history – Ask if they have taken any OTC folic acid. Ask if they have taken any medications that are contraindicated in pregnancy (tetracyclines, gentamicin, trimethoprim, ciprofloxacin, ACEIs, statins, warfarin, sulphonylureas, retinoids, NSAIDs [third trimester], lithium, chloramphenicol, methotrexate and antiepileptics [valproate]).

» Social history – Ask if they are in a current relationship, who lives at home, what their support networks are like, what their occupation is, and if they smoke, drink alcohol and take recreational drugs.

## Examination

» Vitals – BP and BMI.

» Urine – Dipstick the urine (protein indicates HTN, ketones indicate hyperemesis, and glucose indicates gestational DM).

» Obstetric exam

› Inspection – Look for any previous Caesarean scar, skin changes (linea nigra or striae) and FGM.

› Palpation

- Symphyseal fundal height (SFH) (>24 weeks) – Establish the fundus using the ulnar border of your hand. Measure the SFH with the tape measure blindside up from the fundus to the pubic symphysis. Turn the tape measure to reveal the SFH.

- Position – Place one hand on either side of the uterus and palpate. Locate the foetus's back and limbs, and determine if the lie is longitudinal, transverse or oblique.

- Presentation – Press firmly over the pubic symphysis and establish presentation. Check if it is cephalic or breech.

› Auscultation – Use a sonic aid to listen to the heartbeat (normal foetal HR is 110–160).

## Abdominal Pain in Pregnancy

*First trimester*

» Ectopic pregnancy (amenorrhoea, colicky and shoulder-tip pain)

» Miscarriage (passage of the products of conception and a uterus that is normal size)

*Second trimester*

» Miscarriage

*Third trimester*

» Labour (contractions from 5–10 minutes, and their water breaks)

» False labour (irregular, non-persistent contractions)

» Preterm labour (labour <37 weeks)

» Placental abruption (dark, painful bleeding and a woody, hard uterus)

» Uterine rupture (scarred uterus)

## Bleeding in Pregnancy

*Early (<24 weeks)*

» Miscarriage

» Ectopic pregnancy

» Hydatidiform mole

*Late (>=24 weeks)*

» Antepartum haemorrhage

» Placental abruption

» Placenta praevia

» Uterine rupture

*Scheduled Appointments*

| | |
|---|---|
| 25 weeks (nulliparous women) | Measure SFH, BP and urine. |
| 28–34 weeks | Measure SFH, BP and urine. Offer second screening for anaemia and an injection of the antibody against D antigen (anti-D) if they are Rh negative.<br>Ask if she has a labour and birthing plan. |
| 36–38 weeks | Measure SFH, BP and urine. Check the position of the baby. Offer external cephalic version for breech presentation. Review pelvic/TV USS for placenta previa.<br>Discuss breastfeeding and postnatal care (postnatal depression, baby care and vitamin K for the baby). |
| 40 weeks (nulliparous women) | Measure SFH, BP and urine. |
| 41 weeks | If the patient has not given birth, offer a membrane sweep and/or induction of labour. Measure SFH, BP and urine. |

## Investigations

» Urine – Pregnancy test.

» Bloods – FBC, haemoglobinopathies, blood group and Rh status, Hep B status, HIV, rubella immunity, syphilis, and HbA1c for at-risk patients to exclude gestational DM (risk factors are BMI >30, past medical history of gestational DM, previous baby <4.5kg, family history of DM, and ethnicity). Offer a referral for Down's syndrome screening if it has not been offered already through the antenatal care plan.

» USS – Pelvic/TV USS in the form of a dating USS (10–14 weeks) and anomaly USS (18–21 weeks). Additional USSs offered if there are concerns about the baby's growth.

### Screening for Down's Syndrome

» Risk increases with the following:

  › Maternal age – one in 1,500 in their 20s, one in 800 in their 30s, and one in 100 in their 40s.

  › Past medical history of a Down's syndrome baby.

» Combined test

  › This is a blood test (BHCG and pregnancy-associated plasma protein A [PAPP-A]) that is performed with a nuchal translucency scan (11–13 weeks).

  › The results are expressed as a risk score (low risk or high risk). If this is high risk, the mother will be offered a screening test.

  › Amniocentesis is performed at 15–18 weeks. There is a 1% risk of miscarriage.

  › Chorionic villus sampling is performed at 10 weeks, which permits an earlier TOP if required

## Management

### Conservative

✓ Diet – Advise the patient to avoid food-acquired infections:

  › Listeriosis – They should avoid soft cheese, pâté and unpasteurised milk.

  › Salmonella – They should avoid both eggs (mayonnaise) and meat that are uncooked / partially cooked.

  › Toxoplasmosis – They should wash all fruits and vegetables. They should avoid cleaning a cat litter tray.

  › Caffeine – They should avoid more than 200mg a day (about two mugs of coffee).

  › They should ensure that they eat at least five portions of fruit and vegetables a day, and drink plenty of milk for calcium and vitamin D.

› They should avoid liver due to it having an excess of vitamin A.

› They should avoid swordfish and shark due to it containing methylmercury, though they can have up to four cans (140g) of tuna a week.

✓ Smoking – Offer smoking-cessation advice; NRT is safe, but Champix is contraindicated. Continuing to smoke increases the risk of intrauterine growth retardation and miscarriage.

✓ Alcohol – Advise them to avoid drinking, especially in the first three months. Continuing to drink increases the risk of foetal alcohol syndrome, reduces growth and causes mental retardation.

✓ Exercise – Advise them to take moderate regular exercise, but avoid contact/high-impact sports and scuba diving.

✓ Travel – Advise them that there is an increased risk of DVT if a flight is longer than five hours. They should consider compression hosiery and avoid travelling to malaria-endemic and Zika-virus-affected areas. They should position their seat belt above and/or below their bump, not over it.

✓ Morning sickness – Resolves by 16–20 weeks. Advise them to consider ginger or wrist acupressure.

✓ Heartburn – Give them lifestyle advice such as having small, regular meals and increasing the number of pillows they sleep on. Offer antacids.

✓ Constipation – Advise them to modify their diet (adding bran or wheat). Offer bulk-forming laxatives such as lactulose or macrogol if there is no improvement.

### Medical

✓ Folic acid – Initiate folic acid 400mcg, which is to be taken before conception and until week 12 of the pregnancy. Folic acid 5mg should be given if there is any history of neural tube defects, coeliac disease or sickle cell disease, or they are on anticonvulsants.

✓ Ferrous – Do not offer routine iron supplements.

✓ Vitamin D – Offer vitamin D 10mcg for at-risk groups (at-risk ethnicity, poor diet or BMI >30).

✓ Morning sickness – If this is not managed by conservative means, consider promethazine or cyclizine as the first-line treatment. Second-line treatment is prochlorperazine, metoclopramide (for up to five days maximum) or ondansetron.

✓ Heartburn – Consider omeprazole or ranitidine (unlicensed), if it is too severe to be managed by conservative means.

✓ Immunisation – Consider a rubella immunisation if warranted. Offer the annual flu vaccination (available from October to March). Offer a pertussis vaccination from 16–32 weeks.

✓ Inform them regarding being exempt from prescription costs.

## Referral

→  Illicit drug use – Refer them to a multidisciplinary team (MDT). These patients will require detoxification prior to conception.

→  Depression – For severe depression, consider referring them for CBT.

## Safety Netting

»  If a pregnant woman experiences abdominal pain or PV bleeding, seek medical advice. Seek emergency advice if she experiences a severe headache, blurred vision and vomiting (pre-eclampsia).

---

*References*

National Institute for Health and Care Excellence (2008). *Antenatal care for uncomplicated pregnancies.* https://www.nice.org.uk/guidance/cg62

National Institute for Health and Care Excellence (2014). *Antenatal and postnatal mental health: clinical management and service guidance.* https://www.nice.org.uk/guidance/cg192

# Vaginal Discharge and Sexually Transmitted Infections

Vaginal discharge that is clear or white is often a normal physiological finding that may occur at any time during the monthly cycle. The discharge usually becomes clearer when the woman is ready to ovulate. Women on the pill may not notice this change. The most common causes of a change in discharge include bacterial vaginosis and candidiasis, but it is important to exclude other sexually transmitted and non-infectious causes. There are a number of different causes that may lead to changes, such as ectopy and polyps. It is important to take a thorough history and examine the patient to make a clear diagnosis.

## Pathophysiology

» Candida – Yeast-like fungal infection due to *Candida albicans*, which is not an STI. The most common cause of vaginitis.

» Bacterial vaginosis – Caused by *Gardnerella vaginalis*, which is also not an STI. The most common cause of vaginal infection in women.

» Gonorrhoea – An STI caused by *Neisseria gonorrhoea*. Around 50% of patients with this may be asymptomatic.

» Chlamydia – The most common STI, caused by *Chlamydia trachomatis*. It is a common cause of PID, and can also cause ectopic pregnancy and infertility. About 70% of patients with this are asymptomatic.

» Trichomoniasis – Caused by the flagellate parasite *Trichomonas vaginalis*. This may lead to preterm labour.

» PID – This is usually caused by an STI, including chlamydia and gonorrhoea.

## *History*

» Focused questions

› Ask them to describe the discharge.

› Ask if it is it thick and curdy, like cottage cheese, or if it is thin and frothy.

› Ask what colour it is (clear, white, purulent or blood stained).

› Ask if there is any smell associated with it (e.g. fishy smell).

› Ask if they experience any itching or soreness in the groin area.

› Ask if the discharge is related to their menstrual cycle.

» Associated history

› Ask if they suffer from any abdominal pain, and if so, where.

› Ask if they have experienced any pain during intercourse.

› Ask if they have discomfort or burning when passing urine.

› Ask if they have had any fever.

» Sexual history – Ask if they are sexually active; if they have a regular or casual partner; if their partner is male or female; if they have had vaginal, oral or anal sex; if they have used any condoms; if they or any of their partners have been diagnosed with an STI.

» Menstrual history – Ask when their LMP was, and if their periods are regular, light, heavy or absent.

» Obstetric history – Ask if they are pregnant, and if they have any children.

» Past history – Ask if they have had DM.

» Drug history – Ask if they are taking the pill, if they have taken antibiotics recently, or if they have been on any oral steroids.

## RED FLAGS

Weight loss, intermenstrual bleeding, postcoital bleeding.

## Examination

» Vitals – Pulse and temperature.

» Gynaecological exam

  › Always request a chaperone is present.

  › Abdominal exam – Palpate the abdomen for iliac fossa or suprapubic tenderness.

  › Vaginal exam – Inspect for redness, ulceration or irritation. Palpate for adnexal or cervical tenderness.

  › Speculum – Inspect the cervix for lesions, polyps or a strawberry cervix.

## Differential Diagnosis

| | |
|---|---|
| Candida | Thick, white, cottage-cheese-like discharge with severe pruritus, vulval redness and irritation. Can affect the vulva and groin. Occasionally, there is superficial dyspareunia and dysuria. |
| Bacterial vaginosis | Thin, greyish-white discharge with a distinct fishy odour. |
| Gonorrhoea | There may be associated dysuria and frequency, cervicitis, and a greenish-yellow discharge. |
| Chlamydia | Yellowish discharge, often with lower abdominal pain and urethritis. |

| Trichomoniasis | Profuse, frothy, greenish-yellow discharge with an offensive odour. May also have superficial dyspareunia, itchiness and dysuria. May have a strawberry cervix. |
|---|---|
| PID | Pain on sexual intercourse, vaginal discharge and intermenstrual bleeding are common symptoms. |

## Investigations

» Urine – Pregnancy test and MSU for nucleic acid amplification tests (NAATs).

» Vaginal swabs – Endocervical (chlamydia and gonorrhoea) and HVS (candida and bacterial vaginosis).

» Bloods – HIV, syphilis serology (venereal disease research laboratory [VDRL] test) and hepatitis.

» Specialist – Pelvic/TV USS.

## Management

*Conservative*

✓ Barrier contraception – Educate the patient around using condoms and/or diaphragms.

✓ Candida – Advise them to wear loose-fitting undergarments made of cotton and avoid washing them with biological washing powder.

✓ Advise them to not use perfumed soaps or bubble baths, and to not douche the vaginal area. They should use unscented soaps and water to clean only. Natural live yoghurt may be placed inside the vagina.

*Medical*

✓ Contact tracing – Offer contact tracing, which is often performed at a GUM clinic.

✓ Atrophic vaginitis – Vaginal oestrogen for six months.

✓ Antibiotics

› PID – Ofloxacin 400mg bd plus metronidazole 400mg bd for two weeks. Consider IV if severe.

› Candida – Clotrimazole cream or pessary (200mg for three days or 500mg stat). Alternatively, consider oral fluconazole 150mg stat, or itraconazole 200mg bd for one day. For recurrent thrush, consider oral fluconazole 150mg od for three days, then weekly for six months, or use PV clotrimazole 500mg weekly for six months.

› Bacterial vaginosis – Oral metronidazole 400–500mg bd for five to seven days or 2g stat. Alternatively, consider metronidazole gel od for five days or clindamycin 2% cream od for seven days.

› Trichomoniasis – Metronidazole 400–500mg bd for five to seven days, metronidazole 2g stat, or tinidazole 2g stat.

›   Chlamydia – Doxycycline 100mg bd for seven days or azithromycin 1g stat. Alternatively, consider erythromycin 500mg bd for 14 days or ofloxacin 200mg bd for seven days.

›   Gonorrhoea – Ceftriaxone 500mg IM stat plus azithromycin 1g by mouth (PO) stat. Alternatively, consider cefixime 400mg PO stat plus azithromycin 1g PO stat.

## Safety Netting

»   Consider reviewing the patient in a few weeks after receiving all test results or if symptoms persist. Consider a referral to a GUM specialist if there is no response to first-line treatment.

---

## References

British Association for Sexual Health and HIV (2015). *BASHH CEG guidance on tests for sexually transmitted infections*. https://www.bashhguidelines.org/media/1084/sti-testing-tables-2015-dec-update-4.pdf

Lazaro, N. (2013). *Sexually transmitted infections in primary care*. https://www.rcgp.org.uk/-/media/Files/CIRC/RCGP-Sexually-Transmitted-Infections-in-Primary-Care-2013.ashx?la=en

Morris, S. (2020). *Gonorrhoea infection*. https://bestpractice.bmj.com/topics/en-gb/51

# Breast Pain and Lumps

Breast pain and lumps are an extremely common presentation that women of all ages can experience in their lifetime. The most common cause of breast pain is related to the menstrual cycle and may occur a few days prior to a period. The mild pain is usually associated with lumpy breasts within two weeks of the menstrual period, which eases once the period starts. Around one-third of cases are non-cyclical. It is important to recognise that bilateral breast pain is not an early sign nor a risk factor for developing breast cancer, and patients should be reassured accordingly.

## Pathophysiology

» Mastitis is a painful inflammatory condition of the breast that may or may not be accompanied by an infection. It is usually associated with lactation ('lactational' or 'puerperal mastitis'), but it can also occur in non-lactating women. In lactating women, milk stasis is usually the primary cause of mastitis. The accumulated milk causes an inflammatory response, which may or may not progress to an infection. The most common organism associated with infectious mastitis is *Staphylococcus aureus*.

» A breast abscess is a localised collection of pus within the breast. It is a severe complication of mastitis, although it may occur with no apparent preceding mastitis.

» Fibroadenosis causes cysts (fluid-filled lumps) in the breast, which are believed to be caused by the breast responding to hormonal fluctuations within the menstrual cycle.

» Fibroadenomas are often caused by an overgrowth of glands and connective tissue. They are thought to occur due to increased sensitivity to oestrogen.

## Risk Factors for Breast Cancer

➤ Past medical history of breast, endometrial or ovarian cancer

➤ Family history of breast disease

➤ >40 years old

➤ Early menarche

➤ Late menopause

➤ Nulliparity

➤ On COCp or HRT

➤ Smoker

## History

- » Focused questions
  - › Ask if there is any pain or tenderness in their breasts (mastalgia), if it is only in one or both breasts, if it is always there or it comes and goes, and if anything makes the pain better or worse.
  - › Ask if there is any discharge from the nipples, and what colour it is. Ask if there is any blood.
  - › Ask when they first noticed the lump, if the lump has changed in size since then, and if they have noticed lumps elsewhere in the breasts.
  - › Ask how long they have experienced these symptoms for and if they are related to their menstrual cycle.
  - › Ask when their LMP was, at what age they experienced menarche and/or menopause, and if they are breastfeeding, pregnant or have any children.

- » Past history – Ask if they have had any breast problems and any previous investigations of their breasts.

- » Drug history – Ask if they are on the pill or HRT.

- » Family history – Ask if there is a family history of breast disease.

- » Social history – Ask if they smoke.

## Examination

- » Always request a chaperone is present.

- » Inspection – Inspect for skin changes, including *peau d'orange*, eczema, tethered lumps and nipple changes.

- » Palpation – Using the flats of the fingers, feel for any lumps, noting the location, size, consistency (rubbery, firm or soft) and mobility (mobile, fixed or tethered).

- » Request that the patient expresses their nipples if there is any discharge.

- » Examine both axillae, checking for any LNs.

## Differential Diagnosis

### Mastalgia (breast pain)

| Cyclical | Usually in those <35 years. Tenderness around the upper, outer breast; increased breast size; lumpiness; symptoms relieved by menstruation; and often dull, heavy, aching and bilateral. |
|---|---|
| Non-cyclical | Not linked to periods, can be on the chest wall or referred, and other diagnoses should be considered, such as mastitis, an abscess, fibroadenosis or carcinoma. Others can include costochondritis or thoracic spondylosis. |

*Lumps*

| | |
|---|---|
| Breast abscess | Tender lump with pus caused by a blocked duct. There can be a fever; the lump is hot to the touch; red, inflamed skin; and flu-like symptoms. |
| Fibroadenosis | The most common cyst seen in women of reproductive age. Can be single or multiple cysts, which are painful with a lumpiness of the breast. The size and pain are associated with their cycle. |
| Fibroadenoma | A benign tumour occurring in women <35 years. Discrete, non-tender, firm, mobile lump described as a 'breast mouse'. Can grow in pregnancy, shrink in menopause and spontaneously resolve. |
| Carcinoma | Known to be hard and tethered, and cause *peau d'orange*, dimpling, nipple inversion, bloody discharge and non-cyclic breast pain (uncommon). |

## Investigations

»   If there is discharge, consider swabbing for microbiology.

»   These are often performed by secondary care:

  ›   Imaging – Mammogram, USS and MRI.

  ›   Biopsies of lumps and/or fine-needle aspiration for cytology.

## Management

*Conservative*

»   Breast pain

  ›   Cyclical – Reassure the patient, and advise them to wear a better-fitting bra. They should keep a pain diary.

  ›   Mastitis – If they are breastfeeding, they should continue to do so, as there will be no harm to the baby from this. Consider evening primrose oil, though this is not routinely recommended.

*Medical*

»   Breast pain

  ›   Cyclical – Offer topical NSAIDs or oral paracetamol/NSAIDs. The second-line treatment is to refer the patient.

  ›   Non-cyclic – Treat the underlying cause. For example, for mastitis, give oral analgesia, plus flucloxacillin 500mg qds for two weeks or erythromycin 500mg qds for two weeks if the patient is breastfeeding with a penicillin allergy.

> › Offer antibiotics to all women with non-lactational mastitis – Co-amoxiclav 500/125mg tds for 10–14 days, and if they are allergic to penicillin, give a combination of erythromycin (250–500mg qds) or clarithromycin (500mg qds) plus metronidazole (500mg tds) for 10–14 days.

## Referral

→ If a breast abscess is suspected, the woman should be referred urgently to a general surgeon for confirmation of the diagnosis and management.

→ Refer them under the 2WW rule for the following:
  › >30 years with unexplained breast lump with or without pain.
  › >30 years with an unexplained lump in the axilla.
  › >50 years with nipple discharge, retraction or any other changes of concern.
  › Any skin changes suggestive of cancer.

→ Refer them as non-urgent if they are <30 years with a lump with/without pain.

## Safety Netting

» Review in three months regarding their response to treatment.

---

### References

Goyal, A. (2014). *Breast pain. BMJ Clinical Evidence, 2014,* 0812. https://www.ncbi.nlm.nih.gov/pmc/articles/PMC4200534/

# Infertility

Infertility is the inability to conceive or fall pregnant after having regular, unprotected coitus for one year (at least twice weekly), in the absence of any known reproductive pathology. One in every seven couples has difficulty conceiving. However, after one year, 84% of couples will conceive; this increases to 92% within two years. While there are many causes for infertility, in 25% of cases none is found. Causes of infertility include ovulatory disorders (25%), tubal damage (20%), uterine/peritoneal disorders (10%), as well as male infertility issues, such as low sperm count or low sperm quality (30%). Primary infertility is when couples have never conceived; secondary infertility is when couples have previously conceived.

## *History*

» Focused questions

  › Ask how long they have been trying to conceive, how often they have been having sex, and if they have had any problems (retrograde ejaculation, erectile dysfunction or dyspareunia).

  › Ask if they have used any contraception and when they stopped using it.

» Associated history – Ask about menstrual history (regular), PCB, IMB, abdominal pain, galactorrhoea (milky breast discharge) and hirsutism.

» Past history (both) – Ask them about each of the following:

  › If they have any children from previous relationships.

  › What their STI history is.

  › If they have had any relevant medical issues (thyroid problems and DM).

  › If they have had any relevant surgery (appendectomy or pelvic surgery).

» Past history (female) – Ask them about each of the following:

  › If they have had any previous pregnancies, miscarriages or TOPs.

  › What their smear test history is (any abnormal smears).

  › If they have had any relevant medical issues (PCOS, ectopic pregnancy, endometriosis or PID).

» Past history (male partner) – Ask them about each of the following:

  › If they have had any relevant medical issues (varicocele, mumps, measles or testicular trauma).

» Drug history – Ask if they have taken spironolactone, cytotoxic drugs, neuroleptics, metoclopramide or antipsychotics.

» Family history – Ask if there is a family history of similar problems or hypothyroidism.

› Social history – Ask if they smoke, drink alcohol or take recreational drugs; ask if their partner smokes, drinks alcohol or is overweight; ask what their occupation is (chemical exposure, working with x-rays or with metals); ask if they have had any recent stress; and ask if/how they exercise.

## Causes of Infertility

| PCOS | Hirsutism, obesity, acne, irregular periods and fertility problems. |
|------|-----------------------------------------------------------------------|
| Endometriosis | Dysmenorrhoea (>30 years) affecting daily activities, deep dyspareunia, chronic pelvic pain, pain during ovulation, cyclic/premenstrual symptoms affecting the bowel or bladder, and IMB. OE: tender nodules in the pouch of Douglas / uterosacral ligaments, fixed uterus, enlarged ovaries and tender adnexa. |
| Fibroids | Abnormal uterine bleeding, heavy periods, IMB is unusual, abdominal bloating/swelling, and urinary incontinence/ frequency. Pelvic pain can occur. OE: large fibroids that can be palpated, or a firm or irregularly enlarged uterus. |
| Hypothyroidism | Increased BMI, dry skin, thin hair, feeling cold, reduced reflexes, low BP, bradycardia, low mood, constipation and tiredness. |

## Examination

» Vitals – BMI (obesity).

» Inspection (female)

› Inspect for acne, hirsutism, androgenisation, galactorrhoea and abnormal genitalia.

› Pelvic exam – Examine for tenderness (endometriosis or PID).

› Bimanual – Examine for fibroids and ovarian cysts.

» Inspection (male partner) – Check for the presence of testicles, varicocele, abnormal genitalia and gynaecomastia.

## Investigations

Consider investigations when couples have failed to conceive after one year, or sooner if they are less likely to conceive.

» Female

› Swabs for STIs (chlamydia).

› Blood tests – Day 21 progesterone (to confirm ovulation), LH, FSH (if they have irregular periods), TFT, prolactin and testosterone.

> › Pelvic/TV USS – PCOS and fibroids.

> › Specialist – Anti-mullerian hormone (AMH) to check the ovarian reserve (premature ovarian failure is indicated by a very low AMH; if they are postmenopausal, AMH is undetectable). Check tubal patency using a hysterosalpingogram (HSG) and a laparoscopy (endometriosis).

» Male partner

> › First void urine sample for a chlamydia screen.

> › Semen analysis – If it is abnormal, repeat after three months. If there are two abnormal results, refer them to urology.

**Producing a semen analysis**

- Produce a specimen within a pot provided by the surgery or lab. Do not use a sample from a condom.

- Advise them to avoid having sex for at least two days before producing the specimen, but it should be no longer than seven days since last having sex.

- The sample should arrive at the lab within one hour of production.

## Management

*Conservative*

✓ Reassure the patient; 84% of couples will conceive within one year, which increases to 92% within two years.

✓ Recommend having intercourse two or three times a week.

✓ Lifestyle

> › Advise them to stop smoking and/or taking recreational drugs.

> › Advise them to consider reducing their caffeine consumption to <200mg/day.

> › Advise the man to cut his alcohol intake down to less than one unit/day. Advise the woman, to consume no alcohol while trying to conceive. If they are not, then they may have less than one to two units once or twice a week.

> › Advise them to aim for a BMI of 19–30 and to have a balanced diet. Consider referring them to a dietician or exercise programme if their BMI >30.

> › Advise the man to wear loose-fitting underpants and trousers, and to avoid very hot baths or saunas.

✓ Offer them counselling if their mood is affected. Consider referring them to a fertility support group.

### Medical

✓ Preconception – Offer folic acid 400mcg daily (if they have DM or a neural tube defect, then 5mg).

✓ Fertility – Offer clomiphene for up to six months (this may be given by secondary care).

## Referral

→ Refer them to a specialist if they have been trying for more than one year and there is no obvious cause for infertility. Consider referring them earlier if the woman is >36 years and there is a known clinical cause for infertility.

› Intrauterine insemination (IUI) – Consider unstimulated IUI as a treatment option in people who are unable to (or would find it very difficult to) have vaginal intercourse, suffer from a clinically diagnosed physical disability or psychosexual problem, or in people with conditions that require specific conditions (e.g. after sperm washing for an HIV-positive male partner).

› Invitro fertilisation (IVF) – Offer this to women with unexplained infertility who have not conceived after two years of regular unprotected sexual intercourse.

→ Sperm donor – Consider donor sperm in cases of male azoospermia, if there is a high risk of an inherited genetic deformity, or if there is a high risk of passing an infectious disease to the woman or child.

→ Oocyte donor – Consider a donor egg when the woman has suffered premature ovarian failure, failure due to chemotherapy or radiotherapy, or gonadal dysgenesis, or has had a bilateral oophorectomy.

### Access to fertility treatment

» A woman (of reproductive age) who has not conceived after more than one year of unprotected sexual intercourse, in the absence of any known cause of infertility, should be referred for further investigation along with her partner.

» NICE recommend up to three cycles of IVF or intracytoplasmic injection.

» This should be available to 23–39-year-old men with an identifiable cause of infertility (azoospermia or a partner with blocked fallopian tubes), or more than three years of fertility problems.

## Safety Netting

» Review in six months regarding their response to treatment.

### References

National Institute for Health and Care Excellence (2013). *Fertility problems: assessment and treatment.* https://www.nice.org.uk/guidance/cg156

# Combined Oral Contraceptives

The COCP refers to contraception that contains both oestrogen and progesterone as the main components. Although there are numerous different types of COCP, they largely differ based upon the amount of hormone contained (monophasic, biphasic, triphasic and quadriphasic), the type of progesterone and the strength of the oestrogen (low or standard).

When considering a patient for the COCP, it is important to risk assess them thoroughly to see whether they are at a higher risk of side effects; if they are, then they should be offered alternative forms of contraception. Do not forget that the COCP does not protect against sexually transmitted diseases. The COCP can also be taken as a patch or as a vaginal pessary.

## Common COCPs

| Oestrogen | Progesterone | Brand |
|---|---|---|
| Ethinylestradiol 20mcg | Desogestrel 150mcg | Gedarel and Mercilon |
| | Gestodene 75mcg | Femodette |
| Ethinylestradiol 30mcg | Desogestrel 150mcg | Gedarel and Marvelon |
| | Drospirenone 3mg | Yasmin |
| | Gestodene 75mcg | Femodene |
| | Levonorgestrel 150 mcg | Levest, Microgynon and Rigevidon |
| Ethinylestradiol 35mcg | Norgestimate 250mcg | Cilest |

## Definition of Fraser competence

➤ If a child presents and is <16 years old, check if they have sufficient comprehension and understanding of the issues at hand. Respect confidentiality if they are Fraser competent. *Refer to the Emergency Contraception section, page 378* for more information.

## History

» Focused questions

› Menstrual history – Ask when their LMP was, if their periods are regular, and what the length of their cycle is.

› Contraceptive history – Ask if they have used any contraceptives previously, what types have been used and why they want to change to the COCP now.

› Recent sexual history – Ask when their last UPSI was, and if there has been any contraceptive use. If not, ask if there is any chance of pregnancy. If they have had UPSI within the last five days, then offer a form of emergency contraception (EC) if they do not want to fall pregnant.

› Consensual – Ask if they are feeling pressured to have sex.

» Associated history – Ask if they have an STI (a change in vaginal discharge or itching), ask about their obstetric history and if are they breastfeeding.

» Past history – Ask if they have had a DVT (clot in the leg or lungs), breast cancer, migraines with visual symptoms, weakness or numbness in the arms or legs, IHD, HTN, or DM.

» Drug history – Ask if they have used any form of contraceptive pill or the coil, if they have ever taken EC, and if they have taken any other medicines (anticonvulsants, rifampicin or griseofulvin).

» Family history – Ask if there is a family history of DVT or PE (first-degree relatives).

» Social history – Ask if they smoke or drink alcohol.

## Hepatic-enzyme-inducing antiepileptic drugs (AEDs)

» Patients taking an enzyme-inducing AED (e.g. phenytoin or carbamazepine) should start on 50mcg oestrogen. If breakthrough bleeding occurs, the oestrogen content should be increased to 75–100mcg/day and consider tricycling (taking three packs back to back). In addition, they should use condoms or have progesterone depo injections. Sodium valproate is not an enzyme inducer, so it does not interact with a COCP.

## Absolute vs Relative Contraindications for the COCP

| Absolute | Relative |
|---|---|
| Past medical history of DVT or PE | Family history of DVT or arterial disease (<45 years) |
| Migraine with aura | Migraine without aura |
| Breast or cervical cancer | BRCA1 gene carrier or past medical history of breast cancer |
| >35 years and a smoker | |
| BP >160/95 | BP <160/95 |
| IHD, CVA or TIA | Risk factors for CVD |
| Major surgery | BMI >35 |
| Breastfeeding <6 weeks | AF |
| SLE with positive antiphospholipid antibodies | DM with nephropathy, retinopathy or neuropathy |

*Advantages and Disadvantages of the COCP (The Faculty of Sexual and Reproductive Healthcare [FSRH], 2018):*

| Advantages | Disadvantages |
|---|---|
| Halves the risk of ovarian and endometrial cancer. Benefits last >15 years. | A small increase in the risk of breast cancer. Risk becomes normal 10 years after stopping meds. A small increase in the risk of cervical cancer. |
| Effective form of contraception (99.7%). | Three to five times increased risk of DVT. |
| Does not interfere with intercourse. | Two-fold increase in strokes. A small increase in the risk of CHD (HTN and MI). |
| Reduces the severity of acne in some. Normal fertility returns immediately when stopped. | Does not protect against STIs, so condoms are still needed. |
| Regulates periods. | Less effective than a long-acting reversible contraception (LARC). |

## Examination

> » Vitals – BP and BMI.

> » Pelvic examination – If there is persistent PV bleeding for three months or more after starting on the COCP, or they report pelvic pain, dyspareunia or PCB.

## Investigations

> » Urine – If in doubt, perform a pregnancy test.

> » Swab – Screen for chlamydia if there is evidence of bleeding.

## Management

> ✓ How to take – To get the maximum benefit, advise them that it is best to start taking the COCP on the first day of their period. They should take the COCP at the same time every day for three weeks (if it is a 21-day pack) and have a break of seven days, during which time there may be a withdrawal bleed. At the end of the seven days, restart a new pack immediately to continue the effects of the contraception.

> ✓ When to start taking the COCP

> > › Normal – If started on days one to five of their cycle, no additional contraception is required. If it is started at any other time in their cycle (and they are not pregnant), they should use barrier methods for seven days.

> › Amenorrhoea – If the patient is not pregnant, start the COCP at any time. They should use additional contraception for seven days.

✓ Postpartum

> › If they are not breastfeeding – Advise them to start the COCP on day 21 postpartum, and use additional contraception for seven days. If it is >21 days and they are having periods, they should start the COCP as for other women with a menstrual cycle. If >21 days and they have no periods, they should start the COCP as for women who have amenorrhoea.

> › If they are breastfeeding – They must not start the COCP less than six weeks postpartum. If it is between six weeks and six months postpartum, they may start the COCP if they are not breastfeeding.

✓ TOP/miscarriage

> › If it occurred at <24 weeks gestation, they should start the COCP within five days of the TOP, ideally on day one or two. No extra contraception is required. If they start the COCP at any other time, advise them to use a barrier method for seven days.

> › If it occurred at >24 weeks gestation, initiate COCP as per women who are postpartum.

✓ EC

> › Levonorgestrel – Take the COCP immediately and use barrier contraception for seven days.

> › Ulipristal acetate – Start taking the COCP five days after taking the ulipristal acetate. Use barrier contraception for seven days.

✓ Everyday pack – If the COCP preparation is an everyday pack, then continue taking the COCP daily at the same time. There are seven placebo pills that will result in a withdrawal bleed when taking them.

✓ Efficacy – If the COCP is taken correctly, the chances of falling pregnant are less than 0.5%. However, with common errors and missing pills, it's effectiveness is still around 95%.

✓ Side effects – Headaches, nausea, vomiting, breast tenderness, low mood and irregular bleeding (20%). If severe vomiting occurs within three hours of taking the COCP, take another pill. If diarrhoea or vomiting lasts >24 hours, consider using condoms for seven days, and consider each day of vomiting as a missed pill.

*Missed-pill rule*

✓ Missing a single pill (>12 hours late, 48–72 hours since last pill) anytime during a pill pack should not cause any problems. Advise the patient to take a pill as soon as it is remembered and take the next one at the normal time, even if it means taking two pills together.

✓ If two or more pills are missed (>72 hours since last pill), take the last pill that was missed as soon as possible. Continue taking the remainder of the pills as normal and use condoms for the next seven days. If there is any UPSI in the first seven days, this may require EC.

✓ If the number of pills left is seven or more, complete the pack and have the seven-day break as normal. If there are fewer than seven, then complete the pack and start the next pack without the seven-day break.

### Situational Advice When Using the COCP

✓ Pregnancy – When issuing hormonal EC, women should be advised of the following:

› They should avoid a withdrawal bleed. It is not known to be harmful to have back-to-back packs.

› If there is no withdrawal bleed when one would be expected, they should exclude pregnancy or consider a lower strength COCP.

› Breakthrough bleed – This can be normal for three months. Otherwise, exclude STIs, pregnancy and cervical lesions. Consider a different progesterone or higher oestrogen content in the COCP.

✓ Side effects – Consider Gedarel, Femodette or Femodene if the patient suffers side effects such as acne, headaches, depression, breast symptoms and breakthrough bleeding with another COCP.

✓ Changing pills

› COCP to COCP – Start the new COCP on the day after the last active pill. There is no need to wait for the next menstrual period.

› POP to COCP – Start the COC at any time during the menstrual cycle, provided it is certain that the woman is not pregnant.

› Depo injection to COCP – Start the COCP on or before the day that the injection was due.

✓ Pregnancy – If the patient becomes pregnant while on the COCP, stop the COCP. Inform them that there is no evidence of this causing harm to the baby or mother.

✓ Surgery – Advise them to stop taking the COCP four weeks before major surgery. No precaution is required for minor surgery.

### Patch contraception

✓ The combined contraceptive patch (Evra) works in the same way as the pill. The hormones are absorbed into the bloodstream through the skin.

✓ How to use – Advise the patient that, to get the maximum benefit, it is best to put the patch in place on the first day of the period (days one to five). They should change the patch every seven days for the first three weeks, then take a break of seven days, during which time the patient may notice a withdrawal bleed. At the end of the seven days, they should restart a new patch immediately to continue the effects of the contraception. The patch is sticky and can be worn on the body even when showering.

✓ Efficacy – The patch is an extremely good form of contraception. If taken correctly, the chances of falling pregnant are less than 0.5%.

✓ Side effects – Skin irritation, headaches, nausea, vomiting, breast tenderness and low mood.

> › Skin irritation – Some patients suffer with skin irritation due to the patch, and rotating the sites where it is applied may reduce this. It can be placed on the upper arms, thighs or buttocks. However, two out of 100 women suffer quite bad irritation and will not be able to continue using it.

> › Adhesives – Bandages or adhesives should not be used to secure the patch in place. If it is no longer sticky, replace it with a new patch.

### Missed-patch rules

✓ <48 hours – If the patch falls off and is noticed in <48 hours, then re-apply it immediately and continue as normal.

✓ >48 hours – If the patch is detached and is not noticed >48 hours, then apply a new patch and start this as if it were the first week of protection. Use barrier contraception for seven days, and then use two further weekly patches to complete a patch cycle.

✓ UPSI – If there is any UPSI within five days of noticing the patch being detached, then they should consider EC.

### Ring contraception

✓ Explanation – The vaginal ring (NuvaRing) is a flexible, transparent, plastic ring (5cm in diameter) that contains two hormones, namely oestrogen and progesterone, which prevent pregnancy. The hormones are absorbed through the skin of the vagina.

✓ How to use – Insert the ring on the first day of the period while squatting or lying down. Squeeze it between the forefinger and thumb to help to insert it as high up as possible. The exact position does not affect efficacy. You can leave the ring in for three weeks, but do check its position regularly. Remove the ring with a finger (shaped like a hook), and replace it with a new ring exactly one week later.

✓ Efficacy – The ring is effective as the COCP.

✓ Side effects – Headaches, vaginitis and vaginal discharge.

✓ Expelled ring rules – If it falls out for less than three hours, rinse it in water and reinsert it straight away. No extra precaution is required.

## Safety Netting

» Late period – If the next period is later than expected, do a pregnancy test.

» Symptoms – Review as soon as possible if patient has chest pain (pleuritic), SOB, haemoptysis, calf swelling, weakness/numbness in the arms or legs, or unusual or worsening headaches.

» Follow-up – Review in three months, then in 6–12 months.

## NATIONAL EXAM TIPS

When offering your explanation of the oral contraceptive pill, it may appear quite daunting to explain all elements of it in a 10-minute consultation. To save valuable time in the exam, ask the patient what areas they would like to discuss and check their understanding around the other areas, as often patients may already be well acquainted with some elements of the pill. Ensure you risk assess them before deciding which contraception to initiate.

## References

The Faculty of Sexual and Reproductive Healthcare (2016). *UK Medical eligibility criteria for contraceptive use.* https://www.fsrh.org/standards-and-guidance/documents/ukmec-2016/

The Faculty of Sexual and Reproductive Healthcare (2018). *FSRH clinical guideline: combined hormonal contraception.* https://www.fsrh.org/standards-and-guidance/documents/combined-hormonal-contraception/

# Progesterone-Only Contraception

Progesterone-only contraception is a type of contraception that solely uses the hormone progesterone to prevent pregnancy. It is used particularly when the COCP is contraindicated for the patient due to breast feeding, a risk of VTE, liver disease or a migraine with an aura. Progesterone-only contraception comes in three different forms, including orally as a pill, as an IM injection and via an implant. Do not forget that these forms of contraception do not protect against sexually transmitted diseases, so it is important to advise about the possible need for barrier contraception.

*Common Progesterone Contraceptives (Joint Formulary Committee, 2017)*

| Brand Name | Progesterone | Strength (mcg) |
|---|---|---|
| Norgeston | Levonorgestrel | 30 |
| Noriday | Norethisterone | 350 |
| Cerazette/Cerelle | Desogestrel | 75 |

## Ideas, Concerns and Expectations

➤ Ideas – Ask what they know about the POP, and if there is any reason why they wanted this type

➤ Concerns – Ask if they have any worries about taking the pill

➤ Expectations – Ask if they have a specific pill in mind that they want you to issue

## *History*

» Focused questions

› Menstrual history – Ask when their LMP was, if their periods are regular or irregular, how many days they last, and if they are heavy or they have any clots.

› Sexual history – Ask if they have had any STIs, or if there is any change in vaginal discharge or any itching, and ask about their partners.

› Contraceptive history – Ask if they have used any other contraception; if so, what types; and ask why they wish to change.

› Last sexual encounter – Ask when their last UPSI was, if they used any contraceptive, and if not, if there is any chance of pregnancy. If the patient had UPSI <120 hours ago, then offer a form of EC if they do not want to fall pregnant.

- » Associated history – Ask about their obstetric history and if they are breast feeding.

- » Past history – Ask if they have had an ectopic pregnancy, breast cancer within the past five years, or liver disease (cirrhosis or hepatitis).

- » Drug history – Ask if they have taken carbamazepine, phenytoin, itraconazole or St John's wort, or if they have had a coil fitted.

- » Social history – Ask if they smoke or drink alcohol.

## Risk of Breast Cancer from Taking the POP

➤ There is a small increase in the risk of getting breast cancer associated with women using the POP. The most important factor is the age at which the POP is stopped. The risk disappears 10 years after stopping taking it.

## Hepatic-enzyme-including AEDs

Progesterone-only contraception (POP and implants) is not recommended as a reliable form of contraception in women taking hepatic-enzyme-inducing AEDs. Their efficacy is reduced by these drugs, and alternative methods should be sought.

## Examination

- » Vitals – BP and BMI.

- » Urine – If in doubt, request a pregnancy test.

## Management

- ✓ Explanation – The POP is so called as it contains the hormone progesterone, which is similar to the one found naturally in the body. By taking the mini-pill, the hormone balance in the patient's body is altered, creating a thicker mucus in the womb, which prevents sperm from entering it. In some women, it also works to prevent the release of an egg. Women can take this pill until 55 years of age.

- ✓ How to take – Advise the patient that, to get the maximum benefit, it is best to start the pill on the first day of their period. They should take the pill at the same time every day, with no days where they take a break. When they finish a pack, it is important for them to start the next pack immediately (the next day). If they have just given birth and start the POP within three weeks of delivery, then it will work straight away. If it is started on any day other than days one to five of their period, they should use condoms for 48 hours.

- ✓ Efficiency – The POP is a good form of contraception. If taken correctly, the chances of falling pregnant are <1%. However, with common errors and missing pills, the effectiveness is still over 92%.

- ✓ Side effects – Change in weight, transient breast pain and menstrual irregularities.

> › Period – The main side effect is causing irregular menstrual bleeding: 4/10 will have no problems with their periods, a further 4/10 will experience irregular bleeding, and 2/10 will have no periods at all.

✓ Missed-pill rule – Advise them that if they forget a pill, they should take it as soon as they remember and carry on with the next pill at the usual time. If the pill was more than three hours overdue, they are not protected. They should continue with normal pill-taking, but they must also use another method, such as a condom, for the next two days (FSRH, 2015).

✓ EC should be considered if the POP is more than three hours late and UPSI has occurred recently.

## Situational Advice When Using the POP

✓ After childbirth – The POP can be initiated from delivery to day 21 postpartum without any further precautions. If started >21 days postpartum, then use condoms for any intercourse during the next 48 hours.

✓ Changing from the COCP – Start the POP the day after completing the COCP pills without a break (days one to seven of the COCP-free interval). If starting on the first week of the COCP, use condoms for 48 hours.

✓ From IM POP – Start the POP up to 14 weeks from the last injection. If >14 weeks, use condoms for any intercourse during the next 48 hours.

✓ Amenorrhoea – Exclude pregnancy, then the POP can be started at any time, but advise them to use condoms for any intercourse during the next 48 hours.

## Progesterone-Only Injection

✓ Explanation – The progesterone injection contains the hormone progesterone, which is similar to the one found naturally in the body. By taking this injection, the hormone balance of the patient's body is altered, creating a thicker mucus in the womb, preventing sperm from entering it. It is usually given by a health professional and administered into the patient's buttock at regular intervals.

✓ How to use – Advise the patient that, to get the maximum benefit, it is best to have the first injection during the first five days of their period. Then they can have the injection outside this time, but they should make sure they are not pregnant, and then use barrier contraception for the next seven days. They should ensure that they take the next injection after 12 weeks (Depo-Provera) or 13 weeks (Depo Sayana Press).

✓ Side effects – Increase in weight, transient breast pain and menstrual irregularities.

## Progesterone-Only Implant

✓ Explanation – Implanon is a rod-shaped implant that is inserted into the upper arm and prevents pregnancy by releasing a progesterone hormone just under the skin. It works primarily by preventing ovulation, but also increases the thickness of the mucus in the womb, preventing sperm from passing through the cervix.

✓ How to use – If it is inserted within the first five days of their cycle, it provides immediate protection. However, on any other day of their cycle, they must use barrier protection methods (condoms) for the next seven days. It works effectively for up to three years. If you wish to fall pregnant, the device will need to be removed by a trained healthcare professional.

✓ Side effects – Increase in weight, transient breast pain and menstrual irregularities.

## Safety Netting

» Late period – If the patient's next period is later than expected, do a pregnancy test.

» Follow-up – Review in three months, then 12 monthly.

## References

Joint Formulary Committee (2017). *BNF 74 (British National Formulary) September 2017*. Pharmaceutical Press.

The Faculty of Sexual and Reproductive Healthcare (2015). *FSRH clinical guideline: progesterone-only pills*. https://www.fsrh.org/standards-and-guidance/documents/cec-ceu-guidance-pop-mar-2015/

# Emergency Contraception

EC is a form of contraception that is taken to prevent unwanted pregnancy in a case where either no contraception was used during sexual intercourse or in the event of contraception failure, such as a split condom or a missed tablet. There are currently three forms of EC: two tablets and an IUD. EC is only effective if taken within a defined window post-coitus, and it is important that patients understand the risk of failure.

## *History*

» Focused questions

› Ask why they need EC.

› Ask about contraception failure: ask if the condom split, or they missed pills, and if so, how many.

› Last sexual encounter – Ask when it was, with whom, if it was a regular partner or not, and if it was consensual.

› Fraser competence – If a child attends and is <16 years, check if they are Fraser competent and respect confidentiality if they are. Ask if they have spoken to their parents about it, and if not, ask if there is a reason why they have not.

» Associated history – Ask if they have had an STI (discharge, pain or itchiness), what their cycle is like (are they regular and when their LMP was), and about their obstetric history (if they have ever been pregnant or missed a period).

» Past history – Ask if they have had liver problems or porphyria.

» Drug history – Ask if they have taken the pill or had a coil fitted, if they have taken any other medication (warfarin or rifampicin), and if they have ever taken EC before.

» Social history – Ask if they smoke or drink alcohol.

## RED FLAGS

» Rape – If their last sexual encounter was non-consensual, consider referring them to a SARC.

» Vulnerable child – If the child is <13 years, make a referral to the child protection team. If the partner is significantly older than the child, consider contacting the police / child protection services.

» Pregnancy – Ask if they have done a pregnancy test.

## Contraception Failure: When EC Is Indicated

» Condom – If the condom splits.

» POP – If the woman has a late or missed pill (>27 hours, or >36 hours if on desogestrel).

» COCP – If the woman misses two consecutive pills in week one.

» Progesterone injection – If there is a gap of >14 weeks since the last injection.

## Examination

» Vitals – BP, weight and BMI.

» Urine – If in doubt, request a pregnancy test.

## Management

✓ Levonorgestrel – Also known as Levonelle. A 1.5 stat dose of progesterone hormone. It is effective up to 72 hours after UPSI, with the efficacy reducing with time (24 hours is 95%, and 72 hours is 58%). Consider a 3mg dose if their BMI >26 or they are on an enzyme-inducing drug.

  › Side effects – Nausea and vomiting (If the patient vomits within two hours of taking it, they should take a replacement dose). Occasionally causes spotting or light bleeding.

✓ Ulipristal acetate – Also known as ellaOne. It is effective up to 120 hours after an episode of UPSI, with an efficacy rate of around 98%. Contraindicated for repeated use in a menstrual cycle. Avoid in asthmatics on oral glucocorticoids.

  › Side effects – Headaches, nausea and vomiting. If the patient vomits within three hours of taking it, they should take a replacement dose.

✓ Copper IUD – Small, copper-based device that is inserted into the womb. It can be used up to 120 hours after an episode of UPSI, with an efficacy rate of almost 100% if used correctly.

  › Side effects – May make periods feel heavier, longer or more painful, but these may settle down after a few months of use.

  › Contraindicated – Pregnancy, STI, unexplained PV bleeding or copper allergy.

✓ STI risk – Advise the patient that UPSI can expose them to the risk of contracting an STI. Refer them to a GUM clinic or a nurse for swabs.

✓ LARC – Give them long-term contraception advice (e.g. Implanon, coil or injections).

*Advice After Using EC*

✓    Advise the patient of the following:

> ›    Their next period may be early or late.

> ›    A barrier method of contraception needs to be used until their next period.

> ›    They should seek medical attention promptly if any lower abdominal pain occurs.

> ›    They should return in three to four weeks if the subsequent menstrual bleed is abnormally light, heavy, brief or absent, or if they are otherwise concerned (if there is any doubt as to whether menstruation has occurred, a pregnancy test should be performed at least three weeks after UPSI).

## Safety Netting

»    Ectopic pregnancy – If the patient experiences lower abdominal pains or abnormal PV bleeding, a review is needed as soon as possible.

»    Late period – If the next period is later than expected, they should do a pregnancy test.

---

*References*

National Institute for Health and Care Excellence (2019). *Contraception – assessment.* https://cks.nice.org.uk/topics/contraception-assessment/

# Menopause and Hormone Replacement Therapy

The menopause is the period when the female menstrual cycle ceases due to the permanent loss of ovarian activity. The average age this takes place in the UK is between 51 and 52 years old. It is diagnosed when a year has passed since the LMP in women of this age group. Although it usually occurs in women >50 years, it can occur in women much younger – which is known as premature menopause if <40 years, and early menopause if <45 years – usually due to ovarian failure.

Prior to the periods stopping completely, women usually have a period of two years whereby they suffer with a number of symptoms due to the altering levels of hormones. This is known as the climacteric phase (or perimenopause) and is characterised by hot flushes, dry vagina, night sweats, mood swings and problems sleeping.

## History

» Open question – Ask them to tell you more about the symptoms they have been experiencing recently.

» Focused questions

  › Menstrual history – Ask when their LMP was, how regular their periods are, and how their periods have been over last year: shorter, longer or more erratic.

  › Hot flushes – Ask whereabouts they are experiencing hot flushes (chest, face or neck), and how long they last for.

  › Night sweats – Ask how often the bedding has to be changed.

  › Vaginal atrophy – Ask if there is any dryness, itching or dyspareunia.

  › Other – Ask about their mood, if they have difficulty sleeping (insomnia), loss of libido, or joint or muscle pain.

» Associated history – Ask if there is any chance of pregnancy.

» Past history – Ask if they have had DVT, cancer (breast/endometrial), IHD, CVA, BP, liver problems, radiotherapy/chemotherapy on the pelvis or ovaries, or surgery (oophorectomy/hysterectomy).

» Drug history – Ask what medication they have been taking.

» Family history – Ask if there is a family history of DVT.

» Social history – Ask if they smoke or drink alcohol.

## RED FLAGS

Postmenopausal bleeding.

## NICE Guidelines for PMB (NICE, 2015)

» If there is bleeding following 12 months of amenorrhoea, all patients require a full pelvic exam and a speculum exam of the cervix.

› If they are not on HRT – Refer the patient with PMB under the 2WW pathway, including patients on tamoxifen with PMB or an endometrial thickness >4mm on USS.

› HRT-related bleeding – Stop HRT for six weeks and refer them if there is ongoing bleeding.

## Examination

» Vitals – BP and BMI.

» Urine – If in doubt, perform a pregnancy test.

» Blood test – FSH (>40mIU/l is diagnostic).

» USS – For PMB, pelvic/TV USS looking for the thickening of the endometrial lining (>4mm).

## Management

*Conservative*

✓ Exercise – Advise the patient to take regular exercise and lose weight to reduce hot flushes (by up to 50%).

✓ Foods – Advise them to avoid trigger foods (e.g. spicy foods, caffeine and alcohol) to reduce night sweats.

✓ Others – Advise them to wear light clothes, sleep in a cool room and stop smoking.

✓ Vaginal atrophy – Advise them to use lubricant gel if sexual intercourse is painful. They should stop using soap and use clean water instead. They should avoid using lotions and perfumed products on the vulval area.

*Medical*

✓ Non-HRT

› Topical oestrogen – Offer vaginal cream, rings or tablets to reduce atrophy.

› Hot flushes – Offer low dose SSRI, norethisterone 5mg od or clonidine 50mcg bd.

› Mood – Consider referring the patient for counselling, CBT or psychotherapy, or giving SSRI.

✓ HRT

› For a patient without a uterus – Offer oestrogen alone for continuous use, except in cases of endometriosis.

> For a patient with a uterus:

- Cyclical – Comes as monthly or three-monthly cyclical regimens. Consider this if their periods have just stopped or become erratic. Offer oestrogen daily, with progesterone added to the last 10–14 days of the cycle (monthly or every 13 weeks). Advise them that they will experience monthly or three-monthly periods.

- Continuous – Offer if a patient has had no periods for one year. Avoid for those in the perimenopause. Offer a combination of oestrogen and progesterone daily. No monthly periods will be experienced.

- Side effects – Nausea, headaches, migraines, cramps, fluid retention, breast enlargement, weight gain and spotting for the first few months (investigate if longer than six months)

✓ Contraception – Consider adding contraception if a patient is still having periods, as HRT does not act as a contraceptive. There is no need for contraception if the periods have been stopped for more than a year in those >50 years or for more than two years in those <50 years.

✓ Tibolone – Contains oestrogen, progesterone and androgen properties. It is useful for sweats, hot flushes and vaginal dryness. Consider this for a patient without periods for one year. Use in a similar way to continuous HRT. This has a lower breast-cancer risk.

## Safety Netting

» PMB – If the patient has any abnormal bleeding, they are to return as soon as possible.

» Symptoms – Consider stopping HRT if a patient has chest pain (pleuritic), SOB, calf swelling, weakness/numbness in their arms or legs, unusual or worsening headaches, or BP >160/95.

» Follow-up – Review in three months to assess the patient's response.

---

*References*

National Institute for Health and Care Excellence (2015). *Menopause: diagnosis and management.* https://www.nice.org.uk/guidance/ng23

# Premenstrual Syndrome

Premenstrual syndrome (PMS) is a condition that affects women in the luteal phase of their cycle, prior to their menstrual period. It is defined as 'distressing physical, psychological and behavioural symptoms not caused by organic disease which regularly recur during the luteal phase of the menstrual cycle, and significantly regress or disappear during the remainder of the cycle'.

It usually affects middle-aged women between the ages of 30 and 40, and causes physical (fluid retention, breast fullness and bloating), psychological (irritability, depression and loss of libido) and behavioural symptoms (aggression). In most cases, the symptoms are bearable, but in a significant minority (5%), the symptoms may affect day-to-day functioning.

## *History*

- » Focused questions
  - › Physical symptoms – Ask if they suffer from bloating, breast tenderness, headaches, weight gain or changes to their bowel habits.
  - › Psychological symptoms – Ask if they experience mood changes, irritability or loss of libido.
  - › Duration – Ask how long they have been experiencing symptoms for.
  - › Cyclic – Ask if their symptoms are related to their menstrual cycle, and if so, whether they are worse in the second half of the cycle.

- » Past history – Conduct a depression screen, and ask if they have any other medical conditions.

- » Drug history – Ask if they have taken any medications (e.g. the COCP/POP) and if this helps with their symptoms.

- » Family history – Ask if there is a family history of anyone with similar symptoms, or anyone diagnosed with PMS.

- » Social history – Ask what their diet is like (if they drink coffee and if they have a balanced diet), and if they smoke or drink alcohol.

## Examination

- » Vitals – BMI.

- » Examination – Although examination is not necessary to make a diagnosis of PMS, it may be helpful to exclude other potential diagnoses. Offer to examine the relevant areas where the patient presents with symptoms (i.e. a breast exam for breast pain, and an abdominal exam for bloating and/or bowel-habit changes).

## Differential Diagnosis

| Affective disorder | Prolonged low mood, poor concentration, insomnia, anxiety, decreased libido, and feeling hopeless, helpless and worthless. |
|---|---|
| DM | Thirst, weight loss, malaise and an increase in urinary frequency. |
| Hypothyroidism | Weight gain, tiredness, oedema, malaise, cold intolerance and dry skin. |
| Side effect of COCP | Headaches, low mood, breast tenderness and breakthrough bleeding. |
| Perimenopause | Irregular periods, hot flushes, breast tenderness, tiredness, mood swings, insomnia and decreased libido. |

## Management

*Conservative*

✓ Menstrual diary – Advise the patient to keep a symptom diary to check if it correlates with their periods (premenstrual) over two cycles, to use a Daily Record of Severity of Problems (DRSP), and to record their weight as well.

✓ Lifestyle – Recommend that they exercise, advise them on their diet (eat small, regular portions; reduce caffeine intake; and increase fibre intake), and recommend that they get regular sleep and lose weight. Advise them to stop smoking and reduce their alcohol intake.

✓ Psychological - Advise them to seek counselling (CBT) or use relaxation techniques if appropriate.

✓ Vitamins – Consider advising them to take evening primrose oil (breast tenderness), St John's wort or ginkgo biloba. Also consider vitamin B6 (there is evidence for its efficacy), or calcium / vitamin D, magnesium or vitamin A supplements (limited evidence) two weeks before their period starts.

*Medical*

✓ Pain – Offer simple analgesics such as paracetamol or an NSAID to help treat breast or abdominal pains.

✓ COCP – In patients with moderate PMS, consider commencing the COCP, especially if they require contraception. Use it back to back rather than cyclically, or limit it to during the luteal phase (days 15–28).

✓ SSRI – Consider this in cases of unresponsive, severe PMS. This can be prescribed continuously or solely during days 15–28 of the period. Trial for at least three months before continuing for one year.

## Referral

→ Refer the patient to a specialist if there is a poor response or there is underlying psychiatric illness. Surgical options include hysterectomy and bilateral oophorectomy.

## Safety Netting

> » Follow-up – Review in three months regarding their response to the treatment.

---

### References

GPnotebook (2018). *Pre-menstrual syndrome.* https://gpnotebook.com/simplepage.
cfm?ID=1295319095&linkID=41577&cook=no&mentor=1

Royal College of Obstetricians & Gynaecologists (2016). *Premenstrual syndrome, management (Green-top Guideline No. 48).* https://www.rcog.org.uk/en/guidelines-research-services/guidelines/gtg48/

# Termination of Pregnancy

Approximately one in five pregnancies are terminated in the UK (200,000 per year) with most carried out within 13 weeks of gestation (84%). Most (60%) are performed on women <24-years-old. It involves either taking medication or undergoing a simple surgical procedure to remove the pregnancy, depending on the gestation of the pregnancy. It is currently legal in the UK to terminate up to 24 weeks of pregnancy if certain conditions are met, but this can be extended if there is evidence of more serious sequelae to the mother of child, such as permanent harm or death.

Two doctors must give consent, stating that to continue the pregnancy it would do one of the following:

>> Endanger the life of the mother.

>> Endanger the physical or mental health of the mother.

>> Be a risk to the physical or mental health of the siblings.

>> The foetus would have a high chance of having a disability.

The majority of abortions in the UK (97%) fall under the second category. Patients must be referred for a TOP by their GP surgery, family planning centre or private healthcare centre. No doctor is obliged to consent to or participate in an abortion, but they have a duty of care to refer the patient onwards to the correct department.

## Risk Factors

➤ Physically abusive relationship (domestic violence)

➤ Socially isolated individual

➤ Young child or vulnerable adult

## *History*

>> Ask why they would like to have a TOP, and how they found out they were pregnant.

>> Focused questions

> Contraception – Ask if contraception was being used at the time, and if so, what went wrong (split condom, missed pill or a lost patch).

> Menstrual cycle – Ask when their LMP was and if their periods are regular.

> Partner – Ask if they had UPSI with, regular or casual partner, if the partner knows about the pregnancy, and if the UPSI was consensual.

> Fraser competence – If a child attends and is <16 years, check if they are Fraser competent and respect confidentiality if they are. Ask if they have spoken to their parents about it, and if not, ask if there is a reason why they have not.

» Past history – Ask about their obstetric history (gravida and parity, and if they have had any other TOPs or miscarriages), if they have had any surgery (particularly pelvic surgery), and if they have received any psychiatric treatment (depression).

» Drug history – Ask if they take any medications.

» Social history – Ask about their relationships, home life and support networks; ask what their occupation is; and ask if they smoke, drink alcohol or take recreational drugs.

## RED FLAGS

Abdominal pain or a fever.

## Fraser's Guidelines

It is acceptable for PAs to consent to a patient having an abortions without parental consent provided that the following is adhered to:

» The young individual understands the advice.

» They cannot be persuaded to inform their parents.

» Unless they receive treatment, their physical health, mental health or both are likely to suffer.

In such situations, every effort should be made to encourage the patient to speak to their parents.

## Examination

» Vitals – BP and BMI.

## Investigations

» Urine – Pregnancy test.

» Bloods – Hb level, Hb screen, blood group and Rh status (usually performed by the provider).

» USS – Pelvic/TV USS for viability and dating, taken prior to the TOP (routinely unnecessary).

## Management

✓ Counselling – Counsel the patient to make sure that they are certain of their decision.

✓ Explanation – Offer appropriate termination advice to them, depending on the number of weeks of pregnancy:

> Five to 24 weeks – Medical termination involving taking two medications, 48 hours apart, at a clinic. The patient is offered oral mifepristone and then returns two days later for prostaglandin, either as a pessary or orally. The patient can experience pain, vaginal bleeding and the expulsion of the products of pregnancy. The patient may require analgesia and may require repeat doses, depending on the gestation period, to help induce the abortion. They may have to progress to a surgical procedure if it is unsuccessful.

> Seven to 14 weeks – Conventional vacuum aspiration. Tell them that a small plastic tube will be passed through the neck of the womb and the content of the pregnancy is removed by gentle suction.

> >14 weeks – Dilatation and evacuation (D&E) where surgical procedure is required. Tell them that they will be put to sleep under a GA. The neck of the womb will be stretched gently. The pregnancy will be removed using forceps and a suction tube.

✓ Risks – The risks of complications are low (1%), particularly if it is done in early pregnancy (<12 weeks). Common complications include bleeding, damage to the neck and body of the womb, genital-tract infection, and failure.

## Referral

→ As a PA in primary care, it is advised to refer the patient to termination services (e.g. British Pregnancy Advisory Service [BPAS] or Marie Stopes). Offer psychological or emotional support / counselling.

## Safety Netting

» If the patient experiences abdominal pain or fever to seek medical advice (exclude ectopic pregnancy).

**Follow-up post TOP**

> LARC – Discuss long-term contraception (Implanon / Mirena coil) or the pill (COCP or POP) with the patient.

> STIs – Offer the patient an STI screen.

---

*References*

Royal College of Obstetricians & Gynaecologists (2011). *The care of women requesting induced abortion.* https://www.rcog.org.uk/globalassets/documents/guidelines/abortion-guideline_web_1.pdf

# Cervical Smear Test

The cervical screening programme in the UK was established to pick up early signs of changes in the cells of the womb that may lead to cancer. All women ages between 25 and 64 years of age are invited into a regular, rolling programme of cervical smear testing. Those aged between 25 and 49 are recalled every three years, whereas those between 50 and 64 have smear tests every five years. As a result of the programme, 3,000 people are diagnosed with cervical cancer a year, and the number of women dying from cervical cancer has halved. Although all ages of women can get cervical cancer, it is generally rare in women <25 years of age and is most common in women from 30–45 years of age.

## Invitation and Screening Intervals

- Age 24.5 – First invitation
- Ages 25–49 – Three yearly
- Ages 50 to 64 – Five yearly
- Age >64 – Only required if they have had recent abnormal tests, or have not had a smear >50 years of age and have requested one.

### Women 20–24 Years Old

» The programme no longer tests for changes in women <25 years of age, as the prevalence of cervical cancer in this cohort is <50 cases a year. It is hoped that the prevalence of cancer in this age group will drop greatly as a result of the human papilloma virus (HPV) vaccination programme. In addition, it has been determined that the percentage of patients found with abnormal cells was far greater than those who went on to develop cervical cancer.

» HPV is extremely common, with there being >100 different types. Of all the types, HPV-16 and HPV-18 are deemed to be of the highest risk and are implicated in most cases of cervical cancer. If HPV is detected in low-grade or borderline dyskaryosis, then a patient should automatically be referred for a colposcopy.

  › If they are HPV negative – The patient will be discharged for routine recall (every three to five years, depending on her age).

  › If they are HPV positive – Cytology will be undertaken, and if it is normal, the patient will have a recheck for HPV in one year. If this is negative, then they will revert to routine recall. If the cytology is borderline or worse, then the patient will be referred for colposcopy.

## *History*

- » Focused questions
    - › Sexual history – Ask if they are sexually active, and if they have a regular partner.
    - › Gynaecological history – Ask when their LMP was, if their periods are irregular or heavy, how many days they last for, if they have had any clots, and if they have had IMB, PCB or dyspareunia.
    - › STIs – Ask if they have had any abnormal discharge or itching.
    - › Ask if they have lost weight.

- » Past history – Ask about previous smears and any abnormalities in the past, if they have had a colposcopy or cervical stenosis, and if they have had a previous referral for a colposcopy or hysterectomy (to determine if they still have a cervix).

- » Family history – Ask if there is a family history of cervical cancer.

- » Drug history – Ask if they have taken COCP, tamoxifen or EC.

- » Social history – Ask if they smoke or drink alcohol.

## Examination

- » Smear – Obtain consent and then perform a liquid cervical smear test via a speculum examination if one is due, according to the cervical screening programme. If the patient does not give consent, offer further information about the process. If they are still not keen, request written withdrawal or a signed consent confirming their decision.

    **When not to take a cervical smear**
    - › If the patient is pregnant, menstruating, less than three months postnatal, less than three months after a TOP/miscarriage, or when vaginal discharge or a pelvic infection is present (treat and do the smear test later).

## Investigations

- » Smear results – Refer for a colposcopy if there is an abnormal smear (borderline positive HPV, moderate or severe dyskaryosis, or more than three consecutive borderline smears). If, on inspection, you find features of malignancy, refer them under 2WW, not for colposcopy.

    **Interpreting smear results**
    - › Negative – A normal smear with normal endocervical cells and HPV negative requires a normal recall. However, normal cells and HPV positive requires a repeat smear in 12 months' time.

> › Inadequate – An insufficient smear was taken, so repeat the sample after three months to allow the cells to regenerate. If three inadequate samples are found, the patient should be referred for a colposcopy.

> › Borderline – Abnormal nuclei were found, but dyskaryosis could not be confirmed. The results can revert to normal over time. If they are HPV positive, then refer for a colposcopy. If they are HPV negative, then this requires a normal recall.

> › If there are three consecutive borderline changes, recommend a colposcopy. Three consecutive normal results are required six months apart before the patient can revert to the normal routine recall.

» Dyskaryosis – This can be mild, moderate or severe. Patients with mild dyskaryosis with no HPV can be called back as per the routine recall. However, mild dyskaryosis and HPV positive will require a colposcopy. Moderate dyskaryosis warrants a referral for a colposcopy, and severe dyskaryosis needs a referral under 2WW.

» Invasive squamous cell – If invasive squamous cell carcinoma is found, the patient must be referred and seen under 2WW in the colposcopy clinic.

» Glandular neoplasia – The course of action depends on the source. If it is from the endocervix or is unspecified, they must be referred for a colposcopy. If it is from the endometrium or another gynaecological site, then refer them via the 2WW route.

## Explanations

The following will help you explain the results to the patient:

✓ Dyskaryosis – In this case, there were some abnormal changes seen in the cells, known as dyskaryosis. These changes are not cervical cancer or cancerous. In most cases, dyskaryotic cells do not develop into cancer and most will change back into normal cells. However, in a few cases, if left untreated, these abnormal cells may change into cancer in the future.

✓ HPV – This stands for human papilloma virus. It is a very common virus that is spread by sexual intercourse. Once it has been caught, it does not usually cause any symptoms, so most people with it would not know whether they even had it. However, the virus has been found to lead to a few problems, including warts, and it may even lead to cervical cancer.

✓ Colposcopy – This is when a doctor has a closer look at the neck of the womb. It is similar to having a smear test in that a speculum is inserted into the vagina. The doctor will then use a colposcope to get a more detailed view. They will use a special liquid and paint the neck of the womb. This will help highlight the abnormal cells. They may take a small sample of cells, to look at even closer under the microscope. The doctor may treat the abnormal cells using a heat probe (loop diathermy), laser treatment or a cold probe (cryotherapy). A small anaesthetic is given locally before any treatment is undertaken, so that no pain is felt.

## Safety Netting

» Review as per the results, offering a follow-up or repeat smear where needed.

---

### References

Public Health England (2004). *NHS cervical screening call and recall: guide to administrative good practice.* https://www.gov.uk/government/publications/cervical-screening-call-and-recall-administration-best-practice

# Hirsutism

Hirsutism describes the excessive growth of coarse, dark hair with an androgen-dependent (male) distribution where hair would otherwise often be absent in women (i.e. on the face, jaw, chest and nipples). It is caused by an excess of androgens or increased sensitivity to them. It commonly affects one in 10 women, and it varies depending upon ethnicity (less often in Asians, but more common in those of Mediterranean origin). The most common cause is either PCOS or it is idiopathic. If there are signs of virilism, then consider other differentials, such as ovarian or adrenal tumours.

## Causes of Hirsutism

> ➤ PCOS – This is the most common cause (70%).

> ➤ Idiopathic – Familial. Onset from puberty with slow development.

> ➤ Drugs – Steroids, COCP, danazol, metoclopramide, phenytoin, sodium valproate and methyldopa.

> ➤ Menopause – Facial hirsutism. Decreasing oestrogen levels with unopposed androgen effects.

> ➤ Ovarian – Ovarian cancer.

> ➤ Adrenal – Congenital adrenal hyperplasia, Cushing's syndrome (sudden weight gain, and bloating around the chest and stomach) and an androgen-producing adrenal tumour.

> ➤ Endocrine – Hypothyroidism, prolactinoma and acromegaly.

## *History*

> » Focused questions
>> › Ask where they have noticed unusual hair growth (upper lip and chin, chest, nipples, inner thighs, or buttocks).
>> › Ask how long they have had the problem, and if it started recently or has been there for a long time.
>> › Ask if there was a sudden onset (androgen-secreting tumour) or it came on more slowly.
>> › Virilism – Ask if there has been a deepening in their voice or they have noticed a receding hair line from side of the head.

> » Past history – Ask if they have had CVD (raised BP, cholesterol, type 2 DM or a metabolic syndrome), sleep apnoea (problems sleeping at night), epilepsy or bipolar disorder.

> » Drug history – Ask if they have taken any anabolic steroids, COCP, phenytoin, methyldopa, metoclopramide or progestogens.

» Family history – Ask if there is a family history of any similar problems.

» Social history – Ask if they smoke or drink alcohol, what their mood is like, what their occupation is, and about their relationships.

» Questions on differentials

> PCOS

- Periods – Ask if they are irregular, light or absent; how many days they last for; and how long these problems have been going on for.

- Acne – Ask where the spots are, and if they have any whiteheads or blackheads.

- Ask if they have gained any weight.

> Menopause – Ask when their LMP was, and if they have had any hot flushes or excessive sweating.

> Hypothyroid – Ask if they have any intolerance to hot or cold temperatures, have gained or lost any weight, or have any dry skin.

> Cushing's syndrome – Ask if they have gained weight around the face, if they have any stretch marks or bruising of the skin, and if there has been any bloating around the chest or stomach.

> Ovarian cancer – Ask if there has been any weight loss or feeling bloated, any constipation or diarrhoea, or any urinary symptoms.

## RED FLAGS

Cushing's syndrome, virilisation or a pelvic mass.

## Examination

» Vitals – BP (Cushing's syndrome), BMI and weight (obesity).

» Inspection – Observe the distribution of hirsutism on the face, chest, thighs and lower abdomen using the Ferriman-Gallwey score.

> PCOS – Inspect for acne (face, back and chest), and inspect the scalp for alopecia.

> Cushing's syndrome – Look for a moon face, stretch marks and bruises.

» Pelvic exam – To exclude a pelvic mass (ovarian cancer), look for signs of clitoromegaly (virilism).

*Modified Ferriman-Gallwey score*

> » This is a method used to evaluate the severity of hirsutism in women. Hair growth is rated from 0 to 4, where 0 is no growth of hair, and 4 is extensive hair growth over nine areas of the body (upper lip, chin, chest, back [upper and lower], abdomen [upper and lower], upper arms and thighs). The numbers for all the areas are added together to obtain a total score. The maximum score is 36. A score >15 indicates moderate/severe hirsutism.

## Differential Diagnosis

| | |
|---|---|
| PCOS | Hirsutism, obesity and acne. Irregular periods and fertility problems. |
| Cushing's syndrome | Central obesity, facial weight gain (moon face), skin bruises easily, depression, decreased libido, puffy and red face, and purple striae. |
| Prolactinoma | Headaches, double vision, poor peripheral vision, galactorrhoea and infertility. |
| Ovarian cancer | Fifth most common cause of female cancer. Usually affects those >50 years old. Pelvic pain, bloating, decreased appetite and weight loss. |
| Hypothyroidism | Increased BMI, dry skin, thin hair, feeling cold, reduced reflexes, low BP, bradycardia, low mood, constipation and tiredness. |
| Androgen-secreting tumour | Sudden onset of hair growth, severe hirsutism, virilisation (scalp hair loss, deepening voice, muscle bulk and clitoromegaly) and abdominal/pelvic mass. |

## Investigations

> » Bloods – Hormones (hormonal blood test performed in the first week of their menstrual cycle). These are often not needed if the hirsutism is mild and there are no other symptoms.
>
>> › PCOS – LH (10U/l) and FSH. LH-to-FSH ratio is 3:1 with a low SHBG.
>>
>> › Testosterone – Measure this on one of days 4–10 of their cycle. If testosterone is >2.5nmol/l, consider PCOS; if it is >4.8nmol/l, consider the differentials (adrenal hyperplasia, Cushing's syndrome and androgen-secreting tumour).
>>
>> › Others – TFT, prolactin, HbA1c (acromegaly), 17-hydroxyprogesterone (>5 nmol/l indicates congenital adrenal hyperplasia [CAH]).
>
> » Urine – 24-hour urine cortisol to exclude Cushing's syndrome.
>
> » Imaging – Consider a pelvic/TV USS (PCOS), pelvic CT/MRI (ovarian tumour) and brain MRI (pituitary tumour).

## Management

*Conservative*

✓ Lifestyle – Advise them to try to lose weight if they are obese.

✓ Cosmetic – Advise them to consider shaving, depilation (removal of hair through using creams that dissolve hair), plucking, bleaching, waxing or threading to remove the excess hair. More long-term solutions may also be considered:

　› Electrolysis – The removal of hair using electric current. This damages the hair permanently.

　› Laser – Laser and intense pulsed light (IPL) damage the hair at the root. This is performed over a few months. The results are not permanent, but are long lasting.

*Medical*

✓ Dianette – This increases the risk of CVD and DVT/PE (1.5–2 times more than COCP). It is not licenced solely for contraception. This should be taken as per the advice for COCP. Contraindicated for a past medical history of DVT and having several risk factors for arterial disease (smoking, obesity, etc.).

✓ Eflornithine cream – Consider Vaniqa if the COCP is contraindicated or has not worked for facial hirsutism. It slows the growth of hair, making it finer. This takes six to eight weeks for the effects to be seen. Stop it if there are no results after four months. Once stopped, the hair returns to normal after eight weeks. This should be avoided if they are pregnant, breastfeeding or <19 years old.

　› Application – Rub it into the skin and do not wash the treated area for four hours after use. Cosmetics can be applied five minutes later.

　› Side effects – Acne, burning and stinging sensation.

　› Contraindications – Pregnancy and breastfeeding, and is not licenced for those <18 years.

» Specialist – Spironolactone, finasteride, metformin and pioglitazone.

## Referral

→ Consider a referral to an appropriate specialist if there are any red flags (Cushing's syndrome, virilisation or pelvic mass) or a recent rapid progression of symptoms. Refer them if the treatment has not been effective after 6–12 months or if testosterone is >5nmol/l. Refer them urgently if testosterone is >6–7nmol/l.

## Safety Netting

→ Follow-up – Review in three months to Check the patient's response to treatment.

---

## *References*

British National Formulary (n.d.). *Contraceptives, hormonal.* National Institute for Health and Care Excellence. https://bnf.nice.org.uk/treatment-summary/contraceptives-hormonal.html

Royal College of Obstetricians & Gynaecologists (2014). *Long-term consequences of polycystic ovary syndrome.* https://www.rcog.org.uk/globalassets/documents/guidelines/gtg_33.pdf

# Ectopic Pregnancy

A pregnancy that implants outside of the uterine cavity is known as an ectopic pregnancy. This most commonly occurs in the fallopian tube; however, it can also occur in the ovaries, cervix or abdomen. If undiagnosed or untreated, this can lead to maternal death due to rupture and intraperitoneal haemorrhage.

When an embryo is transported within the fallopian tube, an interaction between the tubal epithelium, fluid and contents aids the movement of the embryo towards the uterine cavity. This process can be disrupted, most commonly by abnormal fallopian tube anatomy, which is caused by tubal pathology (such as chronic salpingitis) or tubal surgery (reconstruction or sterilisation). When the ectopic pregnancy grows, the outer layer of the fallopian tube stretches, which can lead to bleeding or rupture.

## Risk Factors

➤ Previous ectopic pregnancy

➤ Previous tubal sterilisation

➤ Smoking

➤ Use of an IUD (particularly if the IUD is still in situ)

➤ Assisted reproductive technology (tubal factor sub/infertility or multiple embryo transfer)

➤ Maternal age >35 years old

### History

» Focused questions

  › Ask if they have had any vaginal bleeding, pelvic or abdominal pain, missed periods or amenorrhoea.

  › Urinary/GI – Be aware that some patients may present atypically with urinary and GI symptoms. Ask if they have any such symptoms, and particularly ask if they have urgency to defecate, which may be a sign of a possible rupture.

  › Ask if they have any shoulder-tip pain. Bleeding from the fallopian tube may irritate the diaphragm causing referred shoulder-tip pain, so this could also be a sign of a possible rupture.

## Examination

» Vitals – BP and HR.

» Examine the abdomen for unilateral lower abdominal pain (which may be generalised), and pelvic and adnexal tenderness.

» Examine for warning signs of a rupture – Cervical motion tenderness, pallor, abdominal distention, shock and hypotension. Blood may be present in the vaginal vault in the absence of a rupture.

## Differentials

➤ Miscarriage

➤ Acute appendicitis

➤ Ovarian torsion

➤ PID

➤ UTI

## Investigations

» Bloods – Serum hCG to confirm pregnancy.

» Urinalysis – Urine dip to confirm pregnancy.

» Imaging

› Transabdominal USS to identify intrauterine pregnancy.

› TV USS to determine the location of the pregnancy. If it is ectopic, a 'donut sign' is present, showing a heterogeneous adnexal mass separate from the clearly identified ovaries, and increased blood flow to the ectopic gestation seen on Doppler USS.

## Management

If an ectopic pregnancy is suspected, always refer the patient to be reviewed by an Early Pregnancy Assessment Unit, which will organise a USS.

### Conservative

✓ The expected management of a patient who is hemodynamically stable with minimal or no clinical symptoms, and decreasing serum hCG is serial hCG monitored.

### Medical

✓ If a patient presents with no significant pain, no intrauterine pregnancy, a low serum hCG (<1,500IU/l) and an unruptured ectopic pregnancy with an adnexal mass <35mm with no visible heartbeat, they can be treated with methotrexate IM, usually in secondary care.

✓ The serum hCG will be monitored. If there is no decrease after two doses of methotrexate, surgical intervention will be considered.

✓ Methotrexate may cause some adverse effects such as hepatotoxicity, nephrotoxicity, pancytopenia, GI symptoms, fever or fatigue. The medication should be stopped if any of the aforementioned occur. If a patient has had a previous adverse reaction to methotrexate, surgical intervention is indicated.

*Surgical*

✓ Laparoscopic surgery (salpingostomy or salpingectomy) should be considered if the patient is haemodynamically unstable.

✓ Serial serum hCG levels are monitored post procedure to monitor the decrease.

✓ If they do not return to undetectable levels, methotrexate can be considered post procedure.

✓ Anti-D immunoglobulin is offered to patients who are Rh-negative post procedure.

---

## References

Pazhaniappan, N. (2016). *Ectopic pregnancy.* https://teachmeobgyn.com/pregnancy/early/ectopic-pregnancy/

The Ectopic Pregnancy Trust (.n.d.). *What is an ectopic pregnancy?* https://ectopic.org.uk/patients/what-is-an-ectopic-pregnancy/

# Prolapse

A prolapse is the herniation of one or more pelvic organs into the vagina. This is usually due to the weakness of the pelvic floor muscles or poor pelvic muscle tone. Genitourinary organs are supported by the levator ani muscles and endopelvic fascia. These supportive structures can be damaged and weakened by direct muscle trauma, disruption and injury.

Prolapses are named based on the organ that is protruding into the vagina, as follows:

» Cystocele – bladder

» Urethrocele – urethra

» Rectocele – rectum

» Enterocele – loops of the intestine

» Uterine – uterus

## Risk Factors

➤ Childbirth

➤ Coughing

➤ Straining

➤ Obesity

➤ Congenital connective-tissue disorder

➤ Menopause

## *History*

» Focused questions

› Ask if they have had a 'dragging sensation' or any abnormal feeling of 'something down below'; for example, a lump.

› Ask if the symptoms are worsened by sitting upright or coughing.

› Ask if they have had difficulty in opening their bowels or having sexual intercourse (as well as a lack of sensation).

» Past history – Ask if they have had recurrent cystitis or polyuria.

## Examination

» Abdominal examination – To rule out a pelvic mass (also do a bimanual examination).

» Speculum examination – This may reveal a prolapse. Ask the patient to cough or bear down.

» Uterine prolapses can be assessed based on their severity, as follows:

> First-degree prolapse – Defined as a prolapse that remains within the vagina.

> Second-degree prolapse – Defined as the prolapse protruding from the vagina when coughing or straining.

> Third-degree prolapse – The prolapse lies outside of the vagina.

## Differentials

➤ Cystitis

➤ Constipation

➤ Urogenital atrophy

➤ Vaginal-wall cysts

## Investigation

» If the result of the examination is no abnormality detected (NAD), a urine dipstick with MSU can be done; otherwise, no further investigation is required in primary care.

## Management

✓ This depends on the patient's preference, severity, past medical history and the interference of the condition in day-to-day life.

✓ Watchful waiting is appropriate when there are mild and minimal symptoms that do not interfere in the patient's life.

### Conservative

✓ Advise them to lose weight (if BMI >30).

✓ Treat the triggers for the exacerbating factors (a cough in COPD, constipation, etc.).

✓ Advise them to do pelvic floor exercises to strengthen the weakened muscles.

✓ Offer ring pessaries. Depending on the local services, this may require referral to urogynaecology specialists. The pessary would need to be changed every three to six months.

### Surgery

✓ Indications for surgery include the failure of the aforementioned management, the presence of urinary or bowel symptoms, the ulceration of the prolapse itself, an irreducible prolapse, the recurrence of the prolapse following surgical repair, and patient preference for surgery. (Note that surgical repair can include a hysterectomy, depending on the type of prolapse).

## References

National Institute for Health and Care Excellence (2019). *Urinary incontinence and pelvic organ prolapse: management.* https://www.nice.org.uk/guidance/ng123/chapter/Recommendations

# 11

# Musculoskeletal

## Systemic Lupus Erythematosus

Systemic lupus erythematosus (SLE) is a multisystem, inflammatory autoimmune disease. The term 'systemic' refers to the involvement of a number of organs in the body. The rash that may develop as a result of SLE is known as lupus erythematosus. The cause of SLE is unknown; however, a genetic component has been found. In addition, environmental factors include some forms of medication, UV light, viruses such as the Epstein-Barr virus and some drugs (methyldopa, isoniazid and hydralazine).

### *History*

»   The history is often non-specific.

»   Associated history

   ›   Ask if they have any general malaise, lethargy or severe fatigue, fever, weight loss, enlargement of the spleen and LNs, mouth ulcers, dry eyes and mouth, headaches and paraesthesia.

   ›   Ask if they also have Raynaud's phenomenon and mild hair loss.

   ›   Ask if they are experiencing joint and muscle pains, often with early morning stiffness. Secondary fibromyalgia is common.

   ›   Ask if they have a malar (butterfly) rash, which is a classic component that is often triggered by sunlight. It may be raised, itchy and erythematous. It spares the nasolabial folds.

   ›   Ask if they have any chest symptoms, such as pleuritic-type chest pain.

### Investigations

»   Urinalysis – To look for any proteinuria/haematuria (initial testing for renal diseases such as glomerulonephritis).

»   Bloods – FBC and ESR (ESR is raised, but CRP may be normal; mild normocytic anaemia is common).

»   Autoantibodies

> Antinuclear antibody (ANA) – This is a screening test with a sensitivity of 95%, but it is not diagnostic in the absence of clinical features. It is a non-specific antibody that is also present in many patients with systemic autoimmune conditions; e.g. systemic sclerosis (scleroderma), polymyositis and primary Sjögren's syndrome

> Anti-double stranded deoxyribonucleic acid (anti-dsDNA) – This is high specificity, but the sensitivity is only 70%. The level reflects disease activity.

> Anti-Smith (anti-Sm) – This is the most specific antibody, but its sensitivity is only 30–40%.

## Management

✓ Treatment for SLE is initiated in secondary care. If it is suspected, order the appropriate investigations if available, then refer the patient to rheumatology.

✓ The main aim of management is to control acute periods of potentially life-threatening ill health, minimise the risk of flares during periods of relative stability, and control the less-life-threatening day-to-day symptoms.

### Conservative

✓ Exercise programmes have been shown to be useful in managing fatigue without causing disease flares.

✓ Lifestyle changes – Advise the patient to avoid sitting in sunlight and to use sun protection, and to avoid using oestrogens (e.g. in COCPs).

### Medical

✓ Management of comorbidities – This requires prompt or prophylactic treatment of infection.

✓ Mild to moderate disease is managed using oral corticosteroids at low-to-moderate doses of antimalarial therapy (hydroxychloroquine).

✓ If symptoms are not controlled by the aforementioned methods, patients would need higher doses of steroids or steroid-sparing agents (azathioprine or methotrexate).

✓ The management of lupus with major organ involvement includes high-dose IV methylprednisolone, immunosuppressant therapies and biological therapies (rituximab or belimumab).

✓ Women with SLE are at greatly increased risk of premature atherosclerosis, and the risk is independent of established cardiovascular risk factors. Monitoring for all cardiovascular risk factors is therefore essential.

---

### References

GPnotebook (2018). Management [Systemic lupus erythematous]. https://gpnotebook.com/simplepage.cfm?ID=295305236

Harding, M (2018). Lupus systemic lupus erythematous. https://patient.info/skin-conditions/skin-rashes/lupus-systemic-lupus-erythematosus

# Joint Pain

Joint pain and musculoskeletal symptoms are very common presentations that patients may attend your clinic with. The key symptoms associated with joint pain include swelling, stiffness and numbness. When taking a history and examining them, it is important to take a clear history from the patient to distinguish whether there is an inflammatory or a degenerative process at play. OA refers to joint pain that is usually accompanied with functional limitation and reduced quality of life. It is usually due to loss of cartilage, remodelling of the bone and local inflammation.

## History

» Focused questions

› Ask which joint(s) and how many, and whether it is symmetrical on both sides or only on one side.

› Ask about the pain, including when it first started, what the site of the pain is, what the character of the pain is (burning, sharp or aching), what the frequency of the pain is, if it comes and goes, and if anything makes it better or worse.

› Ask if it is worse during the day (RA) or at night (OA).

› Ask if there is any radiation of the pain.

› Ask if they have had an injury (a fall or recent trauma).

› Ask how long the joint stiffness lasts (>45 minutes indicates RA).

› Ask if there is any swelling, and if it is always there or comes and goes.

» Associated history – Ask if there is any numbness, pins and needles, Raynaud's phenomenon (their fingers change colour in the cold), dry eyes (Sjögren's syndrome), fever, rash (a facial rash indicates SLE), crepitus or changes in mood.

› Ask about how they are functioning, including if they have any problems when walking up and down stairs, if they are able to comb or do their hair, how far they can walk before experiencing pain, and if they are able to dress themselves or put on their shoes or socks without pain.

» Past history – Ask if they have had IBD, psoriasis or any previous joint operations.

» Drug history – Ask if they have taken any steroids or painkillers (NSAIDs, paracetamol or topical gels). Ask if they have ever taken diuretics, statins, PPIs or olanzapine, which can cause joint pain.

» Family history – Ask if there is a family history of psoriasis or RA.

» Social history – Ask if they have a support network (any close friends, family or any carers), what their occupation is and whether the pain has affected their work, and if they smoke or drink alcohol.

## RED FLAGS

Severe pain, trauma, fever and weight loss.

## Differential Diagnosis

| RA | Mainly affects middle-aged women. Bilateral symmetrical swelling and pain of the small joints of the hands, wrists and feet. Swelling and stiffness is worse in the morning and may improve after exercise. Usually associated with systemic problems such as fever, malaise and weight loss. Patients may have extra-articular symptoms, including eye redness or pain, skin nodules, or fibrosis of the lungs. May have a family history of the disease, raised ESR and CRP, and positive rheumatoid factor. |
|---|---|
| SLE | Autoimmune connective tissue disease that causes inflammation in multiple organs including the skin, kidneys, heart, blood vessels and liver. Ten times more common in women than men. Characteristically, patients have a butterfly facial rash, tiredness and muscle pain. |
| OA | Progressive unilateral or bilateral pain and degeneration, usually in the weight bearing joints of the body (knee and hip), but it may also affect the hands, feet, ankles and spine. Pain increased with activity and reduced with rest. Patient may be obese and are usually middle-aged. Previous falls or trauma may accelerate the development of OA. OE: the patient may have crepitus and knobbly joints. |
| Gout | Unilateral joint pain, usually due to raised uric acid levels. May be as a result of a diet rich in purines (veal, red meat, some seafood, and organ meats such as kidney and liver) or poor hydration / fluid intake. |

## Examination

» Vitals – Temperature, BP, pulse and BMI (weight loss).

» Examination – Look at, feel and move the appropriate joints. Assess for pain and swelling. Perform the metacarpophalangeal squeeze test. A diagnosis is more likely if they cannot make a fist or flex their fingers. Look for rheumatoid nodules over the extensor surfaces.

## Investigations

» Bloods – FBC (anaemia), ESR and CRP (active disease), ANA, CCP (80%), rheumatoid factor (70%) to exclude inflammatory arthritis and a renal profile.

» Other – Bone profile, PSA (elderly), vitamin D (when low, it worsens pain), urate (gout), HLA B27 and IgA for AS, performed in secondary care.

» Imaging

> X-ray – OA of the joint, fractures, hands and feet (RA), and chest (RA)

> MRI – Consider administering for a steroid injection treatment or to exclude a fracture.

> Bone scan – DEXA scan for osteoporosis.

# Management

## OA

### Conservative

✓ Rest – If the pain is due to repetitive movements, advise the patient to rest for up to 12 weeks.

✓ Ice/heat – Advise them to apply an ice or heat pack if it worsens after activity.

✓ Support – Advise them to consider purchasing support bandages, or appropriate footwear (shock absorbing) or insoles.

✓ Exercise – Advise them to continue doing simple exercises (aerobic / muscle strengthening) as the pain eases, to help maintain and improve their range of motion (ROM) and prevent stiffness.

✓ Weight – If their BMI >25, suggest that they lose weight.

✓ Aids

> Walking stick – Offer them a walking stick to reduce the load on the contralateral joint (hip). Suggest a heel raiser to correct unequal leg lengths.

> Assistance devices – Suggest using various assistance devices, including tap turners, enlarged grips for writing, non-slip mats, electric can openers and long-handled reachers/grabbers.

### Medical

✓ Pain

> Simple analgesia (paracetamol) or NSAIDs can be prescribed as topical creams or oral tablets. Ensure there are no contraindications for NSAIDs (ulcers, gastritis or asthma). Consider a cyclooxygenase-2 (COX-2) inhibitor (celecoxib) if there is a poor response.

> Add a PPI with NSAIDs.

> Offer topical capsaicin as an adjunct for knee or hand OA.

> Stronger options include a weak opioid (co-codamol or tramadol). This should be for a short period only. Consider laxatives.

✓ Advise the patient to avoid glucosamine (there is limited evidence for its efficacy).

*RA*

*Medical*

✓ Pain – Offer paracetamol with or without codeine (co-dydramol/co-codamol).

› Consider NSAIDs. Ensure there are no contraindications (ulcers, gastritis or asthma).

› Add PPI with NSAIDS.

› If they have IHD, offer ibuprofen (400mg tds) or naproxen (500mg bd).

✓ Steroids – Do not initiate steroids unless they have been reviewed by a specialist.

✓ Disease-modifying anti-rheumatic drugs (DMARDs) – These help slow the progression of RA and reduce permanent damage (e.g. methotrexate, leflunomide or sulfasalazine, within three months of onset) or consider hydroxychloroquine (for mild or palindromic RA).

› Methotrexate – Once-a-week treatment, given with folic acid.

› Bloods – Every two weeks unless stable, then every two to three months. Check FBC, LFTs and U&Es.

› Toxicity – Advise them that if they develop a rash, mouth ulcer, nausea and vomiting, diarrhoea, SOB or a cough, they are not to take the medication and have a review. If they develop a severe sore throat or bruising, they are not to take the medication and go for an urgent FBC.

› Biological – There are newer drugs that prevent the immune system from attacking the lining of the joints. Examples include infliximab, rituximab and tocilizumab.

✓ Injections – If they have a flare-up, consider an intra-articular or IM steroid injection.

## Referral

*OA*

→ Physiotherapy – Refer them to physiotherapy, which is helpful for strengthening the muscles. They can provide recommendations on strapping and splints.

→ OT – Refer them to speak to an OT about adaptations that can be made (bath aids, putting a chair on bed raisers, raised toilet sets, stair rails, etc.).

→ Chiropodist – This is to assist with foot care or insoles.

→ Pain clinic – Consider referring to MSK or a pain clinic to maximise treatment.

→ Injections – Offer an intra-articular steroid injection for moderate to severe pain.

→ Surgery – Refer them for surgery if the symptoms have deteriorated rapidly or the condition is causing disability.

*RA*

→ Rheumatologist – Refer them urgently within two weeks if there are signs of synovitis affecting their hands or feet (more than one joint). Normal blood tests do not exclude a diagnosis of RA.

→ Physiotherapy – Refer them to physiotherapy, which can offer night-time splints for inflamed joints (to rest the joints). They can demonstrate passive movements when the joints are inflamed and active ones when the joints have improved. The patient can be referred to hand-exercise programmes.

→ OT – Refer them to speak to an OT about adaptations that can be made.

→ Podiatry – Refer them for assessment of their foot needs, and for consideration of insoles or footwear.

→ Surgery – Refer them for joint replacement if it is causing a disability.

## Safety Netting

» Review in four to six weeks regarding their response to treatment, or urgently if there are any red-flag symptoms.

---

*References*

National Institute for Health and Care Excellence (2014). *Osteoarthritis: care and management.* https://www.nice.org.uk/guidance/cg177

National Institute for Health and Care Excellence (2018). *Rheumatoid arthritis in adults: management.* https://www.nice.org.uk/guidance/ng100

# Gout

Gout is a condition in which raised serum uric acid levels lead to the deposition of urate crystals in the joints and allied tissues. It is the most common cause of inflammatory arthritis, and it typically affects the first metatarsophalangeal (MTP) joints (big toe), but can also affect the ankle, knee, wrist and elbow joints.

## Pathophysiology

As crystals build up and solidify, they irritate the joint and cause inflammation, leading to severe pain and swelling. Hyperuricaemia is usually due to the impaired renal excretion of urate. About 90% of people with hyperuricaemia are under-excretors of urate, and about 10% are overproducers of urate. Some people are both under-excretors and overproducers of urate. In many people with hyperuricaemia, the cause is multifactorial.

## Risk Factors

➤ Male

➤ Elderly

➤ High alcohol intake

➤ Diet high in purines (meat and seafood)

➤ Diuretics

## *History*

» Focused questions

› Ask if they have great difficulty with walking or the inability to use the affected joint.

› Ask if they cannot bear to touch or put pressure on the affected joint.

› Ask if there is any reddening (erythema) overlying the affected joint.

› Ask if they have developed acute pain in a joint, which becomes swollen, tender and erythematous, and which reaches its crescendo over a 6-to-12-hour period.

## Examination

» Vitals – Temperature, BP and pulse.

» Inspection – Inspect the affected joint for swelling and redness.

› Chronic tophaceous gout – In this condition, large crystal deposits produce irregular, firm nodules, mainly around the extensor surfaces of the fingers, hands, forearms, elbows, Achilles tendons and ears.

> › Check for tophi on the extensor surface of the elbow, fingers, helixes of the ears and the Achilles tendons.

> › Typically, tophi are asymmetrical with a chalky appearance beneath the skin.

» Palpate – Check for warmth and tenderness.

» Move – Check for active and passive movement (usually reduced due to pain).

## Differentials

➤ Acute attacks – Sepsis and other forms of crystal-related synovitis

➤ Septic arthritis

➤ Chronic tophaceous – RA, generalised nodal OA, xanthomatosis with arthropathy, and multicentric reticulohistiocytosis

## Investigations

» Bloods – Uric acid is not routinely needed. Check four to six weeks after an acute attack, but this can be normal. (Gout may present with normal serum uric acid levels, and those with raised levels do not always have symptoms). Also WCC, ESR and CRP.

» X-ray/imaging – Consider this if you suspect a fracture.

» Specialist – Aspiration (usually performed in secondary care if the diagnosis is in doubt). Joint aspiration if septic arthritis is suspected.

## Management

*Conservative*

✓ Advise the patient to elevate and rest the limb. They should keep the affected area open and uncovered. They should avoid trauma to the joint.

✓ Advise them to apply cold / an ice pack to the area (e.g. frozen peas).

✓ Advise them to reduce their alcohol intake.

✓ Advise them to eat a balanced diet while cutting out purine-rich foods (e.g. liver, kidney, yeast extract, herring and sardines).

✓ Advise them to keep well hydrated (drink at least 2l of water a day).

*Medical*

✓ Acute attack

> › NSAIDs (ensure there are no contraindications; e.g. ulcers, gastritis or asthma <30 eGFR).

> › Colchicine if there are contraindications to NSAIDs or there is no response to treatment. Start with 500mcg bd to qds.

> › Oral steroids if the aforementioned are contraindicated. These can be taken with paracetamol.

✓ Prophylaxis – Consider this if there is more than one attack a year, tophi or urate renal stones. Aim for <300micromol/l if tophi are present, and <360micromol/l if there are no tophi or they have been resolved. Never initiate during an acute attack.

> › Allopurinol. Start one to two weeks after the gout has settled. Start at 100mg daily and increase by 50mcg fortnightly until they are taking 300mg daily. Check serum urate and renal function after three months.

> › Febuxostat if they are intolerant to or have contraindications for allopurinol. Start this one to two weeks after the gout has settled. Start at 80mg daily. Do LFTs before and after regularly. Check serum urate and renal function after three months.

## Referral

→ Refer the patient if there is suspicion of septic arthritis.

→ Refer them to a dietician for more advice regarding a low-purine diet.

→ Refer them to the appropriate specialist if there is suspicion of RA, gout in pregnancy or they are a young patient.

*References*

Hui, M., Carr, A., Cameron, S., Davenport, G., Doherty, M., Forrester, H., Jenkins, W., Jordan, K.M., Mallen, C.D., McDonald, T.M., Nuki, G., Pywell, A., Zhang, W. and Roddy, E. (2017). *The British Society for Rheumatology Guideline for the Management of Gout. Rheumatology, 56*(7), e1–e20. doi: https://doi.org/10.1093/rheumatology/kex156

# Back Pain

Back pain is a common complaint that affects eight out of 10 people at some point in their life. Most cases of back pain are fairly innocuous – mainly caused by a muscle sprain or poor posture – and require mild analgesia. However, a minority of cases may have a serious underlying cause and require immediate intervention to prevent permanent nerve damage (cauda equina). Back pain is usually classified as acute (<6 weeks), subacute (6–12 weeks) or chronic (>12 weeks).

## History

» Focused questions
  › Ask where the pain and tenderness is, and when it first started.
  › Ask about the character of the pain (burning, sharp or aching), the frequency, and if there are any exacerbating or alleviating factors.
  › Ask if it is worse in the day or night, if there is any radiation, and if there is stiffness in the morning or evening.
  › Ask if they have had a recent fall or injury, or if there are any triggers (lifting anything heavy or a road traffic accident [RTA]).

» Associated history
  › Neurology – Ask if there is any weakness, numbness, or pins and needles.
  › Function – Ask if there are any problems walking up or down stairs, how far they can walk, if they are able to dress themself, and if they can put their shoes or socks on.

» Past history – Ask if they have had cancer and if they have had any surgery.

» Drug history – Ask if they have taken any steroids or used anything OTC (NSAIDs, paracetamol or topical gels).

» Social history – Ask if they have any support at home, what their current occupation is, and if the pain has affected their work.

## Yellow Flags

Psychological causes that turn acute back pain into chronic pain, including financial or relationship problems, anxiety, stress or social withdrawal.

## Red Flags

Severe pain at night, thoracic pain, pain in someone <20 years or >50 years, a past medical history of cancer, fever, saddle paraesthesia, urinary retention or incontinence, faecal incontinence, or leg weakness.

## STarT Back Screening Tool

» NICE (2016) recommends using a screening tool to assess and risk stratify back pain at every point of contact with a healthcare professional for each new episode of lower-back pain with or without sciatica.

> If the total score <3 then they are low risk, but if it is >4, they could be medium or high risk.

## Examination

» Vitals – Temperature, BP and pulse.

» Inspection – Observe their gait (antalgic), inspect them for deformity (kyphosis, scoliosis or loss of lumbar lordosis), asymmetry (shoulder or pelvis) or wasting (paravertebral or gluteal).

» Palpate – Check their temperature and for tenderness. Palpate the spine over the spinal processes, paraspinal muscles and sacroiliac joints.

» Move – Check for extension, flexion, lateral flexion and rotation.

» SLR – Have the patient lying supine and get them to lift their foot off the couch, keeping the leg straight, and note the angle when the pain starts (for sciatica this is 30–70°).

» Neurology

> Power – Ask them to walk on their heels to check foot dorsiflexion (L4/L5), and to walk on their toes to check foot plantar flexion (L5/S1).

> Check for sensation.

> Reflexes – Focus the reflex assessment depending on their history. For sciatic pain radiating to the foot, perform an ankle reflex (S1) test. If the pain only radiates to the thigh, perform a knee reflex (L3/L4) test. PR is only indicated if cauda equina is suspected.

*Neurological Signs of Back Pain Based on the Nerve Root*

| Root | Sensory loss | Weakness | Reflex loss | Special test |
|------|--------------|----------|-------------|--------------|
| L3 | Inner thigh | Knee extension | Knee | Positive femoral stretch test |
| L4 | Anterior knee | Knee extension plus foot dorsiflexion | Knee | Positive femoral stretch test |
| L5 | Dorsum foot | Foot plus big toe dorsiflexion | None | Positive sciatic stretch test |
| S1 | Lateral foot | Foot plantar flexion | Ankle | Positive sciatic stretch test |

## Investigations

» Bloods – FBC, ESR, ANA, rheumatoid factor to exclude inflammatory arthritis, bone profile, PSA (in elderly) and vitamin D.

» X-ray – Not routinely done for non-specific back pain. Consider in the young ankylosing spondylitis, elderly (vertebral collapse) or in cases of trauma.

» MRI – Consider for malignancy, infection, cauda equina or fracture.

» Bone scan – DEXA scan for osteoporosis.

## Differential Diagnosis

| | |
|---|---|
| Reactive arthritis | Eye pain (conjunctivitis), urethral discharge and other joints affected. |
| Ankylosing spondylitis | Presents with insidious onset of morning back pain and stiffness that is worsened with inactivity. OE: reduced ROM of the spine, tender sacroiliac joints, loss of lumbar lordosis, Achilles tendonitis and atlantoaxial subluxation. May have neck pain, hip pain, eye symptoms (uveitis), pulmonary fibrosis and amyloidosis. Chronic inflammatory rheumatic disease that commonly affects young Caucasian males. Associated with a family history of the condition. |
| Spinal cord compression from metastasis | Can present in cancer patients, often affecting the thoracic region. Back pain is worse on movement and there is weakness of the legs. If the lesion is above L1, they may have upper motor neurone (UMN) signs (increased tone and reflexes) with the sensory level. If it is below L1, this presents with lower motor neurone (LMN) signs (reduced tone and reflexes) and perianal numbness (cauda equina). Also enquire about weight loss, night sweats, and any past history of prostate or breast cancer. |
| Cauda equina | Compression of the spinal nerve routes, causing lower-back pain, saddle anaesthesia, and urinary or bowel incontinence. Emergency condition that requires urgent admission to prevent permanent damage. |
| Spinal stenosis | Pain when walking only, where the pain moves from the back to the calves of both legs. A narrowing of the spinal canal, which may be congenital or due to acquired spondylolisthesis. |
| Spondylosis | Lower-back pain that may radiate to the buttocks. OA of the spine and damage to the discs. Causes hypertrophy of the superior articular processes of the spinal bodies and may cause osteophyte formation. |

| Sciatica | Reduced SLR raise. A disc pressing on the sciatic nerve due to degeneration and bulging. Can be caused by strenuous activity (lifting). Causes an electric-shock-like pain from the lower back to the ipsilateral leg. May be bilateral. May also cause numbness in the affected dermatomes, foot drop and loss of reflexes if chronic. |
|----------|------------------------------------------------------------------------------|
| Discitis | Infection of a spinal disc. Causes fever, severe back pain and focal tenderness. |

## Management

### Conservative

✓ Advise the patient to avoid prolonged rest. They should return to normal activities, including work, as soon as possible. They should avoid unsupported sitting or heavy lifting. Advise them to increase physical activities over a few days or weeks.

✓ Advise them to apply ice or a heat pack if the pain has worsened after activity.

✓ Advise them to sit down for chores, avoid heavy lifting, and prop up their legs and knees when lying in bed.

✓ If they have not returned to normal activities, they should consider structured exercise programmes.

### Medical

✓ Simple analgesia (paracetamol) and NSAIDs can be prescribed as topical creams or oral medication. Ensure there are no contraindications for NSAIDs (ulcers, gastritis or asthma). Add PPI in the elderly.

✓ Consider a weak opioid (co-dydramol or co-codamol) or tramadol with or without laxatives for constipation. Consider amitriptyline if there is no improvement.

✓ Consider diazepam if back muscles spasm, but for a short period only.

✓ Liaise with the GP to offer a short sick note if they are unable to work. Consider recommending amended duties or altered hours if they are finding it difficult to carry out certain tasks (bending or lifting).

## Referral

→ Patients can consider self-referral to a chiropractor or osteopath for manipulation if they are not able to return to normal activities within the first six weeks, although this may be unavailable under the NHS.

→ Refer them to physiotherapy, which is helpful for strengthening the muscles around the back. Consider referring them to OT for walking aids, a Zimmer frame or a wheelchair if there is severe dysfunction.

→ Refer them for CBT if the back pain is associated with stress or a low mood.

→ Consider referring them for acupuncture, though there is limited availability on NHS. NICE advises against this for lower back pain.

→ Refer them to orthopaedics if their symptoms have deteriorated rapidly or are causing a disability.

→ Refer them to rheumatology if ankylosing spondylitis is suspected.

→ Refer them to ophthalmology urgently if anterior uveitis becomes painful or there is photophobia.

## Safety Netting

» Review in four to six weeks regarding their response to treatment or urgently if there are red-flag symptoms.

---

### References

National Institute for Health and Care Excellence (2016). *Low back pain and sciatica in over 16s: assessment and management.* https://www.nice.org.uk/guidance/ng59

# Chronic Fatigue Syndrome

Chronic fatigue syndrome (CFS) is also called myalgic encephalomyelitis (ME) and it is a clinical condition that is diagnosed when a patient suffers from new onset, persistent (more than four months) fatigue, to the exclusion of other medical conditions. Patients may also suffer with post-exertional malaise, which results in a substantial reduction in activity levels. Patients may present with accompanying problems, such as joint pain, headaches, insomnia, a sore throat and general flu-like symptoms. Although it can affect people of all ages, it mainly affects women between the ages of 25 and 45 years.

## *History*

» Focused questions

  › Fatigue – Ask when the onset was, how often it occurs, if it is there all the time or if it comes and goes. If it is post-exertional, ask when it usually starts and how long it lasts (several days).

  › Function – Ask if it has affected their ability to carry out activities such as walking, cooking, climbing stairs or getting dressed.

» Associated history – Ask if they have had any sleep disturbance (insomnia or early morning waking); joint pain or stiffness, and if so, which ones are affected; cold-like symptoms (headaches or sore throat); dizziness (nausea or vomiting); impaired cognitive function (unable to concentrate, get distracted easily, or find it more difficult to make decisions or complete everyday tasks); or lumps (neck, underarm or groin) and if so, if they are painful.

» Family history – Ask if there is a family history of CFS or ME.

» Social history – Ask about their mood (if there have been any changes recently), about their relationships and support network, what their occupation is (and if they are missing work), what their diet is like, and if they smoke, drink alcohol or take recreational drugs.

## RED FLAGS

Weight loss, night sweats, persistent fevers, haemoptysis, PR bleeding, post-menopausal PV bleeding, dysphagia or swollen LNs.

## Differentials

➤ See *Tired All the Time section, page 226.*

## Examination

» Vitals – Temperature, BP, weight and pulse.

» Do a complete physical exam, focusing on the systems where symptoms may be present.

  › Inspection – Look at their general health, look for any lumps and inspect their throat.

  › Palpation – Palpate any lumps, and examine for LNs in the cervical, axillary, epitrochlear, para-aortic, inguinal and popliteal regions. Palpate for hepatomegaly or splenomegaly.

## Investigations

Perform the following to exclude common differentials.

» Urine – Dipstick for blood, ketones and glucose.

» Bloods – FBC, ESR, CRP, LFTs, U&Es (electrolyte abnormalities), HbA1c, TFT, coeliac screen, vitamin D and a bone profile (if >60 years).

  › If clinically indicated, request vitamin B12 and folate (only if FBC/MCV shows macrocytosis). If FBC suggests iron deficiency, request ferritin.

  › RA – Rheumatoid factor, ANA and anti-CCP.

  › Viral screen – HIV, hep B and C, Epstein-Barr virus (EBV) (if <40 years) and cytomegalovirus (CMV).

  › Myeloma screen – Urine Bence-Jones protein and protein electrophoresis.

» CXR – Consider baseline x-ray (to exclude TB, lung cancer and HF).

» Sputum – Acid fast bacilli (TB) and MC&S (infection).

## Management

*Conservative*

✓ Lifestyle

  › Diet – Advise them to cut down their alcohol intake, eat a balanced diet and eat regularly. Only advise an exclusion diet if supported by a dietician.

  › Nausea – Advise them to eat little and often; to snack on dry, starchy foods; and to sip fluids.

  › Sleep – Advise them to relax in a dark room with minimal distraction, go to sleep at the same time every night and have a light snack beforehand. There should be no sleeping during the day.

  › Exercise: Take low level, regular exercise and try and get out even for a walk.

> › Rest – Ensure any rest periods are <30 minutes. Use breathing techniques or guided visualisation to help relax during a rest period. Use relaxation techniques.

> › Avoid undertaking unsupervised vigorous exercise.

✓ Sickness certificate – Offer them a short fit note if there are severe symptoms. Consider recommending amended duties or altered hours if they are finding it difficult to carry out certain tasks or attend the workplace. Advise them to attend the jobcentre for advice around benefits, income support and disability.

✓ Talking therapies

> › CBT – Consider CBT for mild/moderate depression.

> › Graded exercise – Consider referring them for graded exercise therapies or activity management programmes (slowly increasing the intensity of physical activity).

> › Groups – Suggest that they contact support groups (i.e. an ME support society).

### Medical

✓ Antiemetic – Only consider this if the nausea is severe.

✓ TCA – Consider a low dose of amitriptyline for those with poor sleep or pain. Avoid this if they are taking an SSRI already due to potential side effects.

## Referral

→ OT – Refer them to speak to OT about adaptations that can be made or regarding changes at work to maintain their ability to stay in employment.

→ Pain clinic – Consider referring them to a pain clinic to maximise treatment.

→ Rheumatologist – Refer them to a rheumatologist or specialist CFS service if available locally.

→ Charities – Consider directing them to the ME Association for further information or support about their diagnosis.

## Safety Netting

» Review in four to six weeks regarding their response to treatment or to check the diagnosis.

### References

National Institute for Health and Care Excellence (2017). *Chronic fatigue syndrome/myalgic encephalomyelitis (or encephalopathy): diagnosis and management.* https://www.nice.org.uk/guidance/cg53

# Polymyalgia Rheumatica

PMR is an inflammatory disease that presents with at least two weeks of pain, and morning stiffness affecting the neck, shoulders and pelvic girdle. It often affects elderly (>70 years) women more than men, and it is seen in Caucasians (Northern Europeans) more often than other ethnic groups. Other symptoms include a mild fever, fatigability and weight loss. It is important to diagnose this in order to initiate long-term (one to three years) steroid treatment to prevent complications such as temporal arteritis (or giant cell arteritis) and potential blindness.

## When to Suspect PMR

Consider if the patient is >50 years with at least two weeks of the following:

» Shoulder/girdle pain – This is often bilateral (though it may start as unilateral), worse with movement and affects sleep. It affects the shoulder(s) (it can radiate to the elbows) and pelvic girdle (hip pain can radiate to the knees).

» Stiffness – Occurs in the morning, may last >45 minutes, and is worse after rest periods. It affects the ability to get out of bed or a chair.

» Associated symptoms – Additional symptoms include a low-grade fever, weight loss, anorexia or bilateral upper arm tenderness. It can also be associated with peripheral MSK signs (carpal tunnel, peripheral arthritis, or swelling with pitting oedema of the hands, wrists, feet or ankles).

## *History*

» Focused questions

› Ask if there is any pain or tenderness in both shoulders and when it started.

› Ask about the onset (was it quick), character, frequency, worsening and alleviating factors, radiation (elbow), stiffness (worse in the morning), pain in other joints (hips, pelvis or wrists [carpal tunnel]) and joint swelling.

› Temporal arteritis – Ask if there are headaches (temporal), scalp tenderness (if it hurts to comb their hair), jaw claudication (if it is painful to chew or brush their teeth) or visual disturbances (loss of vision or diplopia).

» Associated history – Ask if they have experienced fatigue, fever, night sweats, weight loss or oedema.

» Past history – Ask if they have RA or OA.

» Family history – Ask if there is a family history of PMR or HLA-DR4.

» Drug history – Ask if they have taken steroids or any painkillers (NSAIDs, paracetamol or topical gels).

» Social history – Ask about their home life, what their occupation is, if they drive, or if they smoke or drink alcohol.

## RED FLAGS

Temporal arteritis symptoms (visual disturbance or temporal headaches).

## Differential Diagnosis

| | |
|---|---|
| PMR | Seen in the elderly. Causes pain (aching) and morning stiffness (they cannot turn over in bed) of the shoulders (bilateral) and pelvic girdle. Has abrupt onset and can last more than weeks. Muscles are tender with no true weakness (only pain). Has raised inflammatory markers (ESR and CRP). Associated with temporal arteritis. |
| Polymyositis | More common in middle-aged women. A connective tissue disease that causes muscular inflammation. Leads to symptoms such as proximal muscle weakness, dysphagia and pain. Often presents with a dermatomyositis. May have a raised CK that is 50 times normal. |
| Multiple myeloma | Bone marrow cancer affecting the plasma cells. Causes tiredness, weight loss, infections, bone pain, and multiple fractures in the spine, skull, pelvis, shoulders and rib cage. May have Bence-Jones proteins in urine. |
| Adhesive capsulitis | Also known as frozen shoulder; it causes pain, stiffness and reduced movements. More common in women from 40–60 and diabetics. Leads to restriction of all shoulder movements (particularly external rotation) whether active or passive. Tends to severely affect activities of daily living (ADLs) such as dressing and washing. |
| Thyroid disease | Underactive thyroid gland. Presents with cold intolerance, hair loss, dry skin, fatigability, heavy periods, increased weight and low mood. |
| CFS | Persistent tiredness and fatigue unrelated to activity and persisting for at least four months. Myalgia, unrefreshing sleep, malaise and arthralgia. |

## Examination

» Vitals – Temperature, BP and pulse.

» Inspection – Look for any muscle swelling or muscle wastage.

» Palpation – Feel for tenderness across the shoulders and pelvic girdle (if indicated). Note any reduction in ROM from pain and stiffness.

> Shoulders – Check abduction, adduction, flexion and extension.

> Hips – Check abduction, flexion and extension.

» Temporal artery – Check for tenderness, thickening or pulselessness of the artery.

» Neurology – Check power against resistance. Note any absence of true weakness.

## Investigations

» Bloods – Request urgent ESR and CRP.

> Other – Consider Hb (WCC), U&E, LFT, CK and TFT, and rheumatoid factor for differentials.

> Myeloma screen – Consider urine Bence-Jones protein and protein electrophoresis.

» USS – Performed occasionally, as it can establish evidence of synovitis, or bursitis within the shoulder and/or hip to support the diagnosis.

## Management

### Conservative

✓ Support groups – Offer the details for patient support groups (Polymyalgia Rheumatica and Giant Cell Arteritis UK).

### Medical

✓ Steroids – Offer a low dose of prednisolone, initiating at 15mg od with a follow-up after one week. If symptomatically controlled, taper the dose to reduce it slowly over a year. Typical treatment lasts one to three years.

> Side effects – Weight gain, dyspepsia, bruising and thinning of the skin, and muscle weakness. Inform the patient not to stop taking the medication abruptly.

> Recommend that they carry a steroid card.

✓ Bone protection – Consider offering protection against osteoporosis when on long-term steroids.

## Referral

→ Rheumatology – Provide them with an early referral if they have atypical symptoms of PMR (young, a lack of stiffness or shoulder involvement, or a normal or high ESR [>100] and CRP) or give them advice regarding steroid use (prolonged use of over two years, poor response or contraindicated).

## Safety Netting

» Refer them urgently to ophthalmology if there are any red-flag symptoms (temporal arteritis).

» Follow-up – If steroids have been initiated, organise a follow-up after one week to assess their response. Review in three to four weeks thereafter to consider lowering the dose, and recheck the inflammatory markers. Check BP and BM at three-monthly reviews. Warn the patient that if they have any headaches, jaw pain or sudden loss of vision, then they are to seek emergency medical advice.

*References*

Dasgupta, B. (2010). *Diagnosis and management of polymyalgia rheumatica.* Royal College of Physicians. https://www.rcplondon.ac.uk/guidelines-policy/diagnosis-and-management-polymyalgia-rheumatica

# Osteoporosis

Osteoporosis is a progressive disease of the bones that casues a decrease in bone density with a subsequent increase in fragility and an increased risk of fracturing. It is painless, and sufferers may not realise they have it until they experience a fracture. Common sites of fracture are the wrist, spine and hip. They become known as fragility fractures if they are sustained when falling from standing height or less. Osteoporosis is defined by the WHO as having a bone density that has a standard deviation of -2.5 (below the mean peak bone mass) and is usually diagnosed on a DEXA scan. Women have a higher risk of osteoporosis resulting from decreased oestrogen production due to the menopause, with up to 2% risk at 50 years and 50% at 80 years.

## High-risk Groups Requiring a Fragility Fracture Risk Assessment

»   Women >65 years and men >75 years.

»   Women who are 50–65 years or men who are 50–75 years with the following additional risk factors:

  ›   Common – A previous fragility fracture or fall, low BMI (<18.5), a smoker or drinks >14 units of alcohol per week.

  ›   Secondary osteoporosis – Hypogonadism or premature menopause (<40 years).

  ›   Endocrine – Hyperthyroidism, hyperparathyroidism, DM or Cushing's disease.

  ›   Rheumatoid – RA or ankylosing spondylitis.

  ›   GI – IBD, coeliac disease or chronic pancreatitis.

  ›   Other – Liver failure, CKD, COPD or immobility.

»   Patients <50 years with one of the following other risk factors: oral steroids, a previous fragility fracture or premature menopause.

»   Patients <40 years with one of the following other risk factors: high-dose steroids (7.5mg prednisolone for more than three months), or previous or multiple fragility fractures.

»   Patients with one of the following other risk factors: SSRI, anticonvulsants (carbamazepine), thyroxine (high dose), SSRI, PPI or pioglitazone.

## History

»   Ask the patient about their understanding of the DEXA results.

»   Focused questions

  ›   Osteoporosis – Ask about recent falls, fractures (spine, wrist or hip), a loss in height, stooping more than before or persistent back pain.

  ›   Risk factors – Ask about hyperthyroid symptoms, bowel symptoms (IBD or coeliac) or menopause symptoms.

» Past history – Ask if they have OA, RA, IBD or other medical problems (type 1 DM, CKD or hyperthyroidism).

» Family history – Ask if there is a family history of osteoporosis or fractures.

» Drug history – Ask if they have taken long-term steroids (for more than three months), pioglitazone, methotrexate or lithium.

» Social history – Ask if they smoke or drink alcohol, what exercise they do, what their diet is like (lack of calcium or vitamin D), what their occupation is, and what their support network is like.

## RED FLAGS

Anorexia, fragility fracture in <50 years, recurrent falls, chronic disease (hyperthyroidism or hyperparathyroidism) or steroids.

## Examination

» Vitals – Weight, height (loss) and BMI.

» Examine the joints (wrists [Colles fracture], vertebrae and hips) for any fractures. Examine the back for kyphosis.

## Investigation

» Risk calculator – Calculate the QFracture score or FRAX (WHO) score that reports the 10-year probability of a major osteoporotic fracture.

» QFracture score – For women >11.1% indicates a high risk, and for men >2.6% indicates a high risk.

» Bloods – FBC, U&Es, TFTs, calcium, PO4, PTH, vitamin D, LFT, ALP, LH, FSH and testosterone (hypogonadism).

» Urine – Bence-Jones proteins if myeloma is being considered.

» Imaging

  › X-ray – Thoracic / lumbar spine can identify osteopenia.

  › Bone scan – DEXA scan for osteoporosis.

    **Indications a DEXA scan is required (NICE, 2014)**

    - >50 years plus a fragility score.

    - <40 years plus the aforementioned risk factors.

    - In all other cases, use the QFracture or FRAX score.

### Interpreting DEXA scans

> Normal – DEXA scan T-score between 0 and -1

> Osteopenia – DEXA scan T-score between -1 and -2.5

> Osteoporosis – DEXA scan T-score <=-2.5 (Severe – T-score <-2.5 plus a fracture)

# Management

*Interpretation of risk of fragility fracture*

✓ High risk – If the T-score <-2.5, treat with bone-sparing medication. If the T-score >=-2.5, treat any underlying cause or modify the risk factors. Repeat the DEXA scan in two years.

✓ Intermediate risk – If the FRAX/QFracture risk is raised, request a DEXA scan and treat with oral agents if the T-score <=-2.5

✓ Low risk – Offer lifestyle advice only and follow up in five years.

*Conservative*

✓ Lifestyle

> Diet – Advise them to eat a balanced diet including calcium (milk, cheese and yoghurt) and vitamin D (salmon, mackerel, tuna and sardines).

> Exercise – Advise them to take regular exercise (outdoor walking in the sun) or strength training (weight training).

> Advise them to stop smoking.

> Advise them to reduce their alcohol intake to the recommended levels (<=14 units/week).

✓ Aids

> Walking stick – Offer a walking stick to reduce the load on the contralateral joint (hip). Suggest a heel raiser to correct unequal leg lengths.

> Assistance devices – Suggest using tap turners, enlarged grips for writing, non-slip mats, electric can openers, and long-handled reachers/grabbers.

✓ Falls prevention

> Advise them to remove/address hazards (e.g. uneven rugs, slippery floor or loose wires).

> Recommend hip protectors to those with a risk of falls.

*Medical*

✓ Supplements

> Adequate calcium – If their calcium intake is adequate (700mg/day), give 400units of vitamin D if they are not exposed to much sun.

› Inadequate calcium – If their calcium intake is inadequate, give 1g calcium daily with 400u vitamin D or 800u if they are housebound / in a nursing home.

› Bisphosphonates – As first-line therapy, offer alendronate (70mg weekly, 10mg od), or risedronate (35mg weekly, 5mg od) if alendronate is not tolerated. Avoid giving with NSAIDs/aspirin (GI). Take >30 minutes before breakfast, medications or another type of drink (milk). Swallow whole with a cup of water. Take in an upright position and remain sitting up for 30 minutes. Side effects are GI symptoms (nausea or oesophagitis), pain (bone, joint or muscle) and atypical stress fractures (femur). Contraindicated in hypocalcaemia, pregnancy, breastfeeding, low eGFR (<35) and ulcers.

✓ Bisphosphonates – Consider prescribing if they are taking a high dose of steroids (prednisolone >7.5mg daily for more than three months).

✓ Analgesia – Offer analgesia (paracetamol/NSAIDs) for vertebral fractures. Add PPI with NSAIDs.

✓ HRT – Consider HRT in premature menopause (<40 years) to reduce the risk of fragility fractures.

## Referral

→ Rheumatologist – If they cannot tolerate bisphosphonates, refer them to a rheumatologist. The treatment includes strontium, raloxifene and teriparatide. Refer all men or premenopausal women with osteoporosis / a fragility fracture to investigate the cause.

→ OT – Refer them to speak to an OT about adaptations to minimise the risk of falls at home (bath aids, chair, raised toilet sets, stair rails, or the removal of rugs and raised carpet edges).

→ Falls clinic – In patients who have had two or more falls in the last year, refer them for falls management.

## Safety Netting

» Review in four to six weeks regarding their response to treatment.

### References

National Institute for Health and Care Excellence (2014). *Osteoporosis – prevention of fragility fractures.* https://cks.nice.org.uk/topics/osteoporosis-prevention-of-fragility-fractures/

Scottish Intercollegiate Guidelines Network (2015). *SIGN 142 Management of osteoporosis and the prevention of fragility fractures.* https://www.sign.ac.uk/media/1741/sign142.pdf

# Hip Pain

Hip pain is a common complaint that usually worsens with aging. The most common cause is due to OA, which may be exacerbated due to a previous fall or trauma. However, when examining a patient, other serious causes must be excluded, such as a hip fracture or the avascular necrosis (AVN) of the head of the femur. Pain felt in the hip joint may not necessarily be as a result of the structures of the hip; back pain and psoas abscess problems may radiate to the hip and cause diagnostic confusion if you are not careful. Similarly, problems with the hip do not necessarily present with symptoms in the hip, rather the hip pain may radiate to the knee, groin, thigh or buttocks.

## History

» Focused questions

  › Ask about the site of the pain (one or both hips, and ask if they can point to it), the onset of the pain (slowly indicates OA, and quickly indicates trauma), the character of the pain, the frequency with which it is felt, if there are any relieving and exacerbating factors, if there is any pain radiation, if there is any swelling, if there is any stiffness of the joint, if there is a grinding noise (crepitus) or if there is a feeling of snapping (tendon problem).

» Associated history – Ask if they have any issue with movements (any problems standing from seated position, when walking up and down stairs, any pain when bending down or turning) or if they have had any falls.

» Past history – Ask if they have RA or SLE, are pregnant (pubic symphysis dysfunction), or have had joint surgery or a hip replacement.

» Social history – Ask about their support network, if they have any carers, what their occupation is and if the pain has affected their work, what leisure activities they take part in, and if they smoke or drink alcohol.

## RED FLAGS

Fevers or sweats (septic arthritis), trauma (fracture), weight loss (malignancy), or acute and sudden onset night pain (AVN of the femoral head).

## Differential Diagnosis

| OA | Progressive unilateral or bilateral pain in the groin or buttocks with radiation to the knee. Pain is increased with activity and reduced with rest. Patient may be obese. Patient may have a limp, and have problems getting out of a chair or require care. OE: antalgic gait, positive Trendelenburg sign, apparent limb shortening, reduction of internal rotation noted (early) and fixed flexion of the hip. |
|---|---|

| Greater trochanteric pain syndrome | Common, self-limiting, causes lateral hip pain and is more common in women and those >40 years. Sharp, intense, outer thigh pain that is worse on lying on the affected side, prolonged standing or running. OE: pain on the greater trochanter and a positive Trendelenburg test. |
|---|---|
| Meralgia paresthetica | Caused by the compression of the lateral cutaneous nerve of the thigh through the inguinal ligament of the fascia lata. Presents with a burning, stinging sensation over the thigh (antero-lateral) that is made worse by standing or walking. OE: pain on hip extensions and paraesthesia over the lateral aspect of the thigh. Risk factors include surgery, pregnancy, obesity, DM and others (sports, tight trousers and seat belts). |
| Pubic symphysis dysfunction | Occurs in late pregnancy or post childbirth. Pain in the pelvic region, usually at the front of the pelvis, but can radiate to the groin and the medial aspect of thighs. Can worsen through pregnancy and with movement. Causes a waddling gait and problems walking up stairs. |
| AVN | Hip pain that is usually sudden onset and unilateral. May be severe enough to cause night-time pain. Patient walks with a limp and may have continuous pain. Risk factors include steroids, SLE, sickle cell disease and excessive alcohol consumption. |
| Psoas abscess | Unilateral pain and swelling, associated with fever and malaise. |

## Examination

» Vitals – Temperature, BP and pulse.

» Inspection – Ask the patient to walk from one end of the room to the other, and inspect for an antalgic gait (limp), Trendelenburg's sign (pelvis tilts down to opposite side) or a short leg gait. Look for a pelvic tilt, scoliosis or increased back lordosis.

» Measure – Have the patient lie flat on the couch. Square their hips and measure from the umbilicus to each medial malleolus (apparent), then from the ASIS to each medial malleolus (true). Inequality suggests limb shortening (fracture).

» Palpate – Locate the pain before starting. Palpate for tenderness over the greater trochanter (bursitis) and for joint tenderness (distal to midpoint of the inguinal ligament).

» Move

  › Flexion – Flex the patient's knees as far as possible (130°).

  › Rotation – Have the hip and knee flexed at 90° while steering the foot laterally for the internal rotation of the hip and medially for the external rotation.

  › Abduction/adduction – Place one hand on the opposite iliac crest to monitor for pelvic movement. Hold the patient's calf in the other hand and abduct the hip. Adduct the hip by crossing the leg over.

» Special tests

> Consider the following if indicated by the history:

- Thomas's test – Place one hand under the patient's lumbar spine. Flex one knee as far as possible and observe the contralateral leg. If the leg is elevated and cannot be fully extended, this is positive for the fixed flexion deformity of the affected side (OA).

- Trendelenburg's sign – Ask the patient to stand on one foot while raising the opposite foot off the ground. Place your hands on the ASIS and check for pelvic tilting on the unsupported side (positive sign). The common cause is hip pain and weakness of the gluteus medius.

## Investigations

» Bloods – Not routinely needed unless septic arthritis or psoas abscess is suspected. If required, Hb, WCC, CRP, ESR, rheumatoid factor and ANA.

» Hip/pelvic x-ray – This is to exclude a fracture and AVN of the femoral head; check for the position of previous hip replacements, and find any evidence of OA (reduced joint space and osteophytes) or osteopenia.

» USS/MRI – This is to look for micro-fractures, tendonitis, bursitis or psoas abscess.

## Management

### Conservative

✓ Diet – Advise them to eat a healthy diet rich in omega-3 fatty acids with fresh fish, fruit and vegetables.

✓ Rest – If the pain is due to repetitive movements, advise them to rest for up to 12 weeks.

✓ Ice/heat – Advise them to apply an ice or heat pack if the pain is worsened after activity.

✓ Splint – Advise them to consider purchasing a splint or clasp to reduce the pressure on the joint/tendon.

✓ Exercise – Advise them to continue with simple exercises (aerobic / muscle strengthening) as the pain eases to help maintain and improve their ROM and prevent stiffness.

✓ OA – If their BMI is >25, suggest that they lose weight, as it puts less pressure on joints. Suggest a heel raiser for unequal leg lengths. Suggest they consider transcutaneous electrical nerve stimulation (TENS).

### Medical

✓ Pain – Simple analgesia (paracetamol or codeine) or NSAIDs can be prescribed as topical creams or oral medication. Ensure there are no contraindications for NSAIDs (ulcers, gastritis or asthma). Add PPI in the elderly. Advise them to avoid taking glucosamine for pain relief (there is poor evidence of its efficacy).

✓ Infection – In septic arthritis, orthopaedic admission is needed for IV antibiotics and drainage.

✓ Sick certificate – Offer a short fit note if they are unable to work. Suggest that they consider amended duties or altered hours if they are finding it difficult to carry out certain tasks.

## Referral

→ Physiotherapy – Refer them to physiotherapy, which is helpful for strengthening the muscles around the hip.

→ OT – Refer them to speak to an OT about adaptations that can be made to their house, such as sock aids, walk-in showers, raised chairs, a stair lift or rails.

→ Injection – Persistent pain may warrant steroid or LA injections to reduce the pain and inflammation in the joint for the short term. The side effects are pain on injecting, atrophy or liponecrosis, loss of skin colour or tendon damage.

→ Orthopaedics – Refer them to orthopaedics if their symptoms have deteriorated rapidly or are causing a disability that impacts their quality of life. Total hip replacement is often recommended for end-stage OA.

## Safety Netting

» Review in four to six weeks regarding their response to treatment.

---

### References

National Institute for Health and Care Excellence (2011). *Hip fracture: management.* https://www.nice.org.uk/guidance/cg124

# Knee Pain

Knee pain is a common symptom that patients may present with. It may be acute or, more commonly, a chronic, worsening condition in the middle-aged. Acute causes include sprain or trauma, and a chronic cause is OA. The knee joint is a hinge joint between three bones – the femur, tibia and fibula – with the patella also providing an articulation point. The joint also consists of two menisci, two cruciate ligaments and two collateral ligaments. Damage or overuse of any of these components may cause pain and stiffness.

## History

» Focused questions

> Ask about the pain or tenderness in the knee, and when it started.

> Ask about the site (if it affects one or both knees, and if they can point to it).

> Ask about the character, frequency, and if there are any relieving or exacerbating factors.

> Ask if there is any radiation (hip).

> Ask if they have had a recent knee injury or trauma, if they were playing any sport when the pain started, and if so, what happened.

> Ask if the joint stiffness is worse in the morning (RA) or evening (OA).

> Ask if there is any locking (meniscal tear or a loose body) or giving way (patella dislocation or a torn ligament).

» Associated history – Ask how their knees are functioning (if there are any problems when walking up and down stairs), how far they are able to walk, and if they have a fever, sweats or rigors.

> Past history – Ask if they have gout, RA, psoriasis or IBD, if they have had any hip problems, or if they have had a patella dislocation before, knee-joint surgery or a knee replacement.

» Drug history – Ask if they have taken steroids or painkillers.

» Social history – Ask if they have a support network and/or carers, what their occupation is and if the knee pain has affected their work, what leisure activities and sports they do, and if they smoke or drink alcohol.

## RED FLAGS

Fever or sweats (septic arthritis), trauma (fracture) or night pain (tumour).

## Knee Pain by Location

➤ Anterior knee

› Patella tendon – Osgood-Schlatter disease, patella tendonitis or a rupture.

› Patella – Chondromalacia, OA, bipartite patella or stress fracture.

› Intra-articular – Meniscal tear or prepatellar bursitis.

➤ Medial knee – Collateral ligament sprain or medial meniscal tear.

➤ Lateral knee – Collateral ligament sprain, lateral meniscal tear or iliotibial band tendonitis.

➤ Posterior knee – Baker's cyst (popliteal), posterior cruciate ligament tear/injury or DVT.

## Differential Diagnosis

| OA | Progressive worsening of knee pain, which may be unilateral or bilateral. Pain increases with activity and reduces with rest. Patient may be obese and have slight stiffness in the morning. OE: crepitus, anterior knee effusion and joint line tenderness. |
|---|---|
| Meniscal tear | Damage to the menisci that stabilise the joint. Often caused by a twisting sprain while flexed (sports) causing knee pain, locking of the knee (particularly extension) or giving way with effusion several hours later. OE: localised joint pain (medial/lateral), limited extension, positive McMurray's or Apley's tests. |
| Osgood-Schlatter disease | Tibial tubercle inflammation due to overuse. Common in teenage boys doing sports. Pain below the patella that is worse during exercise and improves with rest. Settles after two to three months. OE: tender, bony lump below the patella, and pain when resisting knee extension. |
| Housemaid's knee | Prepatellar bursitis caused by chronic friction (bending of the knees), often seen in carpet fitters. Presents with knee swelling and pain that is worse on extreme flexion. |
| Patellofemoral pain | Common cause of knee pain affecting young adults. Anterior dull and aching pain that has a gradual onset. Usually bilateral, and may cause swelling and crepitus. Patient notices a worsening of symptoms when descending the stairs, along with a feeling of instability or giving way. |

| Ligament injury | Damage to the ligaments that support the knee, from an injury (sports). Causes pain effusion and knee-joint instability, and there is a snapping sound at the time of injury. Anterior cruciate ligament (ACL) – Due to a sudden change in direction. Positive for both Lachman and anterior drawer tests. Posterior cruciate ligament (PCL) – Due to a blow to the tibia after a fall on a flexed knee or RTA. Posterior knee pain. Positive posterior drawer test. Medial collateral – Twisting injury or lateral blow to the knee. Tender medial joint line. Positive valgus stress test. Lateral collateral – Twisting injury or medial blow to the knee. Tender lateral joint line. Positive varus stress test. |
|---|---|
| Chondromalacia patella | Overuse of the knee (sports) can result in the softening of the articular cartilage of the patella. Common in teenage girls. Retropatellar pain that is worse on standing from prolonged sitting or using stairs. OE: patella tenderness, effusion and crepitus. |
| Baker's cyst | Fluid-filled sac that can cause posterior knee pain and swelling. More common in females, and may be caused post trauma or due to existing OA. May rupture, causing fluid to leak into the calf. OE: tender, transilluminate, smooth swelling is noted in the popliteal area, which is present on extension of the knee and can disappear on flexion. |

## Examination

»   Vitals – Temperature, BP and pulse.

»   Inspection – Observe the patient standing, to check for deformity (valgus, varus and fixed flexion tests), muscle wastage (quadriceps), scars or effusion. Ask the patient to walk from one end of the room to the other (antalgic gait).

»   Palpation – Check their temperature and for tenderness. Palpate the joint line with the knee flexed (ligaments, bony landmarks, tibial tuberosity and femoral condyles). With the knee extended, feel the patella and popliteal fossa (Baker's cyst).

   ›   Patella tap test – Palpate for effusions by sliding your hand over the suprapatellar pouch, forcing the effusion below the patella. Tap the patella with your index finger (contralateral hand). With moderate effusion, the patella will bounce up.

»   Movement – Check for active and passive flexion, and the extension of the knee.

»   Special tests – Consider the following if indicated by the history:

   ›   Collateral ligaments – Hold the ankle in one hand, and the knee with the other. Apply valgus force by steering the leg medially (medial ligament), then varus pressure by moving the leg laterally (lateral ligament).

> › Cruciate ligaments – Perform Drawer's test by sitting on the side of the foot. Hold the knee with your thumbs over the tibial tuberosity, and your fingers within the popliteal fossa. Check for lag by pulling forward (ACL tear) or pushing backwards (PCL tear).

> › Meniscal – Perform McMurray's test, warning the patient that it may cause pain. Flex the knee as far as possible. Externally rotate the foot, and extend the knee slowly with lateral force (medial meniscus). Repeat, but internally rotate the foot, and extend the knee with medial force (lateral meniscus).

» Referred pain – Examine the hip, ankle and spine for any evidence of pain radiation from these sites.

## Investigations

» Bloods – Not routinely needed. However, consider Hb, WCC, CRP and uric acid (gout).

» Knee x-ray – Do AP/lateral and skyline views to exclude a fracture, and look for OA or haemarthrosis.

**Ottawa rules regarding knee x-rays**

> › Consider an x-ray of the knee to exclude a fracture if one or more of the following applies:

>> - Aged >=55 years.

>> - Tenderness at the head of the fibula or isolated tenderness to the patella.

>> - An inability to flex the knee to 90° or an inability to walk four steps at the time of injury.

» MRI – To look for meniscal and tendon injuries, and bursitis.

## Management

*Conservative*

✓ Rest – If the pain is due to repetitive movements, advise the patient to rest for up to 12 weeks

✓ Ice/heat – Advise them to apply an ice or heat pack if the pain worsens after activity.

✓ Support – Advise them to consider purchasing a knee support and/or insoles.

✓ Exercise – Advise them to continue with simple exercises (aerobic / muscle strengthening) as the pain eases to help maintain and improve their ROM and prevent stiffness.

✓ Weight – If their BMI is >25, suggest that they lose weight.

✓ Housemaid's knee – Advise them to use cushions or knee pads when they are kneeling down.

*Medical*

✓ Pain – Simple analgesia (paracetamol or codeine) or NSAIDs can be issued as topical gels or oral medication. Ensure there are no contraindications for NSAIDs (ulcers, gastritis or asthma). Add PPI in the elderly.

✓ Infection – Septic arthritis needs orthopaedic admission for IV antibiotics and drainage.

✓ Sick certificate – Offer a short fit note if they are unable to work. Advise that they consider amended duties or altered hours if they are finding it difficult to carry out certain tasks.

## Referral

→ Physiotherapy – Refer them to physiotherapy, which is helpful for strengthening the muscles around the knee.

→ OT – Refer them to an OT to discuss the adaptations that can be made. Advise them to consider walking aids, a Zimmer frame, or a wheelchair if there is severe dysfunction.

→ Injections – Persistent pain may warrant steroid injections in the joint to reduce the pain and inflammation for the short term. Side effects are pain on injecting, atrophy, liponecrosis, loss of skin colour or damage to the tendons.

→ Orthopaedics – Refer them to orthopaedics if their symptoms have deteriorated rapidly or are causing a disability that impacts their quality of life. A total knee replacement is often recommended for end-stage OA.

## Safety Netting

» Review in four to six weeks regarding their response to treatment.

*References*

National Institute for Health and Care Excellence (2017). *Knee pain – assessment.* https://cks.nice.org.uk/topics/knee-pain-assessment/

# Shoulder Pain

Shoulder problems affect up to 30% of adults at any given time. Although pain and stiffness are the most common complaints that patients present with, a large number may attend due to a severe reduction in their quality of life. Shoulder pain may be due to problems affecting the joints (acromioclavicular joint [ACJ]), the muscles (rotator cuff tears) or the capsule (adhesive capsulitis). Pain may also be referred to the shoulder from the neck or be due to abdominal pathology (gallstones). The conditions that give rise to shoulder pain and stiffness may have quite non-specific histories with no clear trigger factor. It is important to carry out a full shoulder examination to be able to distinguish between them, and then share a management plan with the patient to help resolve their complaint.

## History

» Focused questions

› Ask when the shoulder pain started.

› Ask about the site (one or both shoulders), and ask if they can point to it (ACJ).

› Ask if they are right or left handed.

› Ask if there has been any recent injury to the shoulder, and if they were lifting or pushing before the pain started.

› Ask about the character of the pain (burning, stinging, sharp or aching).

› Ask about the frequency, and if there are any exacerbating or relieving factors.

› Ask if there is any radiation of the pain (specifically to the neck).

› Ask if they have noticed any swelling (dislocation) or stiffness of the joint.

› Ask if the pain is worse in the evening (OA).

» Associated history – Ask if their shoulder movements are restricted; if it is stopping them from doing everyday things (cleaning, dressing or writing); if they have had any fever, night sweats, numbness, or pins and needles around the shoulder; and if there is stiffness and pain in both shoulders.

» Past history – Ask if they have DM, IHD or epilepsy, or have had a shoulder dislocation, fracture or surgery.

» Drug history – Ask if they have taken any painkillers (NSAIDs, paracetamol or topical gels) or steroids.

» Social history – Ask about their home life, what their occupation is and if the condition affects their work, if they drive, what their hobbies are (cricket, rugby, swimming, weight lifting, etc.), and if they smoke or drink alcohol.

## RED FLAGS

Dislocation, cardiac chest pain and gallbladder disease.

## Differential Diagnosis

| | |
|---|---|
| Impingement disorders | Impingement disorders affect the rotator cuff muscles, which gives rise to pain and shoulder weakness. Usually due to repetitive activities where the arms are overhead, such as skiing, tennis, swimming or those who stack shelves. The pain is usually worse at night, affecting sleep. OE: painful arc between 60° and 120° of abduction. Positive Neer test. |
| Rotator cuff tears | Usually acute following a fall, but may be chronic due to tendonitis. Tears can be full length or partial, and give rise to a painful arc. OE: unable to actively abduct beyond 60°, but can abduct to 90° passively. |
| Adhesive capsulitis | Also known as frozen shoulder, and causes pain, stiffness and reduced movements. Most common in women from 40–60 years and diabetics. Leads to the restriction of all shoulder movements (particularly external rotation), whether active or passive. Tends to affect ADLs severely, such as dressing or washing. Recovery can be from six months to two years. |
| ACJ disorders | Condition affecting the ACJ that is usually found in young males, due to high-impact sports such as rugby, or because of OA. May be secondary to subacromial impingement syndrome. Pain is usually restricted to the ACJ, but may radiate to the base of the neck. OE: painful arc between 90° and 120° of abduction and elevation. Positive scarf test. |
| Cervical radiculopathy | Caused by nerve-root compression in the cervical spine. May be due to disc herniation, OA or injury. Symptoms include pain, numbness and weakness in the affected nerve-root distribution, which may radiate to the scapula bilaterally or unilaterally. |
| Shoulder dislocation | The majority of dislocations are anterior with a small minority (5%) being posterior. Occurs in young males, and is frequently a result of a sporting injury or RTA. Recurrent dislocation may lead to axillary nerve injury with tingling and numbness over the ipsilateral deltoid muscle. |
| PMR | Usually seen in the elderly (>65 years), and causes pain (aching) and morning stiffness (cannot turn over in bed) to bilateral shoulders and the pelvic girdle. It has an abrupt onset and can last more than two weeks. Muscles are tender with no true weakness (only pain). Patient has raised inflammatory markers (ESR and CRP). Associated with temporal arteritis. |

## Examination

» Vitals – Temperature, BP and pulse.

» Inspection – Inspect the shoulder from the front, back and sides. Look for abnormal posture, asymmetry, deformity (winging scapula or prominent ACJ), swelling and muscle wastage.

» Palpation – Feel the temperature, and palpate along the shoulder joint lines (sternoclavicular joint, ACJ, acromion, greater and lesser tuberosity, and glenohumeral joint) for tenderness, effusion or crepitus.

» Movement

> Abduction – Ask the patient to raise both arms to the ceiling from their sides. Notice if the painful arc test indicates pain (60–120° indicates supraspinatus tendonitis / partial rotator cuff tear) or if there is pain at the end of the arc (ACJ OA). If the painful arc test indicates pain, passively abduct the arm further if possible (rotator cuff tear).

> Adduction – Ask the patient to move their arm across their midline and chest.

> Flexion/extension – Ask the patient to lift their arms forwards then backwards.

> Internal/external rotation – Ask the patient to position their elbows flexed at 90° by their sides, then ask them to bend their arms away from body (external) then towards midline (internal).

» Special tests

> Neer test (impingement disorder) – Ask the patient to rotate their arms internally with the thumb facing downwards, and slowly abduct and flex the arm up. Apply downward pressure on the patient's arms (resistance).

» Neurology – Check the patient's power against resistance. Ask them to raise their arms like wings (deltoid) and then like a boxer (biceps/triceps). Ask them to push against a wall (serratus anterior muscle). Check sensation over the deltoid muscle (anterior dislocation of shoulder).

## Investigations

» Bloods – Not routinely performed. Consider CRP and ESR if PMR is suspected, or LFTs if gallbladder disease is suspected.

» Shoulder x-ray – This is to exclude a fracture, calcified tendonitis and ACJ OA.

» USS/MRI – This it to look for micro-fractures, rotator cuff tears, tendonitis and bursitis.

## Management

*Conservative*

✓ Advise them to not sit forwards with their arms held side by side, to support their lower back with cushion when seated, to maintain a good posture when using a laptop or computer, and to avoid heavy lifting and the repetitive movements that cause the pain.

✓ Ice/heat – Advise them to apply an ice pack or heat for 20 minutes every two hours if the worsens after activity.

✓ Sling – Advise them to consider wearing a sling to reduce the pressure on the joint/tendon in ACJ disorders.

✓ Sick certificate – Offer a short fit note if they are unable to work. Advise them to consider amended duties or altered hours if they are finding it difficult to carry out certain tasks.

✓ Exercise – Advise them to continue with simple exercises (aerobic / muscle strengthening) as the pain eases to help maintain and improve their ROM and prevent stiffness.

### Medical

✓ Pain – Simple analgesia (paracetamol or codeine) or NSAIDs can be prescribed as topical creams or oral medication. Ensure there are no contraindications for NSAIDs (ulcers, gastritis or asthma). Consider prescribing a PPI in the elderly for those at risk.

✓ Infection – If septic arthritis is suspected, then they may need an orthopaedic admission for IV antibiotics and drainage.

✓ PMR – Offer a low, tapering dose of prednisolone. Consider bone protection with steroids.

## Referral

→ Physiotherapy – Refer them to physiotherapy, which is helpful for strengthening the muscles around the shoulder joint and reducing stiffness.

→ OT – Refer them to speak to an OT about adaptations that can be made to their house.

→ Infection – Persistent pain may warrant steroid injections to reduce pain and inflammation in the joint in the short term.

→ Orthopaedics – Refer them to orthopaedics if their symptoms have deteriorated rapidly, there is nerve damage or the condition is causing a disability that impacts their quality of life. If there is recurrent shoulder dislocation, this may need surgical correction.

→ Rheumatology – Refer them to rheumatology if RA or PMR are suspected.

## Safety Netting

» Review in four to six weeks regarding their response to treatment.

---

### References

National Institute for Health and Care Excellence (2017). *Shoulder pain.* https://cks.nice.org.uk/topics/shoulder-pain/

# Hand Pain

Hand pain is an important symptom as it usually causes functional problems in the patient. The hand consists of numerous small muscles, nerves, bones and tendons that all may be implicit in the symptoms. A patient presenting following a fall onto an outstretched hand may have simply sustained a sprain or, more importantly, may have fractured a bone in the hand or the wrist. Repeated and repetitive movements as a result of the patient's occupation may result in tenosynovitis or tendonitis causing focal pain in the hand. Systemic conditions such as RA and hypothyroidism may also present with hand symptoms.

## History

» Focused questions

› Ask where the pain affects the hands, and if it is on both; ask if they can point to it.

› Ask about the onset, the character of the pain (burning, sharp, aching or tingling), and if there are any exacerbating or relieving factors.

› Ask if there is any stiffness of the joints, and if it is worse in the morning (RA) or evening (OA).

› Ask if there is any swelling of the joints.

› Ask about their strength and grip.

› Ask if they have had an injury or fall recently.

» Associated history

› Function – Ask which the dominant hand is, if they have any problems with fine movements (holding a pen or doing buttons up) or day-to-day tasks, and if they have felt more clumsy with their hands.

› Sensation – Ask if there is any numbness, or pins and needles in the hand.

» Past history – Ask if they have OA or RA, carpal tunnel syndrome (underactive thyroid or pregnancy), or have had hand surgery or a previous fracture.

» Drug history – Ask if they have taken any medications or painkillers.

» Social history – Ask if they have any support at home (including any carers), what their occupation is and if the condition has affected their work, and if they smoke or drink alcohol.

» Family history – Ask if there is a family history of carpal tunnel syndrome.

## RED FLAGS

Wasting (thenar) of the muscles.

## Differential Diagnosis

| | |
|---|---|
| Carpal tunnel syndrome | Entrapment of the median nerve in the carpal tunnel. Common in women >40 years. Intermittent burning pain, tingling and numbness in the distribution of the medial nerve (radial fingers). Worse at night and may cause the patient to awaken; the pain may improve on shaking the hand. Chronic symptoms may lead to the wasting of the thenar muscle. OE: weakness to thumb abduction, positive Phalen's test and positive Tinel's test. Risk factors are DM, hypothyroidism, RA, obesity and pregnancy. |
| De Quervain's tenosynovitis | Common in 30–50-year-old women and during pregnancy. Causes pain, swelling and tenderness over the thumb. Due to repetitive strain or repeated movements, such as using a mouse or certain manual jobs (carpenter or gardener). OE: radial styloid tenderness and a positive Finkelstein's test. |
| Trigger finger | The flexor tendon becomes trapped in the sheath, resulting in difficulty extending the flexed finger (locking); it is often released suddenly with a snap following assistance from the other hand. Can be associated with DM or RA. Seen in carpenters (screwdriver use). Commonly affects the ring and middle finger and is seen in women >40 years. OE: occasionally a nodule is palpable. |

## Examination

»   Vitals – Temperature, BP, pulse and capillary refill.

»   Inspection

    ›   Inspect for swellings, nail changes, scars, muscle wastage or deformity, and skin changes.

    ›   Nails – Check for psoriatic changes (pitting and onycholysis) and clubbing.

    ›   Deformities – Check for OA changes (Heberden's nodes on the distal interphalangeal joint [DIP] and Bouchard's nodes), RA changes (swan neck deformity, boutonniere deformity, Z-shaped thumb and ulnar deviation), ganglion, tophi and trigger finger.

»   Palpation

    ›   Check the temperature and muscle bulk (thenar and hypothenar), radial pulse and Dupuytren's contracture.

    ›   Joints – Squeeze the radioulnar joint, radial and ulnar styloid, anatomical snuffbox (scaphoid fracture), carpal bones, metacarpophalangeal (MCP) joints and interphalangeal (IP) joints to check for tenderness.

    ›   Tendons – Palpate the radial styloid (de Quervain's tenosynovitis) and ulnar styloid.

» Movement – Also move the wrist joint (to check for pronation, supination, flexion/extension, and radial and ulnar deviation). Ask the patient to make a fist then spread their fingers out. Move each joint individually.

» Special tests – Consider the following if indicated by history:

> Phalen's test – Ask the patient to hold the reverse prayer sign for one minute. Pain or paraesthesia in the medial distribution is a positive result.

> Tinel's test – Tap the medial nerve at the carpal tunnel; if it produces paraesthesia, it is a positive result.

> Finkelstein's test – Ask the patient to make a fist with their thumb inside, then tilt it into ulnar deviation.

» Function – If indicated to be a problem, ask the patient to carry out everyday tasks such as undoing buttons, writing a sentence using a pen or holding a cup.

» Neurological – If indicated to be a problem, test the sensation of the ulnar nerve (little finger), median nerve (index finger) and radial nerve (anatomical snuff box).

## Investigations

» Bloods – Not routinely needed. Consider WCC, CRP and ESR, if an infection is suspected. Request rheumatoid factor if RA is suspected. Request TFT and HbA1c for carpal tunnel.

» Hand x-ray – Required if OA or a fracture is suspected. If a scaphoid fracture is suspected, repeat the scaphoid views in 10 days.

» Specialist – USS of the wrist, and nerve conduction tests.

## Management

*Conservative*

✓ Rest – If the pain is due to repetitive movements, advise the patient to rest.

✓ Ice/heat – Advise them to apply an ice or heat pack if the pain worsens after activity. Advise them to place their hands in warm water for 10–20 minutes, then when dry, to apply moisturising cream and massage it into their hands.

✓ Splint – Advise them to consider purchasing a wrist splint to wear at night for carpal tunnel. A splint with a thumb strap may help reduce de Quervain's tenosynovitis.

✓ Exercise – Advise them to continue with simple exercises (aerobic / muscle strengthening) as the pain eases to help maintain and improve their ROM and prevent stiffness.

✓ Weight – If their BMI is >25, suggest that they lose weight.

*Medical*

✓ Pain – Simple analgesia (paracetamol or codeine) or NSAIDs can be prescribed as topical creams or oral medication. Ensure there are no contraindications for NSAIDs (ulcers, gastritis or asthma). Add PPI in the elderly.

✓ Sick certificate – Offer a short fit note if they are unable to work. Advise them to consider amended duties or altered hours if they are finding it difficult to carry out certain tasks.

# Referral

→ Physiotherapy – Refer them to physiotherapy, which is helpful for strengthening the muscles.

→ OT – Refer them to speak to an OT about adaptations that can be made (to minimise wrist extension, the modification of tools, and an increased diameter handle of spoons or toothbrush).

→ Injection – Persistent pain may warrant steroid or LA injections to reduce the pain and inflammation in the joint in the short term. This is often useful for releasing trigger finger. Side effects are pain on injection, atrophy or liponecrosis, loss of skin colour or damage to the tendons.

→ Orthopaedics – Refer them to orthopaedics if there is thenar eminence wasting for the surgical release of the carpal tunnel or trigger finger. Also to treat Dupuytren's contracture.

## Safety Netting

» Review in four to six weeks regarding their response to treatment.

*References*

National Institute for Health and Care Excellence (2020). *Carpal tunnel syndrome*. https://cks.nice.org.uk/topics/carpal-tunnel-syndrome/

GPnotebook (2018). *de Quervain's tenosynovitis*. https://gpnotebook.com/simplepage.cfm?ID=1301938195

National Institute for Health and Care Excellence (2017). *Dupuytren's disease*. https://cks.nice.org.uk/topics/dupuytrens-disease/

# Elbow Pain

Elbow pain is an extremely common condition. It is usually due to strains or sprains that occur after heavy activity or after a fall. However, the structures of the elbow joint mean that other causes could also be at play, including epicondylitis, bursitis or tendonitis. The elbow is the hinge joint created between the humerus (upper arm) and the two bones of the forearm: the radius and ulna. The outer part of the lower humerus is known as the lateral epicondyle, and the extensor muscles attach via tendons here. The inner humeral bony prominence is known as the medial epicondyle, and the muscles that flex the wrist and fingers attach here via tendons. At the back of the elbow joint is a bursa that allows for the free movement of the joint.

## *History*

- » Focused questions
  - › Elbow pain – Ask if there is any pain or tenderness in the elbow, and if so, when it started.
  - › Ask about the site, and if it affects one or both elbows; ask them to point to it.
  - › Ask about the character of the pain (burning, sharp or stinging).
  - › Ask about the frequency of the pain, and if it is always there or comes and goes.
  - › Ask if anything makes the pain better (medications or rest) or worse (movements).
  - › Ask if there is any radiation of the pain or if it stays in one place.
  - › Ask if there is any swelling, lumps or stiffness (if so, if it is worse in the morning or evening).
  - › Ask if there is any weakness in their grip or difficulty carrying objects.
- » Associated history – Ask if they have had a fall or recent trauma, strain (repeated movements) or fever.
- » Past history – Ask if they have RA.
- » Drug history – Ask if they have taken any painkillers (NSAIDs, paracetamol or topical gels).
- » Social history – Ask what their occupation is, what hobbies they have (tennis, golf, rowing or playing piano), if they smoke or drink alcohol, or if they drive.

## RED FLAGS

Fever or sweats (septic arthritis), trauma (fracture or dislocation), or weakness in the hand.

## Differential Diagnosis

| | |
|---|---|
| Tennis elbow | Often occurs in those >40 years after a history of minor injury or repetitive movements. Worse when straightening the elbow against resistance. Insidious onset of pain, typically of the lateral epicondyle, radiating down the extensor aspect of the forearm. Risk factors include hobbies and occupation (painting, racket sports, plumbing, lifting a baby and gardening). |
| Golfer's elbow | Focal pain over the medial epicondyle from repetitive movements (using a hammer or a ball thrower). Pain can radiate down the flexor surface of the arm. Pain on resisted pronation. Occasional ulnar nerve involvement (paraesthesia affecting the fourth and fifth digits). |
| Olecranon bursitis | Swollen, painful and red bursa over the olecranon process. Usually due to repetitive movements or minor trauma (miners, gardeners and carpet layers), but occasionally due to a bacterial infection. Often affects middle-aged male patients, or patients with RA or gout. |
| OA | Progressive worsening of elbow pain and reduced movements, particularly flexion and extension. May have a history of a previous fall or fracture. May get a grating sensation (crepitus) when testing the range of movement. |
| Cubital tunnel syndrome | Trapped ulnar nerve in the cubital tunnel. Worsened when the elbow is rested on a firm surface. Presents with medial elbow pain and hand weakness. Positive Tinel's test (paraesthesia over the fourth and fifth digits) on tapping over the cubital tunnel (funny bone). |
| Cervical radiculopathy | Referred pain from the cervical spine, which presents with neck pain, numbness or muscle weakness of the C6–8 distribution. |

## Examination

» Inspection – Inspect the carrying angle with the patient's elbows by their side. Look for deformity, bursitis, nodules, swelling or redness.

» Palpation – Locate the pain before starting. Palate the epicondyles (epicondylitis), olecranon process (bursitis) and joint margin for tenderness (OA), effusion or a raised temperature. Feel for rheumatoid tophi. Feel along the common extensor tendon.

» Movement – Assess both the active and passive movements for flexion (flexion deformity) and extension. Assess for pronation (palms facing downwards) and supination (palms facing upwards), with the patient's elbows fixed at the waist and the elbow bent at 90°.

» Special tests

› Tennis elbow – Have the patient's forearm pronated while actively flexing their wrist (resisted extension).

> › Golfer's elbow – Have the patient's forearm supinated while actively extending the elbow and wrist (resisted flexion). Note any pain over the medial epicondyle.

» Neurological – Check sensation over the hand and forearm (ulnar nerve impairment), and check power at the wrist for extension and flexion.

## Investigations

» Bloods – Not routinely needed unless OA is suspected, in which case request Hb, WCC and CRP.

» Elbow x-ray – This is to exclude a fracture and calcified tendonitis.

» USS/MRI – This is to look for micro-fractures, tendonitis and bursitis.

» Electromyography (EMG) – This is to check for cubital tunnel syndrome.

## Management

### Conservative

✓ Rest – If the pain is due to repetitive movements, advise the patient to rest.

✓ Ice/heat – Advise them to apply an ice or heat pack if the pain worsens after activity.

✓ Splint – Advise them to consider purchasing a splint or clasp to reduce the pressure on the joint/tendon.

✓ Exercise – Advise them to continue with simple exercises (aerobic / muscle strengthening) as the pain eases to help maintain and improve ROM and prevent stiffness.

✓ Modifying activities – Advise them to avoid making lifting, gripping or screwing motions. They should take regular breaks. They should speak to a sports doctor or coach regarding how to modify their sporting activity to reduce symptoms.

### Medical

✓ Pain – Simple analgesia (paracetamol or codeine) or NSAIDs can be issued as topical creams or oral medication. Ensure that the patient has no contraindications for NSAIDs (ulcers, gastritis or asthma).

✓ Infection – If there are signs of a local infection (bursitis) then they may need a course of antibiotics. If you suspect septic arthritis, then they may need orthopaedic admission for IV antibiotics and drainage.

✓ Sick certificate – Offer a short fit note if they are unable to work. Advise them to consider amended duties or altered hours if they are finding it difficult to carry out certain tasks.

## Referral

→ Physiotherapy – Refer them to physiotherapy, which may be helpful for strengthening the muscles around the elbow. Other treatments that may be offered include massage or manipulation to help improve the blood flow to the joint. The joint may be strapped over the area that induces pain to help reduce the pressure.

→ OT – Refer them to speak to an OT about adaptations that can be made for occupational-induced elbow pain (carpenters or plumbers).

→ Injection – Persistent pain may warrant steroid or LA injections to reduce the pain and inflammation in the joint in the short term. A maximum of three injections should be offered.

→ Surgery – A small minority who do not respond will need keyhole surgery to remove adhesions or damaged tissue, or for surgical decompression if there is evidence of a trapped nerve.

## Safety Netting

» Review in four to six weeks regarding their response to treatment.

*References*

National Institute for Health and Care Excellence (2017). *Tennis elbow.* https://cks.nice.org.uk/topics/tennis-elbow/

Harding, M. (2015). *Tennis elbow and golfer's elbow.* https://patient.info/doctor/tennis-elbow-and-golfers-elbow

National Institute for Health and Care Excellence (2016). *Olecranon bursitis.* https://cks.nice.org.uk/topics/olecranon-bursitis/

Payne, J. (2015). *Cubital tunnel syndrome.* https://patient.info/doctor/cubital-tunnel-syndrome

# Ankle/Foot Problems

Foot pain is a common problem that patients may present with. The foot carries the body's weight and is put through enormous stresses on a daily basis. It is important to consider the different structures in the foot that may give rise to pain, such as bones, tendons, plantar fascia and ligaments. But also do not forget pain radiating in from outside the foot, such as from the back (sciatica) or the ankle. You should also consider a systemic or metabolic illness that may give rise to foot problems, such as RA and gout, and even causes of a swollen foot such as CCF, CKD and HF. Do not forget that foot problems may be due to poorly fitting shoes or a flattened foot arch.

## History

- » Focused questions
  - › Ask where the foot pain or tenderness is, and when it started.
  - › Ask about the site of the pain, and if it affects one or both feet; ask if they can point to it.
  - › Ask about the character of the pain (burning, aching, sharp or stinging).
  - › Ask about the frequency of the pain, and if it is always there or comes and goes.
  - › Ask if there are any exacerbating (movements) or alleviating (medications and rest) factors, and if it is worse in the morning (fasciitis) or evening (stress fracture or nerve entrapment).
  - › Ask if there is any radiation of the pain (Morton's neuroma).
  - › Ask if there is any swelling or redness of the toes (gout), or any swelling of the ankle or foot (HF, CKD and postural oedema).
  - › Ask if there is any joint stiffness.
- » Associated history – Ask if they have had an injury or fall, any neurology (weakness, numbness, or pins and needles) or any foot drop (the foot dragging along the floor).
- » Past history – Ask if they have DM, RA, OA or gout, or if they have had a recent fracture of the foot (stress fracture).
- » Family history – Ask if there is a family history of pes varus, toe deformity or bunions.
- » Drug history – Ask if they have taken NSAIDs, paracetamol, topical gels or diuretics (thiazide).
- » Social history – Ask what their occupation is (postman, security guard or policeman), what their hobbies are, if they smoke or drink alcohol, or if they drive.

## RED FLAGS

Fever or sweats (septic arthritis), or a significant deformity.

## Differential Diagnosis

| | |
|---|---|
| Morton's neuroma | Benign thickening of the plantar interdigital nerve caused by compression. Common in >50-year-old women. Presents with forefoot pain (between the third and fourth metatarsophalangeal [MTP]) that is described as feeling like they have a pebble in their shoe. Associated with a burning or electric-shock pain along the nerve when walking. OE: pain with pressure over the neuroma, Mulder's click, and loss of sensation in the affected toes. |
| Plantar fasciitis | Inflammation of the ligamentous insertion of the plantar fascia to the heel. Gradual pain, in the sole of heel when standing or walking, which is worse in the morning and relieved upon resting. Common in those >40 years, with a sedentary lifestyle, who wear flat shoes and walk on hard surfaces. OE: tenderness over anteromedial aspect of heel, and a positive Windlass test. |
| Calcaneal spur | Small osteophyte formed on the calcaneus. Associated with plantar fasciitis or ankylosing spondylitis. Heel pain worsens after a period of prolonged rest, with exacerbation from walking or bearing weight. |
| Pes planus | Obliteration of the medial arch of the foot. Common in childhood. Often asymptomatic, but can present with foot pain after prolonged walking. OE: loss of medial arches (medial border and outer heel). |
| Achilles tendonitis | Inflammation of the Achilles tendon. Often caused by overuse, ankylosing spondylitis or medication (ciprofloxacin or steroids). Presents with tenderness and swelling of the tendon. Can cause a rupture (sudden pain and a gap in the tendon) with foot drop. |
| Tarsal tunnel syndrome | Known as posterior tibial neuralgia where the tibial nerve is compressed in the tarsal tunnel. Causes pain and numbness in the foot, especially in the big toe and the adjacent three toes. |

## Examination

» Inspection – Examine the gait by asking the patient to walk normally, then on tiptoes. Inspect the shoes for asymmetrical wear. Check for any deformity (pes cavus, pes planus, hammer or mallet toes, genu valgum or genu varum). Inspect for any bunions (first MTP), corns, callosities, or skin and nail changes (ingrowing). Look for signs of ulceration around the ankle (PVD). Look at the foot arches from the side.

» Palpation – Squeeze the MTP, midfoot, ankle and subtalar joints, and the Achilles tendon. Feel for a raised temperature and tenderness. Palpate the peripheral pulses (dorsalis pedis and posterior tibial).

» Movement – Check the active and passive movement of the ankle, subtalar (inversion and eversion of the ankle), midtarsal (fix the ankle and move the forefoot) and toes.

» Neurological – Check sensation if the patient reports any numbness or paraesthesia.

» Special tests – Consider the following if clinically indicated from their history:

› Mulder's click (Morton's neuroma) – Grip the neuroma between the forefinger and thumb (plantar surface), and squeeze the metatarsal heads with other hand. A click can be heard/felt with pressure.

› Windlass test (plantar fasciitis) – Reproduces heel pain on the extension (passive dorsiflexion) of the first MTP.

## Common Causes of Foot Pain by Location

➤ Heel – Sever's disease (young), plantar fasciitis (older), pes cavus or Achilles tendonitis

➤ Mid foot – Kohler's disease (young), OA (adults) or a stress fracture

➤ Forefoot – Morton's neuroma, pes cavus/planus, RA, gout, Freiberg's disease (second and third metatarsal heads) or march a fracture

➤ Big toe – Gout (first MTP)

## Investigations

» Bloods – Not routinely needed unless osteomyelitis, inflammatory arthritis (Hb, WCC, ESR and CRP) or gout (uric acid) are suspected.

» USS/MRI – If Morton's neuroma is suspected.

» X-ray – Consider this to exclude a fracture or arthropathy (e.g. calcaneal spur) or to determine the degree of a bunion.

**Ottawa rules regarding ankle x-rays**

Consider an x-ray of the ankle to exclude a fracture if one or more of the following apply:

› Bone tenderness along the distal 6cm of the posterior edge of the tibia or the tip of the medial malleolus.

› Bone tenderness along the distal 6cm of the posterior edge of the fibula or the tip of the lateral malleolus.

› An inability to bear weight for four steps, both immediately after the injury and in the emergency department.

**Ottawa rules regarding foot X-rays**

Consider an x-ray of the foot to exclude a fracture if one or more of the following apply:

> Bone tenderness at the base of the fifth metatarsal (for foot injuries).

> Bone tenderness at the navicular bone (for foot injuries).

> An inability to bear weight for four steps, both immediately after the injury and in the emergency department.

# Management

*Conservative*

✓ Rest – Advise the patient to have their foot elevated where possible, and to avoid standing or walking for long periods.

✓ Weight – If their BMI is >25, advise them to lose weight.

✓ Shoes – Advise them to ensure that they wear well-fitted, low-heeled, wide-toed footwear with thick soles. They should avoid high heels and shoes that constrict the toes.

✓ Pad – For Morton's neuroma, suggest that they consider OTC metatarsal pads or orthotic inserts for shoes, which reduce the pressure on the metatarsal heads. For bunions, advise them to consider OTC bunion pads.

✓ Exercise – Advise them to continue with simple exercises (aerobic / muscle strengthening) as the pain eases to help maintain and improve ROM and prevent stiffness.

» Plantar fasciitis – Advise them to avoid walking barefoot or on hard surfaces, and standing for prolonged periods. Suggest they use an ice pack for 15 minutes for pain relief.

> Orthoses – Advise them to use shoes with cushioned heels and arch supports. They may cut a small hole in the pad where the heel is most tender.

> Exercise – Recommend that they roll a drink can or tennis ball under the arch of the foot. They should walk on tiptoe several times a day. They should also stand on the edge of a step with their heels off the edge, then lower their heels down and hold the position for one minute, and then elevate them again.

*Medical*

✓ Pain – Simple analgesia (paracetamol) or NSAIDs can be prescribed as topical creams or oral medication. Ensure that the patient has no contraindications for NSAIDs (ulcers, gastritis or asthma).

## Referral

→ Physiotherapy – Refer them to physiotherapy, which may be helpful for strengthening the muscles, and stretching the Achilles tendon or plantar fascia. This can help to reduce stiffness in the foot and ankle.

→ Orthotics – Refer a patient with Morton's neuroma for a metatarsal dome orthotic.

→ OT – Refer them to speak to an OT about adaptations that can be made for occupational-induced foot pain (shoes for postpersons, security guards, etc.).

→ Injection – Persistent pain may warrant steroid or LA injections to reduce the pain and inflammation in the joint for the short term.

→ Surgery – Consider a neurectomy or decompression of the interdigital nerve for a patient with Morton's neuroma. Consider the release of the plantar fascia and calcaneal spur for a patient with plantar fasciitis.

## Safety Netting

» Review in four to six weeks regarding their response to treatment.

---

### References

National Institute for Health and Care Excellence (2016). *Morton's neuroma.* https://cks.nice.org.uk/topics/mortons-neuroma/

National Institute for Health and Care Excellence (2020). *Plantar fasciitis.* https://cks.nice.org.uk/topics/plantar-fasciitis/

National Institute for Health and Care Excellence (2019). *Heel pain.* https://cks.nice.org.uk/topics/developmental-rheumatology-in-children/background-information/heel-pain/

National Institute for Health and Care Excellence (2020). *Achilles tendinopathy.* https://cks.nice.org.uk/topics/achilles-tendinopathy/

National Institute for Health and Care Excellence (2020). *Developmental rheumatology in children: flat feet.* https://cks.nice.org.uk/topics/developmental-rheumatology-in-children/background-information/flat-feet/

# Raynaud's Phenomenon

Raynaud's phenomenon describes episodic vasospasm attacks of the distal arteries, causing ischaemia (pallor, cyanosis and redness). It is precipitated by cold or a person's emotions. It is often seen in 20–30-year-old women, with 90% having no underlying cause. Secondary causes include connective tissue disorders (SLE, scleroderma, RA and Sjögren's syndrome). It is often characterised by distinctive colour changes of the fingers – white (ischaemia), blue (deoxygenation) and red (reperfusion) – with throbbing pain from rapidly reactive hyperaemia.

## History

- » Open questions
    - › *'How may I help you today? Tell me more about the problems you are having with your fingers/toes.'*

- » Focused questions
    - › Ask if they have noticed a change in the colour of their fingers or toes.
    - › Ask about the site of the issue, and which fingers/toes are affected.
    - › Ask if it affects one or both sides (symmetry).
    - › Ask about the onset of the condition.
    - › Ask about the character, specifically if they have noticed a colour change (white, blue or red).
    - › Ask if there are any triggers that make it worse (cold or stress).
    - › Ask if there is any pain or swelling (reperfusion).

- » Associated history – Ask if it affects other areas (ear lobes, nose, tongue or nipples).
- » Past history – Ask if they have SLE, RA, scleroderma or DM.
- » Family history – Ask if there is a family history of connective tissue disorders (SLE, RA or scleroderma).
- » Drug history – Ask if they have taken any b-blockers, COCP, ergotamine, clonidine or ciclosporin.
- » Social history – Ask what their occupation is; if they work in any cold environments, or with vibrating tools, lead or organic solvents; if they smoke or take recreational drugs; and what their diet is like (tea or coffee).

## RED FLAGS

Underlying connective tissue disorders and digital ulceration.

## Differential Diagnosis

| Raynaud's phenomenon | Vasospasm of the distal arteries. Commonly affects teenage girls. Can resolve by the menopause. Attacks last anywhere from minutes to hours. Causes a colour change (white>blue>red) with a throbbing pain and swelling on reperfusion. Fingers can be cold. Occasionally, it can affect other extremities (nose or earlobes). Secondary causes include CREST syndrome, dermatomyositis, SLE and RA. |
|---|---|
| Chilblains | Skin inflammation of the peripheral digits caused by cold or damp. Common in young women. Appear 12–24 hours after exposure and last up to two weeks. Characterised by an intense itch, a burning sensation and tenderness; typically occur in winter with resolution in summer. Can present with purplish oedematous lesions with vesicles. Can form papules and patches that appear symmetrically and bilaterally. |
| Hypothyroidism | Underactive thyroid presents with fatigue, weight gain, cold intolerance, skin changes (dry, cold, pale complexion and alopecia), hoarse voice and arthralgia. |
| SLE | Connective tissue disorder that is characterised by vasculitis, and it presents with a relapsing, remitting pattern. Non-specific features include fever, oral ulcers, myalgia/myositis, Raynaud's phenomenon and lymphadenopathy. Other features include malar (butterfly) or discoid rash, photosensitivity, and arthritis of the large joints (knee and wrist) and small bones (proximal IP and MCP). |
| Sjögren's syndrome | Associated with keratoconjunctivitis sicca (dry eyes), xerostomia (dry mouth), parotid enlargement, fatigue, myalgia and arthralgia. Often involves other secretory glands (dyspareunia, dysphagia, dry skin, dry cough, chest infection and otitis media). |
| Dermatomyositis | Acute and chronic inflammation of striated muscle fibres with dermatitis. Can cause muscle tenderness, with weakness affecting the proximal (symmetrical and limb girdle) muscles with the preservation of muscle bulk. As a result, the patient presents with difficulty rising from a chair or climbing up stairs. Dermatitis features include a heliotrope rash and papules (Gottron) with telangiectasias (periungual). |

## Examination

» Vitals – Temperature, BP (in both arms) and pulse.

» Inspection – Inspect for colour change (pallor, cyanosis and redness), nail changes (abnormal nailfold capillary), digital ulcers and rashes (SLE or heliotrope).

» Palpation – Check the temperature and for joint tenderness (RA). Check the peripheral pulses.

## Investigations

» Bloods – FBC (polycythaemia), ESR and ANA.

› Other – U&Es, LFTs, TFTs, rheumatoid factor, HbA1c and CK (dermatomyositis).

» Specialist – Use a capillary microscope to examine the nailfold capillaries.

## Management

### For primary Raynaud's phenomenon

#### Conservative

✓ Advise them to keep warm by wearing gloves, socks, fur-lined boots and thermal underwear in cold weather. They should avoid holding frozen foods or cold drinks.

✓ Advise them to avoid caffeine (tea and coffee) where possible.

✓ Advise them to stop smoking and avoid passive smoking.

✓ Advise them to exercise their hands and feet regularly to improve circulation.

✓ Recommend that they minimise stress and consider using relaxation techniques.

✓ Suggest that they consider a change of occupation, or provide a fit note for amended duties, where appropriate.

✓ Advise them to try warming devices for the hands and feet.

✓ Advise them to avoid touching cold objects and carrying bags in their hands (which impairs circulation).

✓ Recommend that they stop taking recreational drugs (amphetamines and cocaine).

#### Medical

✓ Avoid giving b-blockers, COCP, ergotamine and clonidine.

✓ There is some evidence of improvement through using evening primrose oil and fish oils.

✓ Nifedipine – Offer immediate release 5mg tds to 20mg tds, depending on the patient's response. Offer a modified release (MR) preparation if they experience side effects (20mg od increasing to 60mg od). Intermittent prophylactic use, prior to cold exposure, can be adequate. Other CCBs can be considered (nicardipine, felodipine or amlodipine). Side effects are flushing, headaches, palpitations, dizziness and oedema. Advise them to avoid consuming grapefruit.

## Referral

→ OT – Refer them to speak to an OT about adaptations at work.

→ Rheumatology – Refer them to rheumatology for uncontrolled symptoms.

## Safety Netting

» Follow-up – Refer them if there is evidence of secondary causes. Suspect such a secondary cause if the onset is when they are >30 years, the impact is asymmetrical and intensely painful, they have digital ulcers or abnormal nail capillaries, or have a positive ANA or high ESR.

» Admit them if there is evidence of acute or severe ischaemia in one or more digits.

---

### References

National Institute for Health and Care Excellence (2020). *Raynaud's phenomenon.* https://cks.nice.org.uk/topics/raynauds-phenomenon/

# Fibromyalgia

Fibromyalgia is a condition known to cause chronic, widespread pain. Patients will also have multiple muscular tender points, which can be associated with sleep disturbance, fatigue and cognitive dysfunction, with no underlying organic cause. The exact cause of fibromyalgia is unknown. Sleep disturbance is thought to be of major importance (loss of non-rapid-eye-movement [non-REM] sleep).

Possible factors thought to be responsible include the following:

» Altered central pain processing (patients develop a lower threshold of pain).

» Dysfunction of the hypothalamic-pituitary-adrenal (HPA) axis.

» Sleep disturbances, which impairs the healing of microtrauma.

» Genetic factors.

» Psychiatric aspects.

» Trigger factors include infection and physical trauma.

## Risk Factors

➤ Female gender

➤ Age 20–50 years

➤ Stress

➤ Emotional or physical abuse

➤ Genetics – it seems to run in families

➤ Not moving enough

## *History*

» Pain is the primary complaint.

» Focused questions

› Ask how long it has been going on for; the symptoms should be present for at least three months for it to be fibromyalgia.

› Ask about the onset. It is usually gradual, and may start in a localised area. The pain may initially be intermittent and will then progress and become more persistent.

› Ask about the site and intensity of pain, and if it varies from day to day.

› Ask about any trigger factors that modify the pain (weather or stress).

› Ask about other associated symptoms, such as fatigue (in some patients this is more disabling than the pain), non-restorative sleep (impaired daytime function due to sleep disturbance and fragmented sleep), cognitive dysfunction (poor working memory), mood disorder, or pain-related somatic symptoms (IBS, migraine, headaches or TMJ pain).

## Examination

» Palpation – Perform a digital palpation using the thumb to assess the tenderness at tender points. The pressure applied should be just enough to blanch the examiner's thumbnail.

## Differentials

➤ CFS

➤ SLE

➤ PMR

➤ Hypothyroidism

## Investigations

» Bloods – Tests such as ESR, TFTs and ANA to exclude other conditions.

## Management

The ideal plan should include a combination of nonpharmacological and pharmacological treatments.

### Conservative

✓ Advise the patient to take appropriate physical therapies (exercise programmes and balneotherapy).

✓ Advise them to consider acupuncture.

✓ Advise them to utilise appropriate psychological therapies (CBT).

### Medical

✓ The choice of drug should target the patient's most troublesome symptoms.

✓ Advise them to follow the WHO step-up ladder for analgesia (starting with paracetamol and ibuprofen).

✓ Opioids – Tramadol should be reserved for severe pain.

✓ Antidepressants – Amitriptyline, fluoxetine or paroxetine.

---

*References*

Bellato, E., Marini, E., Castoldi, F., Barbasetti, N., Mattei, L., Bonasia, D.E., and Blonna D. (Fibromyalgia syndrome: etiology, pathogenesis, diagnosis, and treatment. *Pain Resolution and Treatment, 2012.* https://doi.org/10.1155/2012/426130

# 12

# Dermatology

## Eczema

The name 'atopic eczema' comes from the Greek word meaning 'to boil' and is characterised by red, flaky and itchy skin, following exposure to triggers such as foods, allergens and irritants. It is increasing in prevalence, currently affecting about 15–20% of children. There is a strong association with a family history of atopy, asthma and hay fever. The condition has a fluctuating course, resolving in about 50% of children by age two. It often presents with around two to three exacerbations per month. Treatment involves avoiding all soaps, and using emollients and ointments instead. Other agents used during a flare-up include topical steroids, antihistamines and antibacterial creams.

### Risk Factors – NICE (2007) Criteria for a High Risk of Atopic Eczema

Itchy skin (scratching) plus three of the following:

➤ Past medical history of dry skin within the last 12 months

➤ Past medical history of flexural eczema (cheeks / extensor surface in those <18 years)

➤ Past medical history of asthma or allergic rhinitis

➤ A family history (first-degree relative) of the condition in those aged under four years

➤ Flexural eczema in those <18 months, affecting the skin creases (elbows and knees)

➤ Symptoms starting at under two years; This is used retrospectively to diagnose older children (over four years)

### *History*

» Focused questions

  › Ask when it started, how long it has been going on for and if it has changed over time.

  › Ask about the distribution (flexor surfaces, including the creases of elbows, knees, neck, wrist and ankles; and extensor surfaces, including the face or cheeks in babies).

> › Ask if the skin is dry or itchy (eczema is unlikely if it is not itchy).

> › Ask if there are any thickened patches (lichenification and chronic signs).

> › Ask is there are any triggers or exacerbating factors (stress, pets, irritants, clothing, latex or topical creams), including dietary ones (milk, egg, soya, peanuts or wheat).

» Associated history – Ask if they have herpeticum (blisters, painful areas or ulcers), bleeding, infection, growth or developmental concerns in children.

» Past history – Ask if they have had hay fever, eczema, asthma or urticaria.

» Drug history – Ask if they have tried any treatments already.

» Social history – Ask what their current occupation is; if they have any involvement with chemicals, animals or dyes; and if they have any pets.

» Family history – Ask if there is a family history of any atopy (eczema, hay fever or asthma).

## RED FLAGS

Eczema herpeticum, bleeding or secondary infections.

## Examination

» Skin – Examine the body for signs of eczema.

» Distribution – Examine the flexural surfaces, including antecubital and popliteal fossae, neck, wrists and ankles (for adult eczema). Look at the face, hands and infra-orbital folds.

» Wrists – Look at the wrists and the neck area for contact dermatitis (from a watch, necklace or bracelet).

» Scalp – Check the scalp area and behind the ears for signs of seborrhoeic dermatitis.

» Hands – Assess the hands for dryness, itching or exposure to irritants.

» Web spaces – Look at the finger and toe web spaces for any evidence of burrows (scabies).

» Skin changes – Look for dry skin, papules, vesicles, crusting, weeping, lichenification, excoriations or scarring.

### Severity of Eczema (NICE, 2007)

➤ Mild – Dry skin area, infrequent itching with or without small areas of redness

➤ Moderate – Dry skin areas, frequent itching, redness with or without excoriation, and skin thickening

➤ Severe – Widespread dry skin, incessant itching, redness with or without excoriation, extensive skin thickening, bleeding, oozing, cracking, and altered pigmentation

➤ Infection – Eczema that is weeping, crusting and has pustules, with a fever

## Differential Diagnosis

| Contact dermatitis | Localised, red, eczematous lesions that come about post contact with an allergen. May include an allergy to cements, soaps, detergents (hands), jewellery (ears, fingers, neck and wrists), nickel (buttons, if in the waist area) or hair dye (scalp and hands). |
|---|---|
| Scabies | Intensely itchy rash over the hands, feet or genital areas. Patients present with a chronic, red rash that is itchy and spares the face. May affect a number of people in the same household. There may be a history of travel or staying in youth hostels. OE: burrows in the web spaces of the hands or toes; the itching is made worse after a bath. |
| Seborrhoeic dermatitis | Mainly affects the face or behind the ears. This is a relapsing condition that can also affect the torso and scalp. Presents with red, scaly, itchy, flaky skin and dandruff. |
| Psoriasis | Typically on the scalp, extensor surfaces (knees and elbows) or lumbosacral area. Has less itchy, well-circumscribed, flat-topped, erythematous plaques (salmon pink) with silvery scales; it is typically symmetrical. Presents in those <35 years. Ask about joint pains and nail changes. |

## Investigations

» Blood tests – Not routinely performed, but FBC and CRP if an infection is suspected.

» RAST IgE blood tests for specific allergens.

» Secondary care – Skin-prick testing (to confirm contact dermatitis or for unknown allergens).

## Management

*Conservative*

✓ Advise the patient to avoid irritants or allergens that are suspected. They should wear cotton clothes and avoid wool. They should avoid excessive heat.

✓ Advise them to reduce the number of dust mites by regular hoovering, removing carpets, increasing room ventilation, and using mite-proof covers for mattresses and pillows.

✓ Advise them to avoid soaps or bubble baths, including perfumes and shower gels.

✓ Advise them to cut their nails short and to avoid scratching their skin. They should consider wearing gloves (or mittens for babies) in bed.

*Medical*

✓ Emollients – Advise them to keep their skin moist using generous amounts of emollients/moisturisers, particularly when washing and bathing. Advise them to avoid perfumed products and aqueous cream. They should apply them to the whole body, and consider applying them at least four times a day. Examples include emulsifying ointment, hydrous ointment and liquid paraffin 50:50. Liberal emollient use should reduce the need for more potent steroid use (250–500g a week).

✓ Topical steroids – Use the weakest cream to the control symptoms. For normal skin (not face, genitals or axillae) use steroids for 7–14 days. For the face, genitals and axillae, use for no more than five days. Avoid using very potent steroids in children unless directed by a specialist. Ointments are the most suitable for dry, scaly eczema, and creams are best for weepy, exudative eczema.

› Mild – Hydrocortisone 0.5–2.5%

› Moderate – Betamethasone valerate 0.025% (Betnovate RD) or clobetasone butyrate 0.05% (Eumovate)

› Potent – Fluticasone propionate 0.05% (Cutivate), betamethasone valerate 0.1% (Betnovate)

› Very potent – Clobetasol propionate (Dermovate)

**Topical steroid volumes (BNF, n.d.)**

- Face and neck 15–30g

- Both hands 15–30g

- Scalp 15–30g

- Groin and genitalia 15–30g

- Both arms 30–60g

- Both legs 100g

- Trunk 100g

✓ Area of skin and fingertip units (FTUs) per dose of steroids:

One FTU equates to 0.5g of steroid, which is sufficient to cover the equivalent of two palms of an adult hand.

› Hands and fingers (front and back) – 1.0

› One hand or foot (all over) – 2.0

› One arm (excluding hand) – 3.0

› Face and neck – 2.5

› One leg (excluding foot) – 6.0

✓ Oral the steroids – If symptoms are severe, consider an oral steroid in adults (30mg prednisolone od for seven days).

✓ If the itching is severe or affecting sleep, consider Piriton, promethazine or hydroxyzine. Non-sedative antihistamines include loratadine, cetirizine and fexofenadine.

✓ If it is infected, try a short course (seven days) of a topical antibiotic (fusidic acid cream) or an oral antibiotic (flucloxacillin or erythromycin). Consider a swab if it is not resolving. Consider acyclovir for herpeticum.

✓ Tacrolimus (immunosuppressant) may be used in moderate or severe cases ofeczema, and should be initiated by a specialist.

✓ Wet wrapping is useful in exudative eczema. Use a Tubigrip bandage with liberal amounts of an emollient. Applications are started and taught by a specialist.

## Referral

→ Refer the patient to dermatology if they have severe eczema that is resistant to treatment; the patient may need an immunosuppressant or phototherapy. Refer them for a same-day admission for eczema herpeticum.

→ Refer them to a counsellor if their eczema is affecting their psychological state.

→ Refer them to a dietician if a diet modification is to be considered.

→ For atopic eczema in children, refer them as follows (NICE, 2017):

› Urgent referral (2WW) if it has not responded to optimal topical therapy after one week.

› If they have bacterially infected eczema that does not respond to treatment.

› If they have facial atopic eczema that does not respond to treatment.

› If they have recurrent severe infections.

› If they require advice on bandaging techniques.

## Safety Netting

» Review in six to eight weeks regarding their response to treatment.

*References*

British National Formulary (n.d.). *Topical corticosteroids.* https://bnf.nice.org.uk/treatment-summary/topical-corticosteroids.html

National Institute for Health and Care Excellence (2007). *Atopic eczema in under 12s: diagnosis and management.* https://www.nice.org.uk/guidance/cg57

# Psoriasis

Psoriasis is a chronic skin condition that is characterised by inflamed, raised, red lesions that develop with silvery scales on the scalp, elbows, knees and lower back. Around 2% of the population have psoriasis, and it mainly affects those <35 years. Alcohol, b-blockers, lithium, NSAIDs and antimalarials can exacerbate the condition. The most common form is called discoid or plaque psoriasis. Symptoms include salmon-coloured plaques with silvery-white scales on the extensor surfaces and the scalp area, which are often itchy in nature. Other types include guttate and pustular psoriasis. Psoriasis can also involve the nails (in 50%) or the joints (7%). Nail features include pitting, ridging, onycholysis (separation of the distal nail from the bed) and hyperkeratosis (a build-up of keratin below the nail bed).

## History

» Focused questions

> Ask when the skin condition started, how long it has been going on for and if there have been any changes over time.

> Ask about the distribution (scalp, elbows, knees, palms and soles of the feet).

> Ask if the skin is dry or itchy.

> Ask if there are any exacerbating (stress, sunlight, trauma, infections, medication or alcohol) or relieving factors.

» Associated history – Ask if they have had any nail changes, arthropathy (joint pain or swelling), streptococcal infection or uveitis (eye symptoms).

» Drug history – Ask if they have taken lithium, an ACEi, b-blockers, antimalarials or NSAIDs (which worsens the condition).

» Social history – Ask what their occupation is and if they have any stress at the moment.

» Family history – Ask if they have a family history of psoriasis.

## RED FLAGS

Generalised pustular psoriasis, erythroderma and severe psoriasis covering more than 10% of the body.

## Differential Diagnosis

| | |
|---|---|
| Erythroderma | Generalised redness to the skin. Refer them urgently to dermatology. |
| Pustular psoriasis | Small pustules that appear all over the body, or just on the palms, soles and other small areas. |
| Guttate psoriasis | Mostly affects teens. Presents with multiple drop-like lesions that are usually preceded by a streptococcal throat infection. |
| Flexural psoriasis | Common in the elderly. Smooth, glazed plaques affecting the axilla or submammary areas. |
| Scalp psoriasis | Common. Well-outlined scaly plaques with thickened scales. |
| Eczema | Very itchy; the patient may have a history of atopy. |
| Tinea infection | Itchy, ring-like lesions; other household members may also have this. |

## Examination

» Skin – Examine the body for signs of psoriasis, and assess the severity using the Physician's Global Assessment (as follows).

» Distribution – Examine the extensor surfaces, including the knees, elbows, scalp, sacrum and hair margin. Examine the axillae (flexural psoriasis), palms and soles of the feet (palmoplantar pustulosis). Look for Koebner phenomenon.

» Skin changes – Look for waxy, salmon-pink plaques or raindrop lesions on the chest/limbs (guttate).

» Nails – Inspect the nails for pitting, onycholysis and oily patch discolouration.

» Joints – Inspect and palpate the hands for arthropathy.

## Physician's Global Assessment of Psoriasis

0: Clear – No signs of psoriasis, but post-inflammatory discolouration may be present

1: Almost clear – Only minimal plaque elevation, scaling and erythema

2: Mild – Slight plaque elevation, scaling and erythema

3: Moderate – Moderate plaque elevation, scaling and erythema

4: Severe – Marked plaque elevation, scaling and erythema

5: Very severe – Very severe plaque elevation, scaling and erythema

## Investigations

»     Rarely performed, but a specialist may perform a skin biopsy.

## Management

### Conservative

✓     Advise them to avoid triggers, such as sunlight and certain medications.

✓     If they smoke, advise them to try to quit.

✓     Advise them to reduce their alcohol intake to a minimum.

✓     If their BMI is >25, suggest that they lose weight.

✓     Advise them to try to mitigate any stress, and to use relaxation or self-help techniques.

✓     Advise them to contact support groups for patients with psoriasis.

### Medical

✓     General – Treat initially with a daily potent topical steroid (clobetasone or hydrocortisone) with vitamin D or vitamin D analogue daily at alternate times for up to four weeks. If it is no better after eight weeks, stop the steroids and continue with vitamin D or vitamin D analogue. If it is no better by eight to twelve weeks, then add a potent steroid bd (clobetasol or diflucortolone) for four weeks, or coal tar.

✓     Topical steroids – Use in the short term to help reduce inflammation. Consider a moderately potent type. A short course may avoid rebound exacerbation when treatment is stopped. Ensure a break of four weeks between treatments. Do not use very potent steroids continuously on any site for longer than four weeks. Avoid giving to children. Do not use potent steroids continuously on any site for longer than eight weeks.

✓     Vitamin D – Vitamin D analogues (Dovonex) reduce the speed of epithelial cell turnover. It causes less irritation, so is suitable for the face or flexures. There are combined forms with steroids available, such as Dovobet.

✓     Dithranol – This is rarely used as it stains clothing (purple) and can irritate the skin. Apply to the chronic extensor plaques only. Avoid using on the face or flexural areas.

✓     Coal tar – This is the least preferred treatment due to the mess and smell. It has anti-inflammatory properties and is useful in the removal of thickened plaques. Different strengths are available.

✓     Salicylic acid – This is useful as an adjunct to remove scales. It is safe for long-term use. It can cause irritation to normal skin.

✓     Emollients – Offer liberal amounts of emollient to keep the skin soft and moist, to avoid irritation. It helps reduce itching, scaling and cracking. *See Eczema section, page 463.*

## Combined Treatments for Psoriasis

|  | Steroid | Vitamin D | Coal Tar | Dithranol | Salicylic |
|---|---|---|---|---|---|
| Steroid | Eumovate | Dovobet |  | Alphosyl HC | Diprosalic |
| Vitamin D | Dovobet | Dovonex |  |  |  |
| Coal Tar | Alphosyl HC |  |  | Psorin | Cocois |
| Dithranol | Scalp gel |  | Psorin |  |  |
| Salicylic | Diprosalic |  | Sebco |  | Lassar's Paste |

## Location-Based Treatment of Psoriasis

| Flexure | Can be managed with the short-term use of a mild- or moderate-potency topical steroid. Tacalcitol can be used in the longer term; calcipotriol is more likely to cause irritation in flexures and should be avoided. Low-strength tar preparations can also be used. |
|---|---|
| Facial | Can be managed with the short-term use of a mild- or moderate-potency topical steroid; if this is ineffective, use calcitriol, tacalcitol or a low-strength tar preparation. |
| Unstable | Widespread unstable psoriasis of the erythrodermic or generalised pustular type requires urgent specialist assessment. The initial topical treatment should be limited to using emollients generously and frequently. More localised acute inflammatory psoriasis with spreading or itchy lesions should be treated topically with emollients or with a moderately potent steroid. |

# Referral

→ Dermatology – Refer the patient for phototherapy (UVB) or photochemotherapy (PUVA and UVA), oral retinoids or immunosuppressive drugs (methotrexate). Refer them in cases where the disease is extensive or they are unresponsive to treatments, where it affects the genitalia, or there is a generalised erythrodermic rash or pustular psoriasis.

→ Rheumatology – Refer them to rheumatology if there is evidence of arthropathy.

## Safety Netting

» Review in six to eight weeks regarding their response to treatment.

## References

National Institute for Health and Care Excellence (2012). *Psoriasis: assessment and management.* https://www.nice.org.uk/guidance/cg153

British National Formulary (n.d.). *Psoriasis. National Institute for Health and Care Excellence.* https://bnf.nice.org.uk/treatment-summary/psoriasis.html

# Acne

Acne is a common skin condition that affects males and females alike. The peak incidence is at 18 years of age; however, it usually begins prior to the onset of puberty when the adrenal gland begins to produce and release increasing amounts of androgen hormones. It is characterised by papules, open and closed comedones (black and whiteheads), pustules, nodules and scars in the sebaceous distribution (face, neck, back and chest). The blockage and colonisation of the pilosebaceous ducts with *Propionibacterium* cause a hypersensitive response that gives rise to inflammatory acne.

## History

» Focused questions

› Ask when the acne started, how long it has been going on for and if it has changed over time.

› Ask about the distribution (face, shoulders, chest and upper back).

› Ask if they have black or white spots, redness, pus-filled pimples, scarring or cysts.

› Ask about aggravating factors.

› Ask about puberty, pregnancy, periods, and if they use oily products or cosmetics.

» Past history – Ask if they have had PCOS or Cushing's disease.

» Drug history – Ask if they have used any OTC products, have been on any special diets, or have used steroids, the POP, the Mirena coil, lithium or cyclosporine, all of which are known to worsen the condition.

» Social history – Ask if they smoke or drink alcohol, and what their occupation is.

» Family history – Ask if there is a family history of acne, endocrine issues or PCOS.

## Differential Diagnosis

| Acne | Bimodal distribution (teenagers and those 30–40 years). Typically occurs over the face (periorbital sparing), upper chest, back and neck area. Presents with comedones (black/whiteheads), papules, pustules, cysts and scarring on a background of greasy skin. |
|---|---|
| Acne Rosacea | Particularly affects women in their 40s, but is often more severe in men. Presents with facial flushing of the nose, cheeks and forehead, along with erythema, papules and pustules. The rash can be sore or itchy in nature. Associated with conjunctivitis or blepharitis, and rhinophyma. |

| PCOS | An endocrine disorder that presents with multiple cysts in the ovaries along with irregular periods (oligomenorrhoea or amenorrhoea) as well as acne and hirsutism. |
|------|------|

## Examination

» Examine the face, back and chest area for signs of acne.

» Look for erythema, open (blackheads) or closed (whiteheads) comedones (the absence of comedones makes acne less likely).

» Look for pustules, papules or cysts.

» Inspect the skin for features of PCOS and hyperandrogenism (hirsutism).

## Severity of Acne

➤ Mild – Open or closed comedones, with some papules

➤ Moderate – Papules, pustules and mild scarring

➤ Severe – Abscesses, nodules and widespread scarring

➤ Conglobate – Burrowing abscesses with scarring

## Investigations

» Bloods – Not routinely performed. If indicated, LH, FSH, testosterone (PCOS) or 17-hydroxyprogesterone (congenital adrenal hyperplasia [CAH]).

» USS – USS of the ovaries if PCOS is suspected.

## Management

### Conservative

✓ Advise them to wash their face at least twice a day with mild soap and water, particularly when sweaty. They should avoid greasy oils, use a water-based moisturising cream and avoid over-cleaning the skin. They should avoid a diet including foods with a high glycaemic index (potatoes and rice).

✓ Advise them to avoid scratching, picking or scrubbing spots.

✓ Advise them to avoid the excessive use of cosmetics. If used, advise them to use water-based products and remove them at night.

### Medical

All treatments require three months of use before considering changing it.

» Topical

› Benzoyl peroxide – Initiate bd for 30 minutes after washing with soap and water. Side effects are skin irritation, it may bleach the hair and clothing, and they must avoid excessive sun exposure. If it causes irritation, reduce the frequency or strength and reapply.

> › Topical retinoid – Apply od or bd. The spots may worsen before they improve (isotretinoin or adapalene). Side effects are burning, erythema, skin peeling and skin dryness. Due to photosensitivity, they should apply it at night, wash it off in the morning and wear sunscreen. Contraindicated in pregnancy (teratogenic) or breastfeeding.

> › Azelaic acid – Available as a cream (Skinoren) or gel (Finacea). Consider using 20% strength, which causes less skin irritation than other topical agents. It may lighten the skin and cause photosensitivity.

> › Topical antibiotics – It is advised to use these with benzoyl peroxide (Dalacin T or Zineryt). Consider clindamycin 1%. Try to limit the usage to 12 weeks.

> › Combinations – Benzoyl peroxide with antimicrobials (Duac or Quinoderm), benzoyl peroxide with a topical retinoid (Epiduo), or a topical retinoid with antimicrobials (Isotrexin or Aknemycin Plus).

✓ Oral

> › Antibiotics – Combine a topical treatment (except antimicrobials) with an oral antibiotic.

> › Tetracycline – Use doxycycline 100mg od or oxytetracycline 500mg bd before food for three months. Use Lymecycline 408mg od as second-line treatment. Side effects are nausea and vomiting, diarrhoea, photosensitivity (doxycycline), oesophagitis and thrush. Contraindicated in pregnancy and when breastfeeding.

> › Erythromycin – Use 500mg bd, but do not offer this routinely due to high resistance. Consider if tetracycline is contraindicated. This is the first-line treatment in pregnancy and in those under 12 years. Side effects are nausea and vomiting, diarrhoea, and indigestion.

> › COCP – Consider co-cyprindiol (Dianette, which has an increased risk of DVT). Stop three months after the acne has been got under control.

## Referral

Refer the patient to dermatology if any of the following apply:

→ Severe acne (nodules, cysts and scarring).

→ There has been the failure of two courses of oral antibiotic regimes.

→ Non-responsive moderate acne, for the consideration of Roaccutane (oral isotretinoin). Side effects are mucosal dryness, nose bleeds, myalgia, high cholesterol, headaches and depression; and it is teratogenic.

## Safety Netting

» Review in six to eight weeks regarding their response to treatment.

---

### References?

National Institute for Health and Care Excellence (2020). *Acne vulgaris*. https://cks.nice.org.uk/topics/acne-vulgaris/

# Rosacea

Rosacea is a chronic inflammatory facial dermatitis that is characterised by erythema and pustules. It is usually limited to the face and scalp. The cause is unknown; however, there are possible associations with face mite *Demodex folliculorum*, H. pylori and migraines.

## There are four phases of rosacea:

1. Pre-rosacea phase
   › Characterised by flushing and blushing with uncomfortable stinging.
   › Tends to be triggered by the sun, stress, weather, alcohol, spicy food and cosmetics.

2. Vascular phase
   › The patient develops facial erythema and oedema.
   › There are multiple telangiectasias present.

3. Inflammatory phase
   › Sterile papules and pustules are present.

4. Late phase
   › This only develops in some patients.
   › There is coarse tissue hyperplasia of the cheeks and nose due to tissue inflammation, collagen deposition and sebaceous gland hyperplasia.

## Risk Factors

➤ Age 30–50 years
➤ Female
➤ Fair-skinned (Northern European)

## *History*

» Focused questions
   › Ask when the rosacea started, how long it has been going on for and if it has changed over time.
   › Ask about the distribution (face and scalp).
   › Ask about aggravating factors (sunlight, stress, weather, alcohol, spicy food and cosmetics).
   › Ask about puberty, pregnancy, periods, and if they use oily products or cosmetics.

» Past history – Ask if they have had H. pylori or migraines.

» Social history – Ask if they drink alcohol, what their diet is like (spicy foods), what their occupation is (outdoor jobs) and if they have been experiencing any stress.

» Family history – Ask if there is a family history of rosacea.

## Differentials

➤ Acne

➤ Contact dermatitis

➤ SLE

➤ Seborrheic dermatitis

## Investigation

» Diagnosis is clinical, based on the findings and examination; there is no specific test.

## Management

### Conservative

✓ Advise them to avoid triggers, use sunscreen, etc. Also review the patient's medications for any triggers.

### Medical

✓ Mild to moderate papulopustular acne rosacea – Metronidazole 0.75% gel or cream bd for six to nine weeks or azelaic acid 15% bd for six to nine weeks.

✓ Moderate to severe papulopustular acne rosacea (extensive papules, pustules or plaques) – Oxytetracycline or tetracycline 500mg bd for six to twelve weeks.

✓ In cases with erythema as the main symptom, with no prominent telangiectasia, consider brimonidine 0.5% gel od.

## Referral

→ For persistent flushing and telangiectasia that does not respond to lifestyle changes – consider referring them to dermatology.

→ Refer them to a plastic surgeon for prominent rhinophyma.

---

### References

National Institute for Health and Care Excellence (2020). *Rosacea*. https://cks.nice.org.uk/topics/rosacea/

# Folliculitis

Folliculitis is an inflammatory condition involving any part of the hair follicle; most commonly, it is secondary to infection. It usually occurs in areas of terminal hair growth (i.e. beard, head, neck, groin, legs and buttocks). There are many different causes of folliculitis (fungal, drug induced and viral), but the most common is infection due to *Staphylococcus aureus*. Depending on the causative agent, different populations of inflammatory cells infiltrate the walls and/or lumens of the hair follicles. Causative agents can infiltrate superficially into the infundibulum portion of the hair follicle, or deeper beneath the infundibulum, causing furuncles and carbuncles. Recurrent and chronic folliculitis can ultimately lead to the destruction of the hair follicle (hair loss), keloids, abscess formation and scarring.

## Risk Factors

➤ Male sex

➤ Adolescence

➤ Acne/dermatitis present

➤ Trauma, including shaving and extraction

➤ Participation in contact sports, such as wrestling

➤ Poor personal hygiene

➤ Treatment with corticosteroids or immunosuppressive drugs, such as DMARDs

➤ Immunocompromised states (including DM and HIV)

➤ Malnutrition

### History

» Patients typically present with painful and erythematous plaques in areas where the skin has suffered from trauma or densely populated hair regions.

» Patients may complain about itching and most commonly that it is unsightly, especially if they present with symptoms on their face.

» Focused questions

  › Ask when the problem started, how long it has been going on for and if it has changed over time.

  › Ask about the site (beard, head, neck, groin, legs or buttocks).

  › Ask if there has been any trauma to the area (shaving or extraction).

  › Ask if there is any itching.

» Associated history – Ask if they have any acne or dermatitis.

» Past history – Ask if they have had any conditions that compromise their immune system (DM or HIV).

» Drug history – Ask if they have taken any corticosteroids or immunosuppressive drugs (DMARDs).

» Social history – Ask what their diet is like (malnutrition), ask about their personal hygiene routines, and ask if they participate in any contact sports (e.g. wrestling).

## Examination

» The diagnosis is commonly made from clinical observation and history.

» Examine all areas affected for erythematous papules, pustules or cysts around the ostia of the hair follicles, with or without a hair shaft present. These can be painful, and large areas may be affected (e.g. the beard or scalp).

» Look for scarring around the affected areas, which indicate an ongoing or previous infection.

## Differentials

➤ Pseudofolliculitis barbae

➤ Acne vulgaris

➤ Acne rosacea

## Investigations

» There are a few tests that can be done if folliculitis persists or if a cause other than bacteria is suspected.

› Gram stain – Performed following recurrent episodes of folliculitis to confirm aetiology.

› KOH preparation – Indicated when the clinical history suggests a fungal aetiology.

› Tissue culture – This is to identify the causative agent.

## Management

*Conservative*

✓ Benzoyl peroxide (topical) – Advise them to apply this to the affected areas bd until it has cleared.

✓ Advise them to use antibacterial soaps or topical antiseptics, such as chlorhexidine.

✓ Advise them to wear loose clothing.

✓ Advise them to practice their shaving technique, avoid shaving in the affected area, to shave less frequently, and apply moisturising lotion after shaving.

*Medical*

✓    First-line treatment – Flucloxacillin 500mg orally for seven days; if the patient is penicillin allergic, prescribe clarithromycin for adults and children >12 years 500mg (in a severe infection) for seven days. Recurrent folliculitis may need prolonged treatment for up to six weeks.

## References

National Institute for Health and Care Excellence (2017). *Boils, carbuncles, and staphylococcal carriage.* https://cks.nice.org.uk/topics/boils-carbuncles-staphylococcal-carriage/

# Fungal infection

Fungal infections are a common presentation in primary care. They are usually caused by dermatophytes, which may lead to tinea corporis (body), tinea cruris (groin / jock itch), tinea capitis (scalp), tinea pedis (athlete's foot), tinea barbae (beard), and tinea unguium (nails). It can be spread through a number of different routes, including via human to human contact, animal to human contact and – less commonly – from the soil.

## Risk Factors

- DM
- HIV
- Obesity
- Humid environments
- Skin folds
- Pregnancy
- Post antibiotics (broad spectrum)

## *History*

- » Focused questions
  - › Ask when the problem started, how long it has been going on for and if it has changed over time.
  - › Ask about the distribution (scalp, feet, web spaces, nails, groin and axillae).
  - › Ask if the skin is dry or itchy, and if there is any bleeding.
  - › Ask about instances of contact (if they have gone swimming recently, have recently used public or shared showers after sports, or visited a farm recently). Ask if anyone in their family or close contacts is also affected.

- » Associated history – Ask about nail changes (discolouration or brittleness), scalp issues (dandruff or hair loss), recurrent infection, HIV (persistent sore throats with white discolouration at the back of the throat), and DM (thirst, weight loss and polyuria).

- » Past history – Ask if they have had DM, HIV or hyperhidrosis.

- » Drug history – Ask if they have taken broad-spectrum antibiotics or steroids.

- » Social history – Ask what their occupation is, if they have been in contact with any animals or done any gardening, if they have had any recent life stresses, and if they have played any sports or been swimming (wearing any occlusive footwear).

- » Travel history – Ask if they have been abroad in any humid climates.

- » Family history – Ask if there is anyone else in the family with a similar rash.

## Differential Diagnosis

| | |
|---|---|
| Eczema | Dry, inflamed skin and a history of atopy. |
| Psoriasis | Mainly on the elbows, knees or scalp areas, and worsened by stress or sunlight. |
| Tinea corporis | Raised plaques on the skin with scaling or erythema of the outer border. Ring-shaped, with a central clearing. |
| Tinea capitis | Scaly area with erythema and possible alopecia. |
| Tinea pedis | Affects the webs between the toes (usually the third and fourth toes). Scaly crusting and white rash. |
| Tinea cruris | Affects the upper thigh and, occasionally, the scrotum. Red, scaly and itchy. |
| Unguium | Affects toenails more than finger nails. Brittle nails with a yellow discolouration and the thickening of the distal edge. |

## RED FLAGS

HIV, recurrent fungal infections or is spreading rapidly.

## Examination

» Skin

› Distribution – Inspect the rash area. Look at the trunk, axillae, scalp, groin, nails and feet. Check under skin folds (neck and submammary). Check the interdigital web spaces.

› Skin changes – Look for scaling or erythema plaques, or a raised annular rash with a central clearing.

» Nails – Inspect the nails for discolouration (yellow), hyperkeratosis or brittleness.

» Scalp – Inspect the scalp for dandruff, scaly plaques and alopecia. Look for a kerion.

» LNs – Consider examining the regional LNs if the rash appears to be infected.

» Groin – Inspect the groin (folds) and inner thigh, as well as the perianal area, buttocks and above the waistline.

## Investigations

» MC&S – Swab if there are signs of a secondary bacterial infection. Perform skin scrapings, nail clippings or pluck hair.

  › Skin scraping – Use a blunt scalpel blade and scrape skin from the edge of the skin lesion. Put it into folded paper.

» Bloods – HbA1c, FBC, HIV test (for recurrent infections), and LFTs if considering oral therapy.

## Management

### Conservative

✓ General advice – Advise them to keep the skin clean and dry, and to avoid scratching the area. They should wear loose garments (cotton clothes) and avoid humid conditions. They should avoid sharing towels, and wash their clothes and bed sheets frequently. They should maintain good hygiene by washing their skin daily.

✓ Athlete's foot – Advise them to wear non-occlusive footwear (open sandals). They should wash and dry their feet daily, including between the toes. They should change their socks daily and alternate between shoes. They should wear cotton socks and leather footwear. They should wear plastic sandals in changing rooms or showers. They should use talcum powder to help dry their feet. Treat athlete's foot early to prevent it spreading.

✓ Tinea cruris – Advise them to change their underwear regularly. They should wash, and keep the groin area clean and dry. They should wear loose-fitting, cotton undergarments.

✓ Tinea capitis – Advise them to dispose of or disinfect (with bleach) contaminated objects (pillows, scissors, combs and hats).

✓ Nail infection – Advise them to cut their nails short and file them down. They should use a separate pair of scissors to shorten the infected nail only. They should wear shoes with a wide toe box. They should replace old shoes (fungal reservoir). Advise them to avoid injuries to their toes.

✓ School – Children with fungal infections can attend school, but should use precautions to prevent it spreading to other children.

### Medical

✓ Topical – Use this for fungal skin infections. Consider imidazole/terbinafine or a steroid adjuvant (hydrocortisone 1% cream for seven days) if the skin is inflamed.

**Generic and trade names**

  › Miconazole – Daktarin

  › Clotrimazole – Canesten

  › Ketoconazole – Nizoral cream

  › Terbinafine – Lamisil

✓ Versicolor – Consider ketoconazole shampoo or selenium sulphide shampoo. Dilute with small amount of water to reduce irritation. Apply to the skin and leave for 10 minutes before washing off.

✓ Oral antifungal – Use in recurrent, persistent or severe fungal or scalp infections (terbinafine, fluconazole, itraconazole or griseofulvin).

  › Tinea cruris – Consider a single dose of oral antifungal (fluconazole 200mg).

  › Tinea capitis – Use oral rather than topical; e.g. oral griseofulvin (contraindicated in pregnancy as it is teratogenic) or terbinafine 250mg od (off label) for four weeks. This can be treated with ketoconazole shampoo, co-prescribed with an oral agent.

✓ Nail infections – Consider amorolfine nail lacquer (Loceryl) twice weekly if it affects one or two nails only. Use for up to three to six months for fingernails and six to twelve months for toenails. Oral antifungals should be used for resistant infections or if more than two nails are affected. Offer terbinafine for six weeks for fingernails and for three months for toenails.

## Referral

Refer the patient to dermatology if any of the following apply:

→ The condition is not improving despite treatment.

→ It is a widespread, recurrent or severe infection.

→ If the patient is immunocompromised.

→ If the patient is drug-resistant.

### References

National Institute for Health and Care Excellence (2018). *Fungal skin infection – body and groin.* https://cks.nice.org.uk/topics/fungal-skin-infection-body-groin/

National Institute for Health and Care Excellence (2018). *Fungal nail infection.* https://cks.nice.org.uk/topics/fungal-nail-infection/

National Institute for Health and Care Excellence (2018). *Fungal skin infection – foot.* https://cks.nice.org.uk/topics/fungal-skin-infection-foot/

National Institute for Health and Care Excellence (2018). *Fungal skin infection – scalp.* https://cks.nice.org.uk/topics/fungal-skin-infection-scalp/

# Scabies

Scabies is a skin disorder that is caused by the human parasite called *Sarcoptes scabiei*. The scabies mite is highly contagious, and it is usually spread by close skin-to-skin contact, and less often by sharing clothes or bedding. Predominant symptoms include a highly intense itch affecting the body, which is a reaction to the saliva and faecal material excreted by the mite. While the head and face are classically spared in adults, this may not be the case in children or in immunocompromised patients. Often, symptoms may start four to six weeks post infestation, and despite treatment, reinfestation is quite common.

## *History*

» Focused questions

› Ask when the rash started and how long it has been going on for.

› Ask about the distribution (feet, fingers, web spaces, wrists, elbows, axilla, umbilicus, areolae and breasts), and if there are any lumps or tracks in the skin.

› Ask about the itching, how intense it is, and if it is worse at night or after a bath.

› Ask if their face has been spared.

» Past history – Ask if they have previously had scabies or any other medical problems (HIV).

» Drug history – Ask if they have already tried any treatments.

» Social history – Ask if they have recently moved into a new home, if they have stayed in a hostel or hotel, and if they have any pets. For an adult, ask what their occupation is. For a child, ask if there have been any recent outbreaks at school.

» Family history – Ask if there is anyone else in the family with similar symptoms.

## Differentials

➤ Eczema

➤ Contact dermatitis

## Examination

» Inspect the interdigital web spaces of the hands, wrists and feet.

» Check the fingers for any burrows or S-shaped tracks.

» Inspect the torso for rashes, vesicles, erythematous papules, pustules or evidence of a secondary infection.

» Look behind the ears, and in the neck and scalp areas.

## Investigations

» Extraction – Isolate and extract the mite from a burrow using a sharp-tipped needle.

» Ink test – Use a special ink to reveal burrows.

» STI – Consider an STI screen if it has been transmitted by sexual contact.

» Bloods – HIV test and FBC if they are immunocompromised.

## Management

### Conservative

✓ Prevention – Advise them to avoid contact with affected individuals and those being treated.

✓ Contacts – Treat all close contacts simultaneously (household), even if they are asymptomatic.

✓ Laundry – Four days before starting treatment, machine wash at 50°C or more all clothes, bed linen and towels. Clothes that cannot be washed should be kept in a plastic bag for three days to kill the mites.

✓ Children – Advise them to avoid school until they have been treated successfully.

### Medical

✓ Permethrin – Use as the first-line treatment. Advise them to apply this to the whole body from the neck and ears downwards. They should cover all creases of the body. They should apply it carefully to toes and fingers. They must not apply it after a hot bath, but rather to cold, dry skin. It should be left on for 8–12 hours before rinsing it off. It should be re-applied to the selected area if the hands are washed. Repeat after one week (Lyclear Dermal Cream 5%).

✓ Malathion – Apply malathion 0.5% to the body in a similar manner to permethrin, but it should also be applied to the scalp, neck, face and ears, and then left on the body for 24 hours. Repeat the application in one week's time (Derbac-M liquid).

✓ Itch treatment – Offer sedating antihistamines at night if the itch is intense. Consider topical crotamiton or a mild steroid (hydrocortisone 1%) to control the itching post treatment. Pruritus may persist for up to six weeks despite successful treatment.

✓ Pregnancy – Start with permethrin 5%, but use malathion if the patient has an allergy. Mums should clear the cream from the nipple before breastfeeding, but reapply thereafter.

## Referral

→ Refer the patient to a dermatologist if the diagnosis is in doubt or it persists despite two treatments.

→ Refer them to Public Health England if an outbreak us confirmed at a school or institution (nursing home).

## References

National Institute for Health and Care Excellence (2017). *Scabies.* https://cks.nice.org.uk/topics/scabies/

# Head Lice

Head lice, otherwise known as *Pediculus humanus capitis*, refers to an infestation of parasitic insects on the human head. Although anyone can catch head lice, they usually affect preschool or primary school children. 'Head lice' refers to the adult parasites, 'nymphs' are the baby lice hatched, while 'nits' refers to the empty eggs. Head lice appear as small, greyish-brown insects, which are often described as being the size of a sesame seed. They spread via close head-to-head contact, and they do not jump like fleas or fly, contrary to popular belief. They are not caught as a result of poor hygiene or dirty hair. They are more likely to affect boys than girls, and especially those with long hair and more siblings.

## History

» Focused questions

> Ask when they started to suspect they have head lice, and how long the symptoms have been going on for.

> Scalp – Ask if the head itches a lot, if it is thicker in a particular area (occipital / post auricular) and how intense the itch is.

> Ask if there is any rash anywhere (nape area).

> Nits/lice – Ask if any white eggs (nits) or greyish-brown insects (lice) have been noticed in the hair.

» Past history – Ask if they have previously had head lice.

» Drug history – Ask if they have tried any medications for the condition.

» Social history – For an adult, ask what their current occupation is; for a child, ask if there have been any outbreaks at school.

» Family history – Ask if they have any siblings, and if anyone at home also has head lice.

## Differentials

➤ Eczema

➤ Psoriasis

➤ Tinea capitis

## Examination

» Scalp – Inspect for any evidence of nits (white specks at the hair roots), faecal matter (black specks) or live moving lice. Witnessing a moving louse is required for a diagnosis (not nits). Inspect the nape area for a rash.

## Investigations

» Combing – Wet or dry combing is used to visualise the lice and confirm the diagnosis. Nits are not proof of an active infection, as they can remain for several weeks after death. It is nearly impossible to tell live and dead eggs apart.

Detection combing

› Spend five minutes combing the hair, detangling and straightening it using a normal comb.

› Use a specialised comb (Bug Buster or Hedrin detection comb) to fine comb the hair.

› Comb from the scalp downwards to the ends of their hair.

› Repeat each area three times before moving to an adjacent area.

› Look for lice caught within the comb as it is passed through the hair.

› If a louse is visualised, catch it between the comb and your thumb.

› Continue combing for lice through the remainder of the hair.

## Management

*Conservative*

✓ Prevention – Advise the patient to plait the hair to prevent the head lice from attaching to it, and to comb the hair regularly. They should avoid sharing pillows or brushes/combs. It is recommended that the school should have whole 'bug busting' days. Check the hair regularly, and check if any eggs or insects are noted. Children do not need to be excluded from school. Bed linen and clothing do not need treatment.

✓ Treatment – Use specialised combs (Bug Buster or Hedrin). The comb can be shared within the family. They should comb the hair methodically to remove the lice. This may take 20–30 minutes. Perform at least four sessions (at three-day intervals) over a two-week period. Continue this until no head lice are seen for three consecutive periods to confirm eradication.

✓ Contact tracing – Consider tracing any contacts over the past month.

*Medical*

✓ Principles – Advise them to ensure that all affected members of the household are treated. All treatments need to be repeated more than once, and none is 100% guarantee of success. They must not go swimming until after the first application. Check the hair for live lice two and three days after treatment. If none are detected, check again nine days after, and if they are clear, then the treatment has been successful.

✓ Dimethicone (Hedrin) – This is available as a lotion or spray. Advise them to apply it and rub it into the scalp. Then leave it overnight for eight hours and wash it out using normal shampoo in the morning.

✓ Malathion (Derbac-M liquid) – Advise them to apply malathion 0.5% to the scalp and dry hair, extending to the neck area and behind the ears. Allow it to dry naturally. Leave it for 12 hours before rinsing it out. Repeat the application in one week's time.

✓ Permethrin (Lyclear creme rinse 1%) – This is not licensed for head lice despite being widely used for this. It is used as a final rinse after using normal shampoo. The hair should be dried with a towel prior to applying the cream rinse to the scalp and hair. Leave for 10 minutes before rinsing. Repeat after seven days. Advise them to avoid using this in pregnancy.

✓ Pregnancy – Recommend wet combing or dimethicone lotion. Malathion is not contraindicated.

✓ Unsuccessful treatment – If the treatment does not work, the other household members should be assessed for head lice. Consider resistance to insecticide and try alternatives. The itching may persist for two to three weeks despite successful treatment. Nits alone on the hair do not represent a failure of treatment.

## References

National Institute for Health and Care Excellence (2016). *Head lice.* https://cks.nice.org.uk/topics/head-lice/

# Alopecia

Alopecia refers to hair loss. Although most people complain of hair loss affecting their scalp, it may occur anywhere on the body. It usually starts suddenly and may present with patchy hair loss initially. It is often a distressing symptom, as it can affect one's self-esteem. There are a number of causes, with androgenic alopecia being the most common, but alopecia areata is the most unpredictable and difficult to treat.

## History

» Focused questions

   › Ask when it started and how long it has been going on for.

   › Ask about the distribution and which areas of the skin are affected (scalp, beard, eyebrows or male/female pattern baldness).

   › Ask if the onset was sudden or gradual over a period of time, and if the hair loss is patchy or affects the whole area.

   › Ask if there has been any scarring of the skin.

» Associated history – Ask if they have any stress or worries, and if they have had a change in diet or are on a specific diet.

» Past history – Ask if they have previously had hair loss, any medical illnesses (thyroid, pernicious anaemia, Down's syndrome or SLE), recent chemotherapy or given birth recently.

» Drug history – Ask if they have tried any medication.

» Social history – Ask if they smoke or drink alcohol, what their occupation is, and how the condition has affected their mood or self-esteem.

» Family history – Ask if there is any family history of hair loss (areata).

## Differential Diagnosis

| Alopecia areata | Unknown aetiology. Peak incidence at 15–30 years. Associated with DM, vitiligo, thyroid disease and pernicious anaemia. Presents with round or oval patches of hair loss, with pathognomonic exclamation mark hairs around the margins. Can affect any area, but the scalp and beard are more common. Associated with pitted nails and Beau's lines. |
|---|---|
| Androgenic alopecia (baldness) | This has a genetic component. Balding over the crown and temples occurs as the hairs become finer. Women have more diffuse hair loss over the crown and frontal scalp, with preservation of the frontal hairline. Often seen in postmenopausal women. |
| Telogen effluvium | Diffuse pattern of hair loss up to three months after a stressful event (stress, illness, fever, etc). Can affect the bi-temporal region in women. |

| Tinea capitis | Fungal infection that typically affects children with pruritus, patchy hair loss and scaling. Can present with a kerion. |
| Trichotillomania | Obsessive-compulsive disorder with patients pulling out their hair. Can affect eyelashes and eyebrows. Pattern is asymmetrical, with unusual patterns of hair loss. Complications include trichobezoar (swallowing hair). |

## Examination

»   Skin – Inspect the hair for signs of scaling, kerion, erythema and pustules. Observe the distribution of the hair and whether the hair loss is symmetrical. Look for signs of exclamation mark hairs.

## Investigations

»   Bloods – If there is male pattern baldness in a woman, consider LH/FSH, testosterone (PCOS), TFTs and ferritin.

»   Skin biopsy – Rarely performed, but a specialist may perform this if necessary.

## Management

*Treat the underlying cause*

### Conservative

✓   Diet – Advise the patient to ensure that they eat a healthy, balanced diet. Advise them to reduce the amount of fast food (animal fats) eaten and avoid excessive vitamin A.

✓   Hair – Advise them to not pull their hair tightly back into a ponytail. They should avoid excessive brushing or heat styling, as this damages the hair.

✓   Cosmetic – Advise them to consider various hair styles that can cover the alopecia. Cosmetic shops may be able to advise about hair extensions.

### Alopecia

#### Conservative

✓   Reassure the patient, and advise them to watch and wait, as most regrows within one year, but it can be difficult to predict. They should wear hats or sun cream to protect the areas from the sun. Consider referring them for counselling. They could consider wearing a wig or a prosthesis.

#### Medical

✓   Consider a trial of potent steroids (Betnovate 0.1% or Dermovate scalp lotion) for three months for non-facial areas. It may take three months to work, and hair growth is initially fine and depigmented.

✓    Refer them to dermatology, who may consider intralesional steroid injections, topical immunotherapy, PUVA light therapy, oral steroids or minoxidil.

## Androgen alopecia

### Conservative

✓    Recommend that they utilise concealment by allowing the lateral hair to grow and combing it over the area. They could also consider a wig or toupee. If there is >50% hair loss, refer them to a dermatologist.

### Medical

✓    Consider minoxidil (2%, 5%) bd (private). It must be used over a longer period of time (nine months) to see benefits. Hair loss is seen once this is stopped. Only use 5% for men.

✓    Consider finasteride 1mg od (private). Improvement may be seen after three to six months of use. Hair loss is seen within 6–12 months once they stop using it. Side effects include loss of libido and erectile dysfunction. An alternative is dutasteride 0.5mg.

## Telogen effluvium

✓    Reassure the patient as hair growth often takes six months. Treat the underlying cause of the trigger. Minoxidil can be trialled.

## Trichotillomania

✓    Refer them for behavioural therapy or CBT. Advise them to consider cropping their hair. A specialist may consider olanzapine or methylphenidate.

---

## References

Blumeyer, A., Tosti, A., Messenger, A., Reygagne, P., Marmol, V., Spuls, P.I., Trakatelli, M., Finner, A., Kiesewetter, F., Trüeb, R., Rzany, B. and Blume-Peytavi, U. (2011). Evidence-based (S3) guideline for the treatment of androgenetic alopecia in women and in men. *Journal of the German Society of Dermatology, 9*(s6), s1–s57. doi: 10.1111/j.1610-0379.2011.07802.x

Messenger, A.G., McKillop, J., Farrant, P., McDonagh, A.J. and Sladden, M. (2012). British Association of Dermatologists' guidelines for the management of alopecia areata 2012. *British Journal of Dermatology, 166*(5), 916–926. doi: 10.1111/j.1365-2133.2012.10955.x

# Melanoma

Melanoma is a form of skin cancer caused by the uncontrolled growth of melanocytes. There is a genetic link in patients who have gene CDKN2A and excessive exposure to UV radiation. Melanocytes produce a protein called melanin, which protects the skin by absorbing UV light. Moles (also known as benign melanocytic naevi) and freckles, which are commonly seen in many individuals, are non-cancerous growths of melanocytes.

There are three forms of melanoma:

1. In-situ melanoma, where the tumour is confined to the epidermis.

2. Melanoma with invasive spread to the dermis.

3. Melanoma with metastatic spread to other tissues (including LNs).

## Risk Factors

➤ Aged 45–64 years (older age group)

➤ Previous melanoma

➤ Previous basal cell carcinoma (BCC) or squamous cell carcinoma (SCC)

➤ Multiple atypical naevi

➤ Family history (first-degree relative) of melanoma

➤ Fair skin (skin type 1 or 2)

➤ Immunosuppression

### History

» Focused questions

› Ask if they have a mole, brown birthmark or flat nevus that has changed, and ask if that change is in colour, shape, ulceration, texture or size.

› Ask about the colour (tan, dark brown, black, red or sometimes even light grey).

» Past history – Ask if they have had previous melanoma, basal carcinoma or SCC.

» Family history – Ask if there is a family history of melanoma.

## Examination

» Examine the suspected melanoma using the following:

› Glasgow seven-point checklist.

› Major features – Change in size, irregular shape and irregular colour.

› Minor features – Diameter >7mm, inflammation, oozing or change in sensation.

› ABCDE of melanoma:

- **A**symmetry

- **B**order irregularity

- **C**olour variation

- **D**iameter >6mm

- **E**volving (enlarging or changing)

## Differentials

➤ Cutaneous SCC

➤ BCC

## Investigation

» For a clinical suspicion, use the aforementioned criteria.

» Diagnostic excision with 2–3mm clinical margin (not done in primary care if there is a suspicion of cancer). Epithelioid cells with fine granules in cytoplasm.

» Staging test – USS or MRI after biopsy confirmation can determine the thickness and spread with possible distant metastases.

## Management

✓ Refer the patient under 2WW to dermatology if there are three points found on the seven-point checklist, although one prominent point can still warrant an urgent referral.

✓ A routine referral can be done for a congenital pigmented naevi that is >=20cm, a family history of three or more cases of melanoma, or if the patient has >100 normal moles or atypical moles present.

✓ Following the confirmation of the diagnosis, a wide local excision is carried out. The extent of the surgery depends on the severity/thickness.

✓ If the local LN is swollen (usually non-tender and hard), it should be removed.

✓ Chemotherapy/biological therapy such as interferon therapy can be considered.

✓ Radiation is recommended for widespread disease.

*References*

National Institute for Health and Care Excellence (2017). *Melanoma and pigmented lesions*. https://cks.nice.org.uk/topics/melanoma-pigmented-lesions/

# Lipomas and Epidermoid Cysts

Lipomas are slow-growing, benign adipose tumours often found in the subcutaneous tissues. They can be found in the intermuscular septa, the abdominal organs, the oral cavity and the thorax. Lipomas may be seen in all age groups, but are usually first seen in those between 40 and 60 years of age. They can be quite large, measuring from 0.5–10cm, and form a smooth, skin-coloured lump. Solitary lipomas are common in women, and multiple lipomas – which are more common in men – are referred to as lipomatosis.

## There are many variants of lipomas, including the following:

➤ Familial multiple lipomatosis

➤ Gardner's syndrome – Multiple cysts, which are often seen in teenagers

➤ Madelung's disease – Benign, symmetric lipomatosis

➤ Post-traumatic lipomas – These appear following blunt trauma

➤ Dercum's disease – The presence of a painful, irregular lipoma

Epidermal cysts are intradermal or subcutaneous benign tumours that can occur anywhere on the body. The most common sites include the face, scalp, neck, back and scrotum. They may present with a painless skin lump, which may contain a discharge of a foul-smelling, cheese-like material. Epidermal and pilar cysts appear firm, round and mobile.

## Differential Diagnosis

| Lipoma and epidermal cysts | Lipoma and epidermal cysts are often misdiagnosed as each other. |
|---|---|
| Neurofibroma | These tend to be hard and are usually multiple. |
| Abscess | These tend to be hot and red. |

## Investigation

» USS – USS all suspected lipomas and epidermal cysts to check for concerning features and to confirm the diagnosis.

## Management

*Conservative*

✓ If the cyst or lipoma is uncomplicated, then, usually, no treatment is advised. The cyst can disappear spontaneously without leaving a trace, and the lipoma's growth will plateau.

*Medical*

✓ If the cyst is red and hot, it is probably infected, and an antibiotic effective against staphylococci (such as flucloxacillin) is used, providing the patient has no allergy to it.

*Surgical*

✓ Lipomas and epidermoid cysts can be removed via minor surgery, but this will leave a scar.

---

## References

MacKenzie Ross, A. (2018). *What is the difference between cysts and lipomas? How lumps under the skin are treated. Top Doctors.* https://www.topdoctors.co.uk/medical-articles/what-is-the-difference-between-cysts-and-lipomas-how-lumps-under-the-skin-are-treated

Harding, M. (2016). *Lipoma.* https://patient.info/doctor/lipoma-pro

Lam, M. (2020). *Epidermoid cyst.* https://dermnetnz.org/topics/epidermoid-cyst/#:~:text=An%20epidermoid%20cyst%20is%20a,Epidermal%20cyst

# Squamous cell carcinoma

SCCs are a non-melanoma skin cancer. There are multifactorial causes, though the most common cause is UV(B) radiation. SCCs tend to occur on exposed areas, such as the hands, face, arms and lips. SCCs that present on areas such as the penis, vulva and the perianal area tend to be caused by the presence of an HPV infection.

## Risk Factors

- Immunosuppression or organ transplantation
- Fair skin or blue eyes
- Sunburn
- Genetic conditions such as albinism
- Tanning beds
- HPV
- Smoking
- Aged >55 years (but also young females)

## History

- The clinical appearance of an SCC is very variable, but is initially a small nodule that enlarges with a red/dark-pink base, and it can present as a scaly plaque with a red/dark-pink base.

- Focused questions
  - Ask when it first appeared, how long they have had it for and if it has changed over time.
  - Ask if it has a scaly/crusted centre (this may develop into an ulcer).
  - Ask if the area is sore and itchy.

- Associated history – Ask if they have been sunburned.

- Past history – Ask if they are immunosuppressed, have had an organ transplant, have a genetic condition (albinism) or have had HPV.

- Social history – Ask if they smoke or have used tanning beds.

## Differentials

- Actinic keratoses
- Non-healing ulcers
- Keratoacanthomas
- BCC

## Investigation

» Within primary care – Investigate any non-healing lesion on sun-exposed surfaces.

» Biopsy - This is essential and is done in secondary care. The whole lesion is excised under LA.

## Management

### Primary care

✓ If SCC is suspected, refer them to dermatology under the 2WW pathway.

✓ Treatment should not be initiated in primary care unless there has been specialist input/investigation.

✓ Prevention – Advise them to stay indoors or in shade away from the midday sun. They should wear clothing that does not expose any areas and should apply high protection sunscreen (>SPF50).

### Secondary care

✓ In most cases, an excisional biopsy is commonly done under LA. This is a full-thickness removal with margins.

✓ If the lesion is large, is in a cosmetically sensitive area or is close to a vital structure, then an incisional or punch biopsy is required.

✓ Curettage and cautery / electrodesiccation may be used on very small lesions (<1cm) or with patients with multiple lesions.

✓ Diagnosis is only confirmed following histology.

✓ Large lesions may require skin grafting.

✓ Cryotherapy is also an option for very small lesions, but histology will not be available with this method.

✓ Topical treatments with creams, such as imiquimod 5%, fluorouracil or diclofenac may be considered for actinic keratoses and SCCs confirmed with a biopsy.

✓ There is also radiotherapy for patients who are not suitable for surgery.

---

### References

National Institute for Health and Care Excellence (2020). *Skin cancers – recognition and referral* https://cks.nice.org.uk/topics/skin-cancers-recognition-referral/

# Basal cell carcinoma

BCCs are common, locally invasive keratinocyte cancers and are also known as a non-melanoma cancer of the skin. The causes could be multifactorial, due to gene malfunction, chronic scarring and sun exposure. Malfunctions within the Hedgehog pathway can lead to the development of BCC due to the non-regulation of cell proliferation.

*The most common BCCs include the following:*

- Nodule BCC – The most common facial BCC
- Superficial BCC – The most common type in younger adults
- Morphemic BCC – Also known as sclerosing BCC

## Risk Factors

- Old age
- Males
- Previous BCC
- Sun damage (e.g. sunburn)
- Fair skin, blue eyes and blond/red hair
- Genetic conditions such as Gorlin syndrome

## History

» Focused questions
  › Ask if the a nodule/plaque has been present for a long time.
  › Ask if it has changed in size, appearance or texture (it may or may not have).
  › Ask if they have concerns about the cosmetic appearance of the nodule.
  › Ask if there is any ulceration of the site (which can be painful).

» Associated history – Ask if they have suffered any sun damage.

» Past history – Ask if they have had a previous BCC or have a genetic condition (Gorlin syndrome).

## Examination

Examine the nodule/plaque and determine if any of the following apply:

» Nodule BCC
  › Shiny/pearlescent appearance with a smooth surface.

> › The edges appear rolled, and it often has a central depression or ulceration.

> › Blood vessels may cross the surface.

> › Jelly-like contents.

> › Most commonly found on the face.

» Superficial BCC

> › Present on the upper trunk and shoulders.

> › Slightly scaly and appears to be an irregular plaque.

> › Has a thin, translucent, rolled border.

> › May contain multiple micro erosions.

» Morphoeic BCC

> › Usually found in mid-facial sites.

> › A waxy, scar-like plaque with an indistinct border.

> › May resemble a scar.

## Differentials

➤ Basosquamous carcinoma

➤ Scar following an injury

➤ Wart

## Investigation

» The diagnosis / suspected diagnosis is usually based on clinical findings.

» Dermoscopy – This should only be done if you are appropriately trained (specialised training is needed).

» Perform a diagnostic biopsy following excision.

## Management

*Primary care*

✓ Routinely refer the patient to dermatology.

✓ If there are any of the following high-risk features, they can be referred under the 2WW pathway:

> › The site is on the nose/paranasal folds.

> › They have a previously treated lesion.

> › The size is >2cm.

› The patient is immunosuppressed.

› The patient has a genetic disorder associated with BCC, such as Gorlin syndrome.

*Secondary care*

✓ Excision – This should include a 2–5mm margin of normal skin around the border.

✓ Cryotherapy – This is better for a superficial BCC on covered areas of the trunk and limbs, as it leaves a permanent white mark.

✓ Imiquimod cream – This is best for a superficial BCC <2cm. This should be applied three to five times per week for around 16 weeks.

✓ Fluorouracil 5% cream – This is best for a superficial BCC. It should be applied for 6–12 weeks.

✓ Radiotherapy – Adjunctive treatments if the margins are not applicable or in young patients where surgery is not suitable.

---

## References

National Institute for Health and Care Excellence (2015). *Suspected cancer recognition and referral.* https://www.nice.org.uk/guidance/ng12

# Urticaria

Urticaria can be acute (resolves within 48 hours) or chronic (persists for more than six weeks). Acute urticaria is associated with viral infections, food/medication allergies and insect bites. Any medication can cause urticaria, but drugs it is commonly associated with include carbamazepine, ACEis, NSAIDs, penicillins, thiazide diuretics and allopurinol. Chronic urticaria can be associated with an unknown cause (idiopathic) or is inducible urticaria (contact with cold, exercise, emotion or sunlight). The underlying mechanism of urticaria involves the activation of mast cells and the subsequent release of histamine. Triggers for mast cell activation can be identified in acute urticaria, but they are difficult to identify in chronic urticaria. Histamine causes vascular permeability and symptoms such as itching and swelling.

## *History*

» The patient may present with swelling and redness of the face, lips and tongue, usually on the back of a known trigger.

» Focused questions

› Ask when it first appeared and how long the symptoms last for.

› Ask about any possible triggers (foods, medications or insect bites).

» Associated history – Ask if they have a history of allergies (if so, what they are), if they have had any SOB (anaphylaxis), if they have a raised skin rash or if they have any associated diarrhoea (food allergy).

» Past history – Ask if they have had a recent viral infection.

» Drug history – Ask if they have taken carbamazepine, ACEis, NSAIDs, penicillins, thiazide diuretics, allopurinol or any other medications.

## Examination

» Vitals – BP, HR, respiratory rate and oxygen saturation.

» ENT – Examine the mouth for any visible obstruction or possible triggers. Lymphadenopathy might be present if it has been triggered by an infection. Listen for stridor.

» Respiratory – Auscultate for a wheeze and reduced air entry.

» Gastro – Palpate the tummy for abdominal pain; a food allergy may also be accompanied with abdominal pain and diarrhoea.

» Dermatology – Examine the skin for rashes and swelling.

## Differentials

➤ Urticarial vasculitis (caused by blood vessel inflammation rather than urticarial)

➤ Eczema

➤ Dermatitis herpetiformis

## Investigations

» The diagnosis is usually clinical. Further investigations are only indicated in recurrent cases or when the patient is hemodynamically stable (after hospital admission).

» Bloods – FBC (may see raised eosinophil / monocytes / white cells), ESR, CRP, IgE for specific allergens, and thyroid antibodies if autoimmune urticaria is suspected.

» Physical provocation tests (e.g. applying ice cubes or warm water to the skin to elicit urticaria) and patch testing for contact urticaria.

## Management

### Conservative

✓ Identify possible triggers and advise the patient to remove them.

### Medical

✓ For acute symptoms

› Follow the ABCDE approach. This is the approach used to assess critically ill patients (look at their airway, breathing, circulation, assess disability and expose the patient's body).

› Non-sedating antihistamines are commonly used (e.g. loratadine or cetirizine 10mg once daily for three to six months) when symptoms are controlled. Loratadine or cetirizine is also preferable in breastfeeding women. During pregnancy, chlorphenamine is preferred (4mg every four to six hours, with a maximum dose of 24mg daily).

› Prednisolone 40mg for seven days can be used in severe cases.

## Referral

Refer them to secondary care (dermatologist or immunologist) in the following scenarios:

→ If symptoms are not well controlled.

→ If an antihistamine is needed to control the symptoms continuously for more than six weeks.

→ If there are signs of angio-oedema or anaphylactic shock.

→ If it is painful or vasculitis urticaria is suspected.

---

## References

National Institute for Health and Care Excellence (2018). *Urticaria.* https://cks.nice.org.uk/topics/urticaria/

# Paronychia

Paronychia is the inflammation of the skin around the nail. There is a disruption between the nail fold and the nail plate, which allows the introduction of organisms. The infection is most commonly caused by *Staphylococcus aureus*.

## Risk Factors

➤ Ingrown nail

➤ Micro/macroscopic injury to nail

➤ Occupational risk

➤ Finger sucking / nail biting

## *History*

» The patient will present with a painful, swollen nail bed.

» There may be discharge.

» Focused questions

› Ask if there has been any recent damage to the nail or loss of skin surrounding the nail.

## Examination

» Vitals – Temperature (to ensure it is stable).

» Inspection – Inspect the area to determine if there is a damaged nail or nail-plate irregularity. There may be disruption between the nail bed and plate.

## Differentials

➤ Bite/sting

➤ Cellulitis

➤ Reactive arthritis

## Investigation

» Usually not needed, but a swab for a gram stain and culture can be considered.

## Management

### Conservative

✓     Advise them to take regular analgesia.

✓     Advise them to soak the nail in salt water.

✓     Advise them to apply a warm compress with vinegar / aluminium acetate.

### Medical

✓     Fusidic acid – Apply tds/qds for seven days.

✓     Flucloxacillin 500mg qds for seven days (for persistent paronychia or possible cellulitis).

✓     Clarithromycin 250–500mg bd for 7–14 days (if they are penicillin allergic).

### Surgical

✓     Incision and drainage when there is a collection of pus or an abscess.

✓     An extensive infection may require the complete removal of the entire nail bed with paronychial elevation.

---

### References

National Institute for Health and Care Excellence (2017). *Paronychia – acute.* https://cks.nice.org.uk/topics/paronychia-acute/

# Cellulitis

The skin is made up of the following layers: the epidermis, dermis and hypodermis. Cellulitis is the infection and/or inflammation of the dermis and subcutaneous tissues. It usually occurs due to skin breakage, but it can sometimes occur spontaneously. Cellulitis is usually associated with a bacterial infection (usually *Streptococcus spp*, but *Clostridium perfringens* is linked with cellulitis post surgery). It can occur anywhere in the body, but commonly appears in the lower extremities.

## Risk Factors

➤ Surgery

➤ IV drug use

➤ Venous insufficiency

➤ Obesity

## *History*

» The patient may present with pain, swelling or itching in the affected area (usually unilaterally).

» Focused questions

› Ask if they have also had a fever, erythema or signs of infection (discharge or weeping).

» Past history – Ask if they have had cellulitis.

» Drug history – Ask if they have used any antibiotics for skin infections.

## Examination

» Vitals – Temperature and HR.

» Palpation – Palpate the affected limb for any warmth or tenderness (pain out of proportion with crepitus might indicate necrotising fasciitis).

» Inspection – Look for ulcers/skin breakage.

» Check the sensation and pulse if distal limbs are affected.

## Differentials

➤ DVT

➤ Lipodermatosclerosis

➤ Necrotising fasciitis

## Investigations

» The diagnosis is usually clinical.

» Bloods – FBC and CRP (to look for raised inflammatory markers), and HbA1c (DM can complicate cellulitis). You can use the laboratory risk indicator for necrotising fasciitis (LRINEC) score to differentiate cellulitis from necrotising fasciitis based on the blood results. A score of 6 is indicative of necrotising fasciitis.

» X-ray – X-ray of the affected part to rule out osteomyelitis if it is suspected.

## Management

### Conservative

✓ Advise the patient to rest and elevate the limb(s).

✓ If they are obese, advise them to lose weight.

### Medical

✓ Advise them to take analgesia (e.g. paracetamol).

✓ Antibiotics – Consider oral flucloxacillin 500mg qds in uncomplicated cases. Erythromycin 500mg qds can be used if they are penicillin allergic.

✓ Patients with complicated cellulitis may require IV antibiotics for up to 14 days.

### Surgical

✓ Patients with necrotising fasciitis will require an urgent surgical review for debridement. If the fasciitis is on the limbs, refer them to an orthopaedic surgeon, and if it is on any other body part, refer them to a urologist / general surgeon / plastic surgeon as appropriate.

## Referral

→ Refer the patient to secondary care if they have/are any of the following:
  › Systemic illness
  › Immunocompromised
  › Lymphoedema
  › Children under one year old
  › Orbital cellulitis
  › Evidence of a deep infection

### References

National Institute for Health and Care Excellence (2019). *Cellulitis – acute.* https://cks.nice.org.uk/topics/cellulitis-acute/

# Bites

In this topic we will cover insect, animal and human bites.

An insect bite is a puncture of the skin by an insect. Following a bite, the surrounding area can become inflamed, leading to the commonly seen papules. Insect saliva can also cause a hypersensitivity reaction to the affected site, which in turn can lead to erythema as well as pruritus. Bacteria can also invade the area via the puncture site, which can lead to a secondary infection. In extreme cases, an allergic reaction can lead to anaphylaxis.

An animal bite is an injury caused by the mouth and teeth of an animal. The most common animal bites in the UK are from dogs and cats. Infected animal-bite wounds are more common from cat bites than dog bites; however, the common causative species are *Pasteurella multocida, Staphylococcus, Streptococcus, Moraxella, Corynebacterium* and *Neisseria*. Over 50% of dog and cat bites involve mixed aerobic and anaerobic species.

A human bite is an injury caused by the mouth and teeth of another human. Human bites are more deliberate in nature and can occur during fights, child abuse or sexual crimes. Accidental incidents are associated with school activities, consensual sexual activity and occupational hazards, such as dental health professionals. Occlusal injuries are inflicted by actual biting, whereas clenched-fist injuries occur when a clenched fist hits a person's teeth, causing small wounds over the metacarpophalangeal joints or dorsal aspect of the hand.

## Risk Factors for Insect Bites

➤ Being outdoors – countryside

➤ Exposed skin

➤ A lack of insecticide in specific environments

## *History*

### *Insect bites*

» Focused questions

› Ask if they have been outside in the woods recently, where they may have been exposed to ticks (to asses the risk of Lyme disease).

### *Animal bites*

» Focused questions

› Ask about the circumstances surrounding the bite to determine the risk of developing rabies.

› Ask about the animal species, and whether it was domestic or feral in status.

› Ask them to describe the wound, including the precise location and dimensions, such as size and depth.

» Associated history – Ask if the patient has an up-to-date tetanus immunisation, and determine whether the wound is tetanus prone.

### Human bites

» Focused questions
  › Ask who was involved in the situation (who bit whom), whether the skin was broken or blood was involved, and ask about the nature of the bite (clenched fist or occlusal).
  › Ask them to describe the wound, including the precise location and dimensions, such as size and depth.

## Examination

### Insect bites

» Examine the bite to check if any of the following are present:
  › Urticated papules; there may be a central punctum.
  › Occasionally, blisters are present.
  › They are often symmetrical in a cluster/group pattern.
  › The skin may be erythematous.

### Animal bites

» Vitals – Temperature and HR.

» Examination – Assess the type of wound, the degree of crush injury, if there is nervous damage, and if any muscles, joints or the vascular system are involved.

» Inspection – Check for any signs of superficial infection, such as erythema and discharge.

» Neurovascular status – Check the pulses and sensation distal to the bite.

» Joints – Assess the ROM of the joints in the area.

» Foreign bodies – Check for any foreign bodies and remove them accordingly if it is safe to do so.

## Differentials

➤ Allergic reaction
➤ Hives
➤ Cellulitis

# Investigation

*Insect bites*

»	A clinical diagnosis is made for insect bites.

*Animal and human bites*

»	Bloods – FBC (elevated WCC and low Hb). Refer the patient for blood cultures if an infection is suspected.

»	Wound swab – Swabs should be taken from the wound and sent for MC&S if any signs of infection are present.

»	X-ray – Refer them to hospital if a bone injury is suspected, such as a fracture, or if there is air in the soft tissues or joints. Also refer them if there are any visible foreign bodies, dental fragments or teeth visualised.

# Management

*Insect bites*

✓	If a stinger is visible, remove it by scraping it sideways with piece of card or a fingernail.

✓	If the tick is present – as long as the patient is not known to be allergic to ticks – remove it by grasping the tick (as close as possible to the skin) with forceps, tweezers or a specialised tick remover, and pull gently. Do not twist. Do not use any form of lubricant to dislodge the tick. Clean the area and use cold compresses on it. Do not routinely offer testing for Lyme disease.

✓	If the bites are thought to be due to an infestation, advise them to contact pest control, use a flea treatment, etc.

✓	Localised bite

	›	Advise that they take simple analgesia and oral antihistamines.

	›	Hydrocortisone 1% can be used, but this is unlicensed and there is a lack of evidence to prove it is effective.

	›	Advise them that OTC preparations that contain a low dose of hydrocortisone and chromatin can aid in easing symptoms.

	›	Advise them that calamine lotion can also ease symptoms.

✓	Secondary infection

	›	Treat cellulitis as per local guidelines; in most cases, flucloxacillin 250–500mg qds.

	›	Consider referring the patient to an allergy specialist if they have had a large local reaction to an insect bite; that is, if there is a large area of erythema, oedema and pruritus >10cm in diameter.

	›	Refer the patient to the emergency department for admission if there is systemic hypersensitivity or a toxic reaction is suspected. Treat them for shock, angioedema and anaphylaxis while they are awaiting transfer.

*Animal bites*

✓ Prescribe prophylactic oral antibiotics for any of the following:

› Animal bites to the face, feet, hands or genitalia.

› All cat bites.

› Puncture or crush wounds.

› Any wound involving surgical debridement.

› Any bite on a limb with impaired circulation.

› Wounds that have undergone primary closure.

› A patient who is at risk of serious wound infection (immunocompromised).

› A patient with a prosthetic valve or joint.

› A patient with a delayed presentation (>8 hours but <24–48 hours).

✓ If the wound is infected:

› Take a wound swab to send for culture before cleaning the wound.

› Treat them empirically with oral antibiotics.

› Admit anyone who is systemically unwell.

✓ For dog and cat bites, offer prophylaxis such as co-amoxiclav for seven days. For adults who are allergic to penicillin, prescribe doxycycline plus metronidazole for seven days.

*Human bites*

✓ Even if there is no sign of infection, offer prophylactic antibiotics for all bite wounds in <72 hours.

✓ If the wound is infected:

› Take a wound swab to send for culture before cleaning the wound.

› Treat them empirically with oral antibiotics.

› Admit anyone who has a severe infection or who is systemically unwell.

✓ For both prophylaxis and the treatment of an infected human bite, prescribe co-amoxiclav for seven days. For people who are allergic to penicillin, prescribe clarithromycin plus metronidazole for seven days.

Give follow-up advice if the person has not been referred to hospital:

✓ If the bite wound is not infected, advise them to check for signs of infection, and if these develop, they should attend urgently for review.

✓ If the wound is infected, review at 24 and 48 hours to ensure the infection is responding to treatment.

✓ Advise them to attend urgently for review if the infection worsens or if they feel increasingly unwell.

## References

National Institute for Health and Care Excellence (2020). *Insect bites and stings*. https://cks.nice.org.uk/topics/insect-bites-stings/

National Institute for Health and Care Excellence (2018). *Bites – human and animal*. https://cks.nice.org.uk/topics/bites-human-animal/

# Lichen Planus

Lichen planus is an idiopathic inflammatory condition that affects the skin, hair, nails and mucous membranes. It is usually self-limiting. Lichen planus is defined as pruritic in nature, causing chronic inflammatory dermatosis due to keratinocyte apoptosis.

## Risk Factors

➤ Hep C

➤ Vaccinations such as hep B and influenza

➤ Psychosocial stressors

➤ Oral allergens, such as flavouring agents, plastics and metals

## *History*

» Patients will usually present with spontaneous intensely pruritic lesions.

» Focused questions

› Ask about the location of the lesions (usually on the ankles, trunk, flexor aspect of the wrists, and extremities).

› If the patient does not have lesions, ask if they have painful erosions or ulcerations (oral or genital lichen planus).

## Examination

Examine the patient and determine if any of the following apply:

» Cutaneous lichen planus

› Violaceous polygonal papules and plaques.

› An overlying lacy, white network, also known as Wickham's striae, is an identifiable feature.

› Bullae may also be seen and likely form on previous lichen planus lesions.

» Oral lichen planus

› White reticulation of the buccal mucosa.

› Painful desquamative gingivitis and tongue erosions.

» Genital lichen planus

› Introital erosions edged by a lacy border.

› Scarring and violaceous polygonal papules.

› Plaques may also be seen in the vulval area.

»     Ungual lichen planus (nails)

>     Lateral thinning of the nail plate.

>     Longitudinal ridging and scarring.

»     Lichen planopilaris (scalp)

>     Follicular keratotic plugs with perifollicular inflammation seen.

>     In a progressive disease, scarring alopecia may be seen.

## Differentials

➤     Lichenoid keratosis

➤     Lichen sclerosus

➤     Psoriasis

➤     Lichen simplex chronicus

## Investigations

»     Clinical characteristics are sufficient for the diagnosis of cutaneous lichen planus.

»     Consider a biopsy for a histopathological investigation to establish a diagnosis.

»     Histopathology will show a band-like lymphocytic infiltrate at the dermo-epidermal junction, necrotic keratinocytes, hyperkeratosis and hypergranulosis.

## Management

*Medical*

✓     Treatment for lichen planus depends upon the form of the disease, and is usually in the form of topical corticosteroids and various adjunct treatments for symptomatic relief. Corticosteroids should be tapered down to avoid adverse reactions.

✓     For cutaneous lichen planus, the first-line therapy is a topical corticosteroid, such as clobetasol 0.05% bd (maximum 50g/week) or betamethasone dipropionate 0.05% bd (maximum 45g/week). Oral antihistamines, such as chlorphenamine 4mg oral every four to six hours, can be used for relief of pruritus.

✓     For oral or gential lichen planus, topical corticosteroids can be used, such as triamcinolone 0.1% bd to tds, or clobetasol 0.05% bd. Oral corticosteroids, such as prednisolone 30–60mg oral od for four to six weeks, can be considered in more severe cases. Benzydamine mouthwash or topical lidocaine can be considered for symptomatic relief.

✓     For ungual lichen planus (nail), the first-line therapy is again a topical corticosteroid, such as clobetasol 0.5% applied to the nail fold bd (maximum 50g/day) or betamethasone dipropionate 0.05% applied to the nail fold bd (maximum 45g/day). Oral corticosteroids, such as prednisolone 30–60mg oral od for four to six weeks, can be considered in more severe cases.

✓     For lichen planopilaris (scalp), a topical or oral corticosteroid is the first-line treatment, such as clobetasol 0.5% bd (maximum 50g/day) or betamethasone dipropionate 0.05% bd (maximum 45g/day).

✓     Intralesional treatment can include the use of triamcinolone acetonide 10–20mg as a single dose PRN. Oral corticosteroids, such as prednisolone 30–60mg oral od for four to six weeks, can also be considered in more severe cases.

### References

National Institute for Health and Care Excellence (2017). *Scenario: management of pruritus vulvae*. https://cks.nice.org.uk/topics/pruritus-vulvae/management/management/#dermatological-conditions

Clark, C. (2010). *Lichen planus and its management*. https://www.pharmaceutical-journal.com/files/rps-pjonline/pdf/pj20100612_cpd.pdf

# 13

# Haematology

## Lymphoma

Lymphomas are cancers of the lymphatic system. They mainly affect the lymphocytes in the body, resulting in the hyperproliferation of lymphoid tissues. Lymphomas are broadly classified into Hodgkin's and non-Hodgkin's (which is more common than Hodgkin's). Hodgkin's lymphoma is characterised histologically by the presence of multinucleated giant cells (Reed-Sternberg cells). Non-Hodgkin's lymphomas are a group of lymphoproliferative malignancies with differing patterns of behaviour and responses to treatment.

### Risk Factors

➤ EBV, human T-cell lymphotropic virus (HTLV) and hep C

➤ Gender – More common in males than females

➤ Ethnicity – More common in those who are Caucasian than those who are black or Asian

➤ Immunosuppressio

➤ HIV / Kaposi's sarcoma

➤ Family history of lymphoma

➤ Smoking

### *History*

» Focused questions

   › Ask if they have any lumps or masses anywhere, usually on the neck, armpit or groin (enlarged LNs, which may be painless).

   › Ask if they have any SOB.

   › Ask if they have itchy skin.

   › Ask if they have any night sweats, fever, weight loss or persistent fatigue.

   › Ask if they have any abdominal masses.

» Associated history – Ask if they have EBV, HTLV, hep C, HIV, Kaposi's sarcoma or are immunosuppressed.

» Family history – Ask if they have a family history of lymphoma.

» Social history – Ask if they smoke.

## Examination

» Inspection – Inspect for lymphadenopathy (especially in the lower neck or supraclavicular) and inspect the abdomen for organomegaly (liver/spleen).

» Palpation – Palpate the abdomen to check for an abdominal mass.

## Differentials

➤ Leukaemia

➤ Infectious mononucleosis

➤ Lymphadenopathy that is secondary to an infectious origin (TB)

## Investigation

» Bloods – FBC (anaemia, thrombocytopenia and neutropenia), serology (HIV and EBV), LFTs (hepatitis), ESR and lactate dehydrogenase.

» CXR – Mediastinal masses are frequent and are sometimes discovered on a routine CXR.

» Specialist – LN biopsy; CT scans of the chest, neck, abdomen and pelvis, which are required for staging; and positron emission tomography (PET).

## Management

*Specialist*

✓ Refer to oncology urgently (2WW) if lymphoma is suspected.

✓ Treatment is initiated by a specialist MDT team (chemotherapy, radiotherapy or bone marrow transplant).

✓ The patient should be made aware that they are at an increased lifetime risk of secondary neoplasms, CVD, pulmonary disease and infertility.

✓ Follow-up – The patient usually has follow-up in the form of intermittent outpatient clinical reviews for two to five years following first-line therapy.

*Conservative*

✓ Regular lifestyle advice should be offered to reduce the risk of secondary neoplasms and cardiovascular complications, including advice on smoking cessation and the management of cardiovascular risks such as HTN, DM and raised cholesterol.

## References

Tidy, C. (2015). *Non-Hodgkin's lymphoma*. https://patient.info/doctor/non-hodgkins-lymphoma-pro

Tidy, C. (2019). *Hodgkin's lymphoma*. https://patient.info/doctor/hodgkins-lymphoma-pro

# Folate Deficiency

Folate (vitamin B9) is an essential vitamin for cell processes that include DNA and ribonucleic acid (RNA) synthesis, and metabolising amino acids for cell division. Folate deficiency can be characterised by large, megaloblastic red blood cells, which are formed by inadequate supplies of folate in the body. This normally occurs when the absorption or dietary intake is inadequate, or when the body gets rid of more than normal. There are other reasons why folate may be deficient, which can be due to malabsorption, some drugs (nitrofurantoin, sulfasalazine and methotrexate) and alcohol intake.

In normal, healthy adults, the body's store of folate comprises 10–15mg. The daily requirement is 0.1–0.2mg. The absorption of folate is rapid and takes place in the jejunum. The major sources of folate are vegetables, nuts, liver and yeast. Cooking food can reduce the folate content, and although Western diets contain 0.5–0.7mg, this may be reduced by cooking.

## Risk Factors

➤ Poor diet

➤ Pregnancy

➤ Malabsorption – Coeliac disease and Crohn's disease

➤ Drugs – Valproate, barbiturates and phenytoin

➤ Alcohol – In addition to a poor diet, this can precipitate a deficiency

## History

» Focused questions

 › Ask if they have had any fatigue.

 › Ask if they have had any chest symptoms such as SOB, angina and palpitations.

 › Ask if they have had any neurological symptoms (decreased sensation, paraesthesia, ataxia, visual disturbances and loss of proprioception).

 › Ask if they have noticed any mouth ulcers.

 › Ask if they have had any GI symptoms such as diarrhoea.

 › Screen them for depression and confusion.

» Associated history – Ask if they are pregnant, or if they have Coeliac disease or Crohn's disease.

» Drug history – Ask if they take methotrexate, sulfasalazine or nitrofurantoin.

» Social history – Ask what their diet is like and if they drink alcohol.

## Examination

- » Vitals – HR (bounding pulse).
- » Inspection – Inspect for any signs of anaemia, such as pallor, and check the mouth for any mouth ulcers or glossitis.
- » Cardiac exam – Check for a systolic flow murmur.

## Investigations

- » Bloods – FBC (shows macrocytosis), MCV (>110FL), low serum folate level, red cell folate level, LFT (to exclude alcoholism), serum B12 level and TFTs (hypothyroidism).

## Differentials

- ➤ Vitamin B12 deficiency
- ➤ Acute leukaemia
- ➤ Excessive alcohol intake
- ➤ Vitamin C deficiency
- ➤ Congenital intrinsic factor deficiency (lack of intrinsic factor)

## Management

*Conservative*
- ✓ Provide dietary advice – Advise them that good sources of folate are broccoli, asparagus, Brussels sprouts, brown rice, chickpeas and peas.

*Medical*
- ✓ Folic acid 5mg/d PO, ideally for four months.
- ✓ Folic acid may need to be taken longer term (sometimes for life) if the underlying cause of the deficiency is persistent.
- ✓ If the vitamin B12 deficiency accompanies a folate deficiency, the vitamin B12 deficiency must be treated first, as there is a risk of it causing spinal cord degeneration.

*Prevention*
- ✓ Folic acid 400mcgs for pregnant women (5mg daily until term) if they have had a neural tube defect (NTD) or a family history of NTD, coeliac disease, DM or the thalassaemia trait.
- ✓ For those on methotrexate – 5mg folic acid weekly.

### References

National Institute for Health and Care Excellence (2018). *Anaemia – B12 and folate deficiency.* https://cks.nice.org.uk/topics/anaemia-b12-folate-deficiency/

# Vitamin B12 Deficiency

This is a deficiency in vitamin B12, which is also known as cobalamin. It is defined as having a serum vitamin B12 of <200picograms/ml. The majority of our vitamin B12 supply is derived from foods such as meat and dairy, and hence the most common cause is due to a vegetarian or vegan diet.

When vitamin B12 is ingested, it is bound to a molecule released from the parietal cells, called the intrinsic factor. The B12 intrinsic factor molecule then binds to transcobalamin in the small intestine, which can then be utilised by cells. Pernicious anaemia (an autoimmune disorder that results in a reduced production of the intrinsic factor) is the most common cause of severe vitamin B12 deficiency in the UK.

*Other causes of a vitamin B12 deficiency are rare, but include the following:*

➤ Drugs – Colchicine, metformin, nitrous oxide, long-term PPI and H2-receptor antagonists

➤ Gastric causes – A total or partial gastrectomy, a congenital intrinsic factor deficiency or abnormality, and Zollinger-Ellison syndrome

➤ Inherited causes – An intrinsic factor receptor deficiency or Imerslund-Gräsbeck syndrome

➤ Intestinal causes – Malabsorption, ileal resection and Crohn's disease

## Risk Factors

➤ Elderly

➤ Vegan or vegetarian

➤ Past history of gastric or intestinal surgery

➤ Crohn's disease or coeliac disease

## *History*

» Focused questions

› Ask if there are any symptoms of anaemia, such as pallor, fatigue and hair loss.

› Ask if they have any chest symptoms, such as SOB and chest pain.

› Ask if have any GI symptoms, such as diarrhoea or constipation.

› Screen for cognitive impairment, including any issues with memory or irritability.

› Ask if they have any neurological symptoms, such as paraesthesia, numbness or delayed reflexes.

› Ask if they have lost any weight.

» Past history

 › Ask if they have had a total or partial gastrectomy.

 › Ask if they have had congenital intrinsic factor deficiency or abnormality, Imerslund-Gräsbeck syndrome, ileal resection or Crohn's disease.

» Drug history – Ask if they have taken colchicine, metformin, nitrous oxide, long-term PPI or an H2-receptor antagonist.

» Pernicious anaemia is indicated by megaloblastic anaemia, GI symptoms and neurological symptoms.

## Examination

» The patient may appear normal on examination.

» The patient may appear pale.

» Neurological – Check for delayed reflexes.

» Inspection – Inspect for oral glossitis, mouth ulcers or petechiae.

## Differentials

➤ Folic acid deficiency

➤ Alcoholic liver disease

➤ Hypothyroidism

➤ Diabetic neuropathy

➤ Depression

## Investigations

» Bloods – FBC (elevated MCV and low haematocrit), serum vitamin B12 (<200picograms/ml), and reticulocyte count (used to differentiate from haemolytic anaemia).

» Peripheral blood smear to check for macrocytes and hyper-segmented polymorphonuclear cells (this may be normal).

» If a vitamin B12 deficiency is found, serum anti-intrinsic-factor antibodies should be checked.

## Management

Management depends on the symptoms present:

✓ No neurological symptoms

 › Initially, 1mg hydroxocobalamin three times a week for two weeks.

> › Maintenance dose based on the cause: if it is not diet related, consider giving 1mg IM every three months for life; and if it is diet related, consider 50–150mcg of oral cyanocobalamin daily between meals or a 1mg hydroxocobalamin injection twice a year.

> › If the cause is dietary, treatment can stop when the bloods have been corrected.

✓ Neurological symptoms

> › Seek advice from haematology – Management will be guided by them in most cases.

> › Consider hydroxocobalamin 1mg IM on alternate days until no more improvement can be seen, and then IM every two months for life (do not give oral cobalamin).

✓ Monitoring

> › Perform a FBC and reticulocyte count within seven to ten days of starting treatment (a rise will indicate it is working). If there is no improvement, do a serum folate test (if it has not already been done).

> › At eight weeks, test for iron and folate. The MCV should have normalised.

## Referral

→ If the patient is not responding to treatment, refer them to haematology.

→ If malabsorption or IBD is suspected, refer them to gastroenterology.

*References*

National Institute for Health and Care Excellence (2018). *Anaemia – B12 and folate deficiency*. https://cks.nice.org.uk/topics/anaemia-b12-folate-deficiency/

# 14

# Infectious Diseases

## Human Immunodeficiency Virus

HIV is a complex disease that affects the immune system, and if untreated, it can lead to acquired immunodeficiency disease (AIDS). It is caused by a retrovirus: either HIV-1 or HIV-2. It infects and replicates within CD4+ cells and macrophages. The virus is transmitted via infected bodily fluids.

### Routes of Transmission

➤ Unprotected sex – There is a higher risk for male to male sex, and a reduced risk for circumcised men

➤ Parenteral transmission – Through needle sharing/injuries and blood transfusion

➤ Vertical transmission – Through breastfeeding and childbirth

*The WHO classifies individuals with a confirmed HIV infection according to clinical features and diagnostic findings:*

» Primary HIV infection – Acute retroviral syndrome or asymptomatic.

» Clinical stage 1 – Persistent generalised lymphadenopathy (PGL) or asymptomatic.

» Clinical stage 2 – Symptoms such as unexplained moderate weight loss (<10%) and recurrent fungal/viral/bacterial infections.

» Clinical stage 3 – Symptoms such as unexplained severe weight loss (>10%), unexplained chronic diarrhoea (for more than one month), unexplained persistent fever ($\geq 36.7°C$, intermittent or constant for more than one month), persistent/severe fungal/viral/bacterial infections, and unexplained anaemia (<8g/dl) and/or neutropenia (<500 cells/µl) and/or chronic thrombocytopenia (<50,000/µl) for more than one month.

» Clinical stage 4 – AIDS-defining conditions (e.g. Kaposi's sarcoma).

## Risk Factors

➤ Aged 20–30 years

➤ Needle-stick injuries/use

➤ Unprotected sexual activity

➤ Breastfeeding or childbirth

## *History*

» Focused questions

› Ask if they have a fever, fatigue, myalgia and arthralgia, headaches, nausea, or diarrhoea.

› Ask if they have lost any weight, and if so, how much.

› Ask if they have had a sore throat or any ulcerations anywhere.

› Ask if they have had chronic sub-febrile temperatures.

› Ask if they have had chronic diarrhoea (for more than one month).

› Ask if they have any skin conditions, such as molluscum, warts or shingles.

» Associated history – Ask if they have had a needle-stick injury or a blood transfusion.

» Social history – Ask if they have shared any needles or had unprotected sexual activity.

## Examination

*The examination may be unremarkable.*

» Inspection

› Check for a generalised rash. It is often maculopapular, but the appearance is variable. It usually develops on the second or third day after infection, and it lasts for five to eight days. Also look for molluscum, warts and shingles.

› Oral hairy leukoplakia – Check for lesions located on the lateral borders of the tongue.

› Examine for generalised non-tender lymphadenopathy.

› Check for localised opportunistic infections, including oral candidiasis and vaginal infections.

## Differentials

➤ Infectious mononucleosis

➤ Cytomegalovirus infection

➤ Influenza infection or common cold

➤ Hepatitis

➤ COVID-19

## Investigation

» Bloods – HIV serology, such as enzyme-linked immunoassay (ELISA) and rapid serology tests; and CD4+ count to assess the overall immune function and stage progression.

» Screen for coexisting STIs.

## Management

*Conservative*

✓ If the patient is well in themselves:

  › Refer them to either GUM or an HIV specialist, ideally to be seen within 48 hours.

  › Advise them on the support services available and risk prevention.

  › Arrange a follow-up in one to two days to ensure the referral has been received and offer further support.

✓ If there has been exposure to HIV via sexual activity or a needle-stick infection:

  › Refer them urgently to an HIV specialist, GUM or the emergency department to be considered for prophylactic drug treatment.

*Medical*

✓ The treatment is initiated by specialists within secondary care, and it is commonly a combination of three or more drugs (to reduce drug resistance):

  › Nucleoside/nucleotide reverse transcriptase inhibitors (NRTIs) (e.g. zidovudine, lamivudine, emtricitabine and abacavir) – These inhibit the reverse transcription of RNA to DNA.

  › Non-nucleoside reverse transcriptase inhibitors (NNRTIs) (e.g. nevirapine and efavirenz) – These are non-competitive inhibitors of viral reverse transcriptase.

  › Protease inhibitors (PIs) (e.g. indinavir, ritonavir, nelfinavir and lopinavir) – These inhibit the viral protease, which leads to the inability to cleave viral polypeptides, and therefore the generation of viral proteins is impaired. As a result, only immature (non-infectious) virions are produced.

  › Integrase inhibitors (IIs) (e.g. raltegravir and dolutegravir) – These inhibit the viral integrase.

*References*

National Institute for Health and Care Excellence (2020). *HIV infection and AIDS.* https://cks.nice.org.uk/topics/hiv-infection-aids/

# Syphilis

Syphilis is caused by a gram-negative, spiral-shaped bacterium called Treponema Pallidum. It is transmitted via sexual contact, such as vaginal or anal contact. It can also be transmitted by oral contact with an infective lesion. In addition, it can also be spread in utero from mother to foetus, through contact with infectious lesions and broken skin, or spread via blood transfusions.

## The Four Stages of Syphilis

1. Primary – A small, painless sore called a chancre, which develops several weeks after the bacteria has entered the body. It usually heals on its own.

2. Secondary – Typically, a non-itchy rash develops either in one area or across the whole body. This is also followed by symptoms such as fever, fatigue, muscle aches, pains and lymphadenopathy.

3. Latent – This phase is usually reached if treatment has not occurred in phases 1 and 2, or if the patient has skipped this phase and gone straight to the tertiary phase. Patients are asymptomatic during this stage and may remain in this stage for several years before progressing to the tertiary phase.

4. Tertiary – It is not infectious at this stage; however, the infection has started to affect major organs. It is also known as neurosyphilis. The patient starts to experience dementia symptoms, paraesthesia, an abnormal gait, vision defects, impotence, bladder weakness, muscular weakness, and a loss of coordination and reflexes. Meningitis is also a common occurrence in this phase.

## Risk Factors

➤ HIV positive

➤ Unprotected sexual intercourse

➤ Multiple partners

➤ Contact with an infected person

➤ Sharing of needles for IV drug use

## Examination

» Vitals – Temperature (fever).

» General appearance – Look for a rash and examine for lymphadenopathy.

» Neurology

› Examine the lower limbs to look for an irregular gait or muscle weakness.

› Consider a CN exam, assess visual acuity and check for hearing loss.

» Mini mental-state examination (MMSE) – Check for issues with memory.

## Differentials

➤ Pityriasis rosacea

➤ Ulcers

➤ HIV

➤ HZV

## Investigation

» Bloods – FBC, U&E, LFT, CRP, HIV serology, syphilis serology, hep B and C screens, and gonorrhoea and chlamydia screens.

» Swabs – Virology swab from an active lesion.

» Specialist – CT if organs are affected, and a lumbar puncture (tertiary phase).

## Management

✓ Refer the patient to a GUM clinic / tertiary centre.

*Medical*

✓ First-line treatment – Benzathine penicillin 2.4 mega units IM single dose (this is not licenced in the UK).

✓ Second-line treatment – Azithromycin 2g PO stat or doxycycline 100mg bd for 14 days.

✓ For a patient with neurosyphilis – Procaine penicillin 1.8–2.4 units od IM for 14 days with oral probenecid 500mg qds.

✓ Testing should be repeated after two years.

---

*References*

National Institute for Health and Care Excellence (2019). *Syphilis.* https://cks.nice.org.uk/topics/syphilis/

# Measles

Measles is a highly infectious disease that is caused by a spherical, heat-labile RNA virus. This means that its natural hosts are commonly humans. The virus is transmitted via droplets, and it infects the epithelial cells of the nose and conjunctiva. The virus then goes on to extend to the regional LNs. The prodromal phase of symptoms is between two to four days, with respiratory tract involvement on days seven to eleven. After about two weeks of infection, a maculopapular rash develops. The maculopapular rash usually starts on the head and spreads to the extremities over several days. The key feature is the resolution of the fever soon after the rash appears. This infection is preventable by immunisation, and there is no specific treatment available.

## Risk Factors

> Exposure to the measles virus

> Not receiving the measles vaccine

> Failure to respond to the measles vaccine

## *History*

» Focused questions

> It is important to ask whether a patient has travelled to a measles-endemic area and if there is a risk of exposure to individuals infected with the virus.

> Ask if they have had a fever, cough, coryzal symptoms or conjunctivitis.

> Ask if they have had any rashes (maculopapular rash).

» Past history – Ask about their vaccination history (this is vital). If a patient has not been immunised against measles, the risk of infection is much greater.

## Examination

» Vitals – Temperature and pulse.

» Conduct a complete ENT and respiratory examination.

» Examine the mouth to look for Koplik's spots. They are red in colour with a blue-white central dot and are found on the erythematous buccal mucosa.

» Inspect the eyes for any signs of conjunctivitis.

» Examine the patient for a maculopapular rash, which starts on the head and spreads to the trunk and extremities over several days.

## Differentials

➤ Rubella

➤ Parvovirus B19 infection

➤ Roseola

➤ Mononucleosis

## Investigations

The diagnosis is mainly clinical; however, the following investigations are all sensitive to the measles virus:

» Bloods – Measles-specific IgM and IgG serology (false positive IgM is possible in rubella and parvovirus B19 infections).

» Throat / nasopharyngeal swab MC&S – Measles is RNA positive (the best yield is on days one to three of the rash).

» Urine sample MC&S – Measles is RNA positive.

## Management

### Conservative

✓ Symptom control with paracetamol or ibuprofen is the treatment of choice, alongside vitamin A replacement in all serious cases of infection. Doses are as follows:

› Paracetamol – Children should take 10–15mg/kg every four to six hours PRN (maximum 75mg/kg/day), and adults should take 500–1,000mg every four to six hours PRN (max 4g/day).

› Ibuprofen – Children should take 5–10mg/kg every six to eight hours PRN (maximum 40mg/kg/day), and adults should take 400–800mg every six to eight hours PRN (maximum 2,400mg/day).

› Vitamin A – Those under six months should be given 50,000 units od for two days, then repeat this in four weeks if required; those six to eleven months should be given 100,000 units od for two days, then repeat this in four weeks if required, and those >12 months should be given 200,000 units od for two days, then repeat this in four weeks if required.

### Medical

✓ The MMR vaccine is a combined vaccine against measles, mumps and rubella. The full course requires two doses, and it should be offered to all children as a part of the routine vaccination schedule. The vaccination regime is as follows:

› The first injection is given within a month of their first birthday.

› The second injection is given before they start school at the age of approximately three years and four months old.

> › Patients over six months old who are at risk of exposure or where there is a local measles outbreak should be offered a vaccination.

## References

National Institute for Health and Care Excellence (2018). *Measles*. https://cks.nice.org.uk/topics/measles/

# Varicella Zoster Virus

The VZV infection is known to cause two different diseases. The first is varicella (chickenpox), which is a common, highly contagious disease that mainly affects children. The second condition is herpes zoster (shingles), which is a reactivation of the latent virus.

Chickenpox is infectious, from a few days before the rash develops to no more than six days after the first lesion appears. (This period is longer in immunocompromised patients.) The lesions can scar if they are scratched excessively. The condition is highly contagious, and it infects up to 90% of people who come into contact with it. Usually, recovery from chickenpox results in lifetime immunity, although recurrence as shingles can happen, albeit rarely.

Those at risk of this second virus are often the elderly and those with compromised immune systems. The transmission is respiratory and conjunctival. Replication takes place in the nasopharynx and regional LNs, followed by the infection of the spleen, liver, sensory ganglia and skin. The patient may have one to two days of fever and malaise prior to the onset, but a rash is often the first sign of the disease. The vesicular eruption of shingles is usually unilateral in distribution of a sensory nerve, and is very painful.

## *History – Chickenpox*

» Focused questions

  › Ask if they have a rash and what it is like (the rash begins as macular lesions that develop into papular or vesicular [fluid-filled] lesions).

  › Ask if there is any redness (erythema) and if the lesions are intensely itchy.

  › Ask if the vesicles dry and crust over.

  › Ask about the distribution of the vesicles (mostly on the face and trunk, and sparsely on the limbs).

## *History – Shingles*

» Focused questions

  › Ask about the distribution of the rash (most often, it follows the distribution of a dermatome in the trunk or CN5).

  › Ask if there was paraesthesia or pain two to four days prior to the eruption (this may or may not occur).

## Examination

» This is diagnosed mainly based on the history and clinical examination.

» Vitals – Temperature (fever).

» Inspection – Inspect for a vesicular rash, vesicles on the mucous membranes and a sore throat.

## Differentials

➤ Smallpox

➤ Stevens-Johnson syndrome

➤ Monkeypox

## Investigations

» The clinical findings are usually enough to make a diagnosis.

» Investigations to consider include a viral culture and PCR.

## Management

### Chickenpox

✓ Management of a child aged two months onwards:

› Aciclovir is not recommended for otherwise healthy children with chickenpox. Treat symptomatically with paracetamol (for pyrexia), emollient lotions and antihistamines (to assist with pruritus).

› If there are serious complications – such as encephalitis, pneumonia or dehydration – or these are suspected, admit them to hospital.

› Consider oral aciclovir 800mg five times a day for seven days for an immunocompetent adult or adolescent with chickenpox who presents within 24 hours of the rash onset, particularly for people with increased risk of complications.

✓ Management of an immunocompromised, pregnant or breastfeeding woman with chickenpox:

› If a patient has any respiratory symptoms, neurological symptoms (other than headaches), haemorrhagic rash or significant immunosuppression, seek urgent advice from a specialist. Only prescribe oral acyclovir on the advice of said specialist.

› Offer treatment of the symptoms.

### Shingles

✓ Admit the patient to hospital if any of the following apply:

› There are any complications – such as encephalitis, meningitis or myelitis – or these are suspected.

› The patient has presented with a rash on the ophthalmic distribution of the trigeminal nerve (Hutchinson's sign, which is a rash on the tip or side of nose).

› They have visual symptoms.

› They have an unexplained red eye.

> › The patient is a severely immunocompromised person.

> › They are systemically unwell.

✓ NICE (2020) recommends prescribing an oral antiviral within 72 hours of the rash onset for patients who meet the following criteria:

> › They are immunocompromised.

> › There is non-truncal involvement (such as shingles affecting the neck, limbs or perineum).

> › The rash or pain is moderate or severe.

> › The patient is >50 years (the antiviral is to reduce the incidence of post-herpetic neuralgia, which is most common in this age group).

✓ If a patient is pregnant or breastfeeding, seek specialist advice before prescribing any antiviral treatment.

✓ Refer the patient to dermatology, or seek specialist advice if new vesicles are forming after seven days of antiviral treatment or if healing is delayed.

---

## References

National Institute for Health and Care Excellence (2018). *Chickenpox.* https://cks.nice.org.uk/topics/chickenpox/

National Institute for Health and Care Excellence (2020). *Shingles.* https://cks.nice.org.uk/topics/shingles/

# Herpes Simplex Virus

The HSV can cause a mild, self-limiting infection of the lips, cheeks or nose, which is also known as a cold sore (herpes labialis) or gingivostomatitis (oropharyngeal mucosa). The most common causative agent is HSV-1. Most HSV-1 infections are usually asymptomatic. The transmission of the virus is via direct contact with a person actively infected with and shedding the virus, with the infective secretions entering the skin via mucous membranes. An oral HSV infection can be severe or life-threatening in immunocompromised patients.

## Risk Factors

- HIV
- Immunosuppression through medication
- High-risk sexual behaviour
- Stress
- Sun exposure
- Infection or fever
- Menstruation

## *History*

» Patients will present with a 2–14 day history of typical crops of vesicles that rupture, crust then heal (usually with no scarring).

» Focused questions

- Ask if they have been exposed to any trigger factors and ask if they have any of the red flags for oral malignancy.
- Ask if they have had a high fever or sore throat alongside painful ulcers.
- Ask if they have had such an infection beforehand, and where it was (patients presenting with a recurrence of the infection usually present with symptoms affecting the same area).
- Ask about any prodromal symptoms of tingling and burning, followed by the development of lesions at the vermillion border. These symptoms will usually last for 6–48 hours and do not typically manifest with systemic symptoms. These lesions usually crust and heal within 10 days.

## Red Flags

Persistent unexplained head and neck lumps for >3 weeks, An ulceration or unexplained swelling of the oral mucosa persisting for >3 weeks, All red or mixed red and white patches of the oral mucosa persisting for >3 weeks, persistent, particularly unilateral, discomfort in the throat for >4 weeks.

## Differentials

- ➤ Syphilis
- ➤ Contact dermatitis
- ➤ Behcet's disease
- ➤ SCC
- ➤ Lymphogranuloma venereum

## Examination

» Inspection – Inspect for painful vesicles and ulcers (the vesicles rupture and form ulcers) in the pharyngeal and oral mucosa, which are a classic symptom. Immunocompromised patients may present with severe atypical lesions anywhere in the oral cavity. Patients suffering from HSV gingivostomatitis often present with crops of painful lesions.

## Investigations

» A diagnosis of an oral HSV infection is usually made based on clinical judgement, and investigations are not usually necessary in the primary care setting; however, swabs can be taken from active lesions (lesions that have not crusted) for HSV culture.

## Management

✓ The treatment for the first presentation of an HSV-1 infection is the most important, and each patients should commence treatment within 48–72 hours of onset. Alongside providing symptomatic relief, this reduces the risk of neurological complications.

✓ First-line treatment includes offering the patient analgesia for pain and fever management, along with the prompt initiation of antiviral treatment with oral antivirals:

   › Paracetamol 500–1,000mg qds or ibuprofen 400–600mg qds. In addition, if required, apply topical lidocaine 5% ointment to the affected areas bd/tds.

   AND

   › Aciclovir 200mg five times a day for 7–10 days or valaciclovir 2,000mg bd for one day.

✓ Topical antiviral preparations, mouthwashes and lip barriers are not routinely recommended according to NICE (2016) guidelines; however, patients may benefit from such symptomatic relief and they can be advised to obtain these OTC. Topical antiviral preparations include the following:

   › Docosanol 10% topical cream PRN

> › Penciclovir 1% topical cream PRN

> › Aciclovir 5% topical cream PRN

✓ Offer supplementary self-care advice such as using sunscreen and sunblock lip balm for patients with recurrent infections triggered by sunlight, and that they should avoid trigger factors.

✓ Hospital admission should be considered if the patient is unable to swallow or is clinically dehydrated, or if the patent is immunocompromised with a severe HSV infection or a serious complication – such as a central nervous system (CNS) infection – is suspected.

## References

National Institute for Health and Care Excellence (2016). *Herpes simplex – oral.* https://cks.nice.org.uk/topics/herpes-simplex-oral/

National Institute for Health and Care Excellence (2017). *Herpes simplex – genital.* https://cks.nice.org.uk/topics/herpes-simplex-genital/

# Impetigo

Impetigo is a superficial skin infection. It can be categorised into bullous and non-bullous. It can also be divided into primary (which occurs in intact skin) and secondary (which occurs in damaged skin). The non-bullous type is usually associated with *Staphylococcus aureus* or *Streptococcus pyogenes*.

## Risk Factors

➤ Atopic eczema

➤ Poor hygiene

## *History*

» Focused questions

  › Ask if they have any blisters or itching (commonly on the face, but this can also occur on the buttocks or extremities).

  › Ask if they have a fever.

» Associated history – Ask if they have atopic eczema.

» Social history – Ask about their personal hygiene.

## Examination

» Vitals – Temperature.

» Inspection – Check the skin for blisters/rashes noting the size, shape, site and exudates. Impetigo may appear as crusted, yellow/gold vesicles/blisters.

» Palpation – Feel the local LN area for lymphadenopathy.

## Differentials

➤ Burns

➤ Contact dermatitis

➤ Scabies

## Investigations

» The diagnosis is usually clinical.

» Bloods – Not usually required. If in hospital, perform routine bloods such as FBC and CRP.

» Swab – A swab of the area can be taken in the following scenarios:

› If there is recurrent/severe impetigo.

› If it doesn't respond to treatment.

› If methicillin-resistant *Staphylococcus aureus* (MRSA) is suspected.

## Management

### Conservative

✓ Encourage good hygiene. Advise them to avoid sharing towels, to wash their hands after touching the affected area, and to keep their fingernails short and clean.

✓ Patients with impetigo should be advised to avoid going to school or work until the lesions have dried or the patient has been on antibiotics for 48 hours.

### Medical

✓ Topical fusidic acid tds for seven days is used as the first-line treatment.

✓ Mupirocin tds for up to 10 days for MRSA impetigo.

✓ Oral antibiotics (e.g. flucloxacillin 500mg qds for seven days) is used if there are extensive symptoms or it is not responding to topical antibiotics.

### References

National Institute for Health and Care Excellence (2020). *Impetigo*. https://cks.nice.org.uk/topics/impetigo/

# 15

# Mental Health

## Depression

Depression is the most common mental health disorder faced in primary care, with over one in 20 adults experiencing an episode of depression in a year. It can vary in intensity, ranging from a single mild episode to a severe, recurrent, chronic disorder. The average length of a depressive episode is just over six months, with a risk of recurrence of at least 50% after the first episode, which rises to 70% after a second episode. Patients may present predominantly with biological symptoms known as 'somatic depression'. Patients with severe depression may even harbour 'mood congruent' delusions or auditory hallucinations. In approximately 4% of cases, the depression will be severe enough to lead them to take their own life, and hence it is important to always screen for suicidal ideation.

### History

Approach the topic sensitively in a non-threatening, non-judgemental manner. It can be quite difficult to approach the subject initially, so begin by using your first few questions to put the patient at ease.

» Open questions

› *'What would you like to talk about today? Can you tell me about how you are feeling?'*

› Cues – If the patient is reluctant to talk or appears withdrawn, and is displaying little eye contact, reflect this non-verbal cue to them by saying something like *'You look upset. Is anything bothering you?'*

» Focused questions

› Depression – Ask when they first started feeling like this and how long it has been going on for.

› Core symptoms – Ask if they have a low mood, anhedonia or fatigue.

› Cognitive symptoms – Ask if they have the ability to concentrate on things (TV/newspaper), are easily distracted or have low self-esteem.

› Biological symptoms – Ask about their sleep (initial insomnia, middle insomnia or early morning waking), their appetite, if they have lost or gained weight, and how their libido is.

» Associated questions

  › Delusions – Ask if they have had any unusual or new ideas that they have struggled to convince others about, and if so, what they are.

  › Hallucinations – Ask if they have seen or heard anything when no one else was around or that others have not noticed. If they heard voices, ask if the voices were talking about them.

  › Suicidal ideation – Ask if they have made any plans for committing suicide, if they have ever acted upon these thoughts, if they have ever harmed themselves, and how they feel today.

» Past history – Ask if they have any history of psychiatric issues such as low mood, anxiety or psychosis; and if they have had any medical issues such as hypothyroid, CVA, DM or IHD.

» Family history – Ask if there is a family history of psychiatry involvement.

» Drug history – Ask if they have taken steroids, COCP, ranitidine, b-blockers, opioids or St John's wort.

» Social history – Ask about their relationships, what their support network is like, what their occupation is (if they are studying or have any financial worries), and if they smoke, drink alcohol or take recreational drugs.

## RED FLAGS

Suicidal ideation, nihilistic delusions or hallucinations (posing a risk to others and themselves), and children.

## Differential Diagnosis

| Subthreshold depression | Have a few symptoms of depression, but able to cope with every-day life. Dysthymia when symptoms go on for two years. |
|---|---|
| Seasonal affective disorder (SAD) | Symptoms of depression occur annually each year, often in winter and resolve in spring. |
| Bereavement reaction | Abnormal reaction to a bereavement (more than two months). Feelings of guilt, a preoccupation with worthlessness, and with psychomotor retardation. Can have thoughts of death. |
| Bipolar | Two contrasting emotional states (i.e. depression/mania). In the elevation phase, the patient is overactive, irritable, distracted, disinhibited, suffers from insomnia, or has flights of ideas or pressure of speech. Can also have grandiose ideas. |

| Anorexia | Affects young girls >16 years. Low BMI (<17.5). Missing meals, vomiting or using laxatives. Obsessed with body image and looking in the mirror. OE: thin, pale conjunctiva, calluses on the knuckles, pallor, low BP and bradycardia. |
|---|---|

## Diagnosing Depression

The diagnosis of depression requires one or two core symptoms, with five or more associated symptoms

➤ Core symptoms

  › Feeling down, depressed or hopeless during the past month.

  › Having little interest or pleasure in doing things during the past month.

➤ Associated symptoms – Disturbed sleep (more/less), changes to appetite and/or weight, fatigue, agitation or slowing of movements, poor concentration, feeling worthless or guilty, or having suicidal thoughts.

## Levels of Depression

➤ Subthreshold – Two to five associated symptoms with one core symptom

➤ Mild depression – More than five associated symptoms with mild impairment to function

➤ Moderate depression – The symptoms or functional impairment are between 'mild' and 'severe'

➤ Severe depression – Experiencing most symptoms with marked interference to daily function, with or without psychotic symptoms

## Examination

» Vitals – BMI.

» Questionnaire – Patient Health Questionnaire 9 (PHQ-9) (a score >11 requires intervention), Hospital Anxiety and Depression Scale (HADS), or Mood and Feelings Questionnaire (MFQ) (child).

## Investigations

» Bloods – Often not indicated. If required, FBC, ESR, HbA1c, U&Es, LFTs, TFTs and vitamin D.

## Management

*Conservative*

✓ Exercise – Advise the patient to take regular exercise and try to get out of the house, even if it is only for a walk.

✓ Diet – Advise them to cut down their alcohol intake, to eat well and regularly, and to stop any recreational drug use (e.g. cannabis).

✓ Sleep – Advise them to relax in a dark room with minimal distractions, go to sleep at the same time every night and get up at the same time every day (including at weekends), to only use the bed for sleeping (and sex), and to avoid excessive eating, smoking or drinking alcohol before sleeping.

✓ Sick certificate – Offer them a short fit note, and advise them to consider amended duties or altered hours if they are finding it difficult to carry out certain tasks or attend work in the morning.

✓ Befriending – Advise them to consider a befriending service or a rehabilitation programme if the condition has resulted in the loss of work.

✓ Self-help

  › Material – Consider offering books or leaflets to help guide patients with their symptoms. The Royal College of Psychiatry (RCPsych) recommends the *Overcoming* series.

  › Online – Advise them to consider online programmes or internet-guided treatments such as 'Beating the Blues' or 'FearFighter', which are recommended by NICE.

✓ Talking therapies

  › Counselling – Refer them to a counsellor or therapist for mild depression.

  › CBT – Consider recommending CBT for mild/moderate depression.

  › Others – Consider referring them for specific therapies such as couples therapy, bereavement counselling, interpersonal psychotherapy, computerised CBT, physical-activity programmes or group therapy, as appropriate.

*Medical*

✓ Titration – Consider prescribing medication for those with moderate to severe depression, especially in combination with psychological intervention. It may take two to four weeks before they feel any improvement. The medication must be used for six months following the remission of symptoms to reduce the relapse risk.

✓ SSRI – For the first episode, offer an SSRI (e.g. citalopram, fluoxetine or sertraline). Second-line treatment includes mirtazapine.

  › Side effects – GI symptoms, GI bleed, increased anxiety and agitation for the first two to four weeks, or serotonin syndrome if taking high doses or two agents (agitation, tremors, fever, tachycardia, restlessness and confusion).

  › Interactions – NSAIDs (add PPI), warfarin (avoid SSRI, but consider mirtazapine), aspirin and triptans.

  › Discontinuation – Gradually taper usage over four weeks (not required for fluoxetine). If stopped suddenly, the patient may experience discontinuation symptoms (restlessness, difficulty sleeping, mood change, sweating, nausea and vomiting, diarrhoea and paraesthesia).

✓ Serotonin and norepinephrine reuptake inhibitor (SNRI) – Consider venlafaxine or duloxetine if there is a poor response to SSRIs or they are in severe depression. This is a second-line treatment. Check BP after initiating.

> Side effects – Nausea, dizziness and a dry mouth.

> Contraindications – Uncontrolled HTN, and CVD.

✓ TCA – This is not to be used if there is a risk of OD, nor is it to be used as first-line treatment. Consider if they have severe depression or have failed to respond to SSRIs. TCAs (e.g. amitriptyline, clomipramine or lofepramine) are only to be prescribed by a specialist.

> Side effects – Dry mouth, drowsiness, blurred vision, constipation and urinary retention.

> Contraindications – Immediately after an MI, or arrhythmia (block).

✓ Specialist – Consider adding lithium, another antidepressant such as mirtazapine, or an antipsychotic such as olanzapine or risperidone if there is a poor response to a single agent.

✓ Electroconvulsive therapy (ECT) – Consider this only as a last resort in severe, treatment-resistant depression.

✓ Pregnancy – Consider if the benefits outweigh the risks. Fluoxetine is the only SSRI licensed in pregnancy. There is a small risk of CHD from giving this in early pregnancy, and neonatal withdrawal symptoms in the third trimester.

### Switching antidepressants

✓ SSRI to SSRI – Cross taper (i.e. reduce one and increase the other), but start the new SSRI at a low dose.

✓ SSRI to TCA – Cross taper (i.e. reduce one and increase other), except for fluoxetine.

✓ SSRI to venlafaxine – Cross taper, but start venlafaxine at 37.5mg od and increase slowly.

✓ Fluoxetine to venlafaxine – Withdraw fluoxetine, then start venlafaxine 37.5mg od and increase slowly.

✓ Fluoxetine to SSRI – Withdraw gradually, and leave a seven-day gap before starting the SSRI.

✓ Fluoxetine to TCA – Withdraw fluoxetine gradually, and leave a seven-day gap before starting TCA.

## Safety Netting

» Suicide risk – Review the patient frequently in primary care. Consider contacting the crisis resolution and home treatment team for an urgent assessment.

» Sectioning – Try to persuade them to go voluntarily, but if they are not compliant, consider compulsory admission (if there is a risk to themselves or to others).

» Safeguarding – Follow the local safeguarding pathways for child protection or vulnerable adults.

» Follow-up – Offer a series of appointments in primary care, with short gaps in more serious cases. Patients started on SSRI should be reviewed in two weeks, then two-to-four-weekly for three months. If they are <30 years old, then see them in one week (increased suicide risk).

## References

National Institute for Health and Care Excellence (2009). *Depression in adults: recognition and management.* https://www.nice.org.uk/guidance/cg90

# Insomnia

Sleep disorders affect one in three people at some time in their life. There are characterised by an inability to fall asleep for a sufficient enough time to feel refreshed in the morning. A lack of sleep may present with symptoms such as forgetfulness, daytime tiredness, irritability or anxiety. It may present as a primary disorder or, more usually, as a symptom of another mental health illness, such as mania, depression, anxiety or post-traumatic stress disorder (PTSD). It is more common in women and with increasing age.

## *History*

Approach the topic sensitively in a non-threatening, non-judgemental manner. It can be quite difficult to approach the subject initially, so begin by designing your first few questions to put the patient at ease.

» Open questions

› *'What problems have you had with your sleep? Give me an account of a typical night's sleep.'*

› Cues – If the patient is reluctant to talk or appears withdrawn, and is displaying little eye contact or spontaneity, reflect this non-verbal cue to them by saying something like, *'You look upset. Is anything bothering you?'*

› Screening – Ask patients who suffer from anxiety or depression if they experience difficulty sleeping, and if they have problems falling or staying asleep, or get up earlier than they want.

» Focused questions

› Sleep – Ask when the sleep problem started, how long it has been going on for, and if it affects them every day or just occasionally. Ask them how they would rate their quality of sleep. Ask them to talk you through how they go to sleep. Ask when they go to sleep, what time they wake up, if they wake up in the middle of the night, if they nap during the day, and how many hours of sleep they get.

› Triggers – Ask if there is anything that could be causing the poor sleep, such as their occupation (stress at work, studying or night shifts), financial worries (losing their job, their mortgage or debt), relationships (if they have any children, and if so, whether they sleep okay), environmental factors (any changes in their environment, a noisy neighbour or jetlag), and their diet (coffee, consumption of energy or fizzy drinks, and what time they have their last drink before sleeping).

» Associated questions

› Depression screen – Ask if they are feeling low or feeling disinterested in life, and what their eating habits are.

› Anxiety – Ask if they are feeling anxious, are worried a lot or have had any panic attacks.

› Psychosis – Ask if they have seen or heard things they cannot explain, or feel that someone is out to harm them.

> › Suicide – Ask if they have ever felt so low that they wanted to end it all.

» Past history – Ask if they have had similar psychiatric issues in the past, such as depression, mania, anxiety, panic attacks or childhood disorders (e.g. attention deficit hyperactivity disorder [ADHD]). Ask if they have restless legs syndrome or an overactive thyroid.

» Family history – Ask if they have a family history of any mental illnesses (anxiety or panic attacks).

» Drug history – Ask if they have taken methylphenidate, NRT or fluoxetine.

» Social history – Ask if they are suffering from any stress, and if they smoke, drink alcohol or take recreational drugs.

## RED FLAGS

Depression, alcohol, recreational drugs and obesity.

## Differentials

➤ Sleep apnoea

➤ Heart failure

➤ Panic disorder

## Examination

» Vitals – BMI, BP and pulse.

» Examination – Perform a cardiac or thyroid exam if indicated.

» Epworth sleepiness scale – Offer this sleepiness questionnaire to assess the severity of OSA.

## Investigations

» Bloods – Not routinely performed. Consider TFTs and pro-BNP.

» Diary – Suggest they keep a diary of sleep and naps over a two-week period to record their sleep-wake patterns and variability. They should record the times they go to bed and wake up, and how long it took to get to sleep. They should rate the quality of their sleep. They should also record significant events, such as consuming caffeine, alcohol and meals, and stressors.

» Sleep studies – Secondary care may refer them for a polysomnogram and the multiple sleep latency test to check for the presence of insomnia or sleep apnoea.

# Management

*Conservative*

✓ Lifestyle

› Diet – Advise them to avoid caffeine for six hours before bedtime, and consider stopping all caffeine intake. They should not eat a heavy meal before sleeping nor sleep on an empty stomach.

› Alcohol and smoking – Advise them to stop or cut down on alcohol and smoking.

› Drugs – Advise them to stop taking any recreational drugs.

› Exercise – Advise them to take regular daytime exercise (jogging, swimming or cycling), which helps reduce stress and will make them feel tired. However, they should avoid exercise for four hours prior to bedtime.

› Relaxation techniques – Recommend that they use relaxation techniques, such as deep-breathing exercises, taking a warm bath before sleeping or listening to calming music.

› Driving – Advise the patient not to drive if they feel drowsy/sleepy.

✓ Sleep hygiene

› Environment – Advise them to ensure they are lying in a dark room, and to use thick blinds or curtains, or an eye mask. They should ensure that the room is quiet with a normal ambient temperature. They should switch off any electronic devices (such as TVs, smartphones or tablets) and close any books.

› Routine – Advise them to go to sleep and wake up at fixed times every day. They should avoid napping during the day and relax prior to sleeping.

✓ Self-help – Offer leaflets on understanding sleep disorders and managing them (*Overcoming* series).

✓ Talking therapies – Suggest CBT, stimulus control, sleep-restriction therapy, biofeedback or paradoxical intention.

*Medical*

✓ Hypnotics – Consider this in cases of short-term insomnia where daytime sleepiness is severe. Offer a maximum of two weeks of medication. Consider a short-acting BDZ (temazepam or lorazepam) or non-BDZ (zopiclone or zolpidem). Do not recommend diazepam (unless it is accompanied by daytime anxiety).

› Side effects – Warn the patient about the risk of drug tolerance and dependence. They should avoid driving or operating machinery. It may also cause drowsiness or confusion.

✓ Melatonin – Consider this in those >55 years old with persistent insomnia (more than four weeks). Initiate for three weeks and continue for 13 weeks in total if they are responding.

✓ Antidepressants – Some have sedative effects, such as amitriptyline and mirtazapine. Consider this if they have concurrent depression and anxiety only.

## Referral

→   Consider referring them to a psychiatrist if their symptoms persist for more than four weeks.

---

*References*

Riemann, D., Baglioni, C., Bassetti, C., Bjorvatn, B., Dolenc Groselj, L., Ellis, J. G., Espie, C. A., Garcia-Borreguero, D., Gjerstad, M., Gonçalves, M., Hertenstein, E., Jansson-Fröjmark, M., Jennum, P. J., Leger, D., Nissen, C., Parrino, L., Paunio, T., Pevernagie, D., Verbraecken, J., Weeß, H. G., ... Spiegelhalder, K. (2017). European guideline for the diagnosis and treatment of insomnia. *Journal of Sleep Research, 26*(6), 675–700. https://doi.org/10.1111/jsr.12594 European guideline for the diagnosis and treatment of insomnia

# Psychosis

Psychotic disorders encompasses a range of mental disorders, including schizophrenia, that are characterised by difficulties in reality testing; fixed, unshakeable, unusual beliefs (i.e. delusions); unusual perceptual experiences (hallucinations in any modality); and changes in behaviour that are significantly different to their own and cultural norms. It can affect anyone at any age, but it most commonly starts in those aged 16–35 years. Psychosis can be a feature of a wide range of disorders, including bipolar disease, a brain tumour, substance abuse and encephalitis, but is most commonly due to schizophrenia.

## Definitions of Types of Psychosis

➤ Hallucinations – This is where perception cannot be distinguished from reality. It occurs in the absence of external stimuli.

› Auditory – False perceptions of sound (e.g. voices heard as a running commentary, command or thought echo).

› Visual – False visual perceptions that are similar to real perceptions projected in the external world.

› Other – Tactile or smell.

➤ Delusions – False beliefs that are unshakeable and fixed, despite evidence to the contrary.

➤ Thought disorder – Disorganised thinking made apparent by disorganised speech (e.g. derailment, poverty of speech or thought blocking).

➤ Negative symptoms – Social withdrawal, self-neglect, reduced speech or loss of motivation.

## *History*

Approach the topic sensitively in a non-threatening, non-judgemental manner. It can be quite difficult to approach the subject initially, so begin by designing your first few questions to put the patient at ease.

» Open questions

› *'Can you tell me more about how you are feeling?'*

› If the patient is reluctant to talk, or appears suspicious or fidgety, reflect this non-verbal cue to them by saying something like, *'You look preoccupied. Is there something on your mind?'*

» Focused questions

› Psychosis – Ask when they first started feeling like this, how long it has been going on for, what they think caused it and how it has affected them.

*Delusions*

» Persecutory – Ask if they think that someone or something is trying to harm them.

» Grandiosity – Ask if they believe that they have special powers that others do not possess.

» Reference – Ask if they have ever felt that the TV/radio was communicating directly to them.

» Perception – Ask if they interpret things differently compared to other people.

» Passivity – Ask if they believe that they are being controlled like a puppet by an outside force.

» Nihilistic – Ask if they believe the world is in a state of destruction, and how they view themself.

» Ekbom's – Ask if they believe they have been infested by an organism.

» Cotard's – Ask if they believe their insides are rotten.

» Fixed – Ask how certain they are about these thoughts.

*Hallucinations*

» Auditory – Ask if they hear any sounds when no one else is around. If so, ask them to tell you about the voices and how many people there are.

» Third person – Ask if the voice speaks about them (third person – a running commentary).

» Second person – Ask if the voice speaks to them directly (second person indicates depression).

» First person – Ask if they ever hear their own thoughts being repeated like an echo (*écho de la pensée*).

» Location – Ask if they hear the voices from inside (pseudo) or outside (real) their head.

» Content – Ask what they hear, what the voices say (derogatory/praiseworthy), or if the voices tell them to harm themself (present in severe depression).

» Visual/olfactory – Ask if they have seen or smelled things that others have said were not there (head injury, organic or temporal lobe epilepsy).

» Formication – Ask if they have felt something walking on their skin like a bug (alcohol or cocaine).

*Thought disorder*

» Insertion/withdrawal – Ask if they have felt that someone is putting thoughts in their head or taking them out.

» Broadcasting– Ask if they think that others can hear what they are thinking.

» Negative symptoms – Lack of motivation, asocial (not mixing with friends or family) and self-neglect (ask how often they are washing or cleaning themself).

## Risk Factors for Developing a Psychotic Disorder (NICE, 2014)

> ➤ Suspect this if the patient is distressed or has had a deterioration in social functioning, including one or more of these:
>> › A first-degree family history of schizophrenia / a psychotic disorder.
>>
>> › Altered behaviour suggestive of psychosis (e.g. suspicious and with a perceptual change).
>>
>> › A short history of low-intensity psychotic symptoms.
>>
>> › Examples of deteriorating social functioning include social withdrawal (no contact with friends), poor personal hygiene and unusual behaviour.

> ➤ Past history – Ask if they have had any previous psychiatric issues, including schizophrenia, depression or similar issues; if they have ever been admitted to a mental health ward; or if they have / have had HIV, TB, dementia or a brain tumour.

> ➤ Family history – Ask if they have a family history of schizophrenia or other mental illnesses.

> ➤ Drug history – Ask if they have taken steroids, levodopa or opioids.

> ➤ Social history – Ask about their relationships (partners and children, including who looks after them), what their support network is like (who lives at home with them, and if they have any close friends or family), what their occupation is (if they are studying or working, and if they have any financial worries), and if they smoke, drink alcohol or take recreational drugs (particularly lysergic acid diethylamide [LSD], cocaine, amphetamines or ketamine). If they do take recreational drugs, for each one, enquire about the quantity, frequency and pattern of use.

## RED FLAGS

Suicidal ideation, persecutory delusions or hallucinations (risk to others), and children.

## Differential Diagnosis

| Schizophrenia | Schneider's first rank symptoms (auditory hallucination, thought disorder, and delusions of perception and control). Negative symptoms include asocial behaviour, lack of motivation, poor concentration and lack of self-care. One-month history of symptoms. |
|---|---|
| Depression | Persistent low mood and effects – with cognitive and biological symptoms, including delusions (worthlessness) and hallucinations (derogatory auditory) – for at least two weeks. |

| Puerperal psychosis | Onset two to four days after delivery, with effects including clouding of consciousness, delusions (paranoid) and hallucinations (depressed or hypomania). Risk of infanticide. |
|---|---|
| Bipolar disorder | Contrasting emotional states (depression and mania). In the elevation phase, the patient is overactive, irritable, distracted, disinhibited, suffers from insomnia, and has flights of idea or pressure of speech. Can also have grandiose ideas. |
| PTSD | Exposure to a traumatic life event. Impairing symptoms are re-experiencing the event as flashbacks or nightmares, avoiding thoughts or places, and emotional numbness with a hypervigilant state. The symptoms must be present six months after the event. |

## Diagnosing Schizophrenia

Schneider's first rank symptoms, which are used to diagnose schizophrenia, include the following:

➤ Auditory hallucinations (third person, running commentary or *écho de la pensée*)

➤ Thought disorder (insertion, withdrawal or broadcasting)

➤ Delusions of perception

➤ Delusions of control

➤ Somatic hallucinations

Patients suffering with psychosis usually lack insight and are unable to recognise that they are unwell. When assessing the patient's symptoms, it is important to challenge their perception to test for insight. If this is not done in a non-judgemental way, they may get angry and disengage from the consultation, particularly if they think you consider that they are mentally unwell. You should practice how you would explain to a patient that they need to see a psychiatrist without causing undue angst or anxiety in the patient.

## Examination

» Vitals - BMI, weight and BP.

## Investigations

» Bloods – FBC, HbA1c, lipid profile and LFTs.

» Specialist – MRI scan to exclude organic psychosis (temporal lobe epilepsy) and a urine drug screen to exclude drug-induced psychosis (LSD or amphetamines).

# Management

*Conservative*

✓ Lifestyle

› Smoking – Offer cessation advice. Consider offering NRT (bupropion and varenicline increase the risk of neuropsychiatric symptoms, particularly in the first two to three weeks).

› Alcohol – Advise them to cut down their alcohol intake

› Exercise – Give them exercise advice. Refer them to healthy-eating or physical-exercise programmes (obesity is a side effect of the medication).

› Comorbidities – Offer interventions for abnormal glucose and cholesterol levels (there is a higher incidence of DM and CVD).

› Diet – Advise them to eat well and regularly.

› Others – Offer support for carers, and direct them to support available from Carers UK.

✓ Work – Offer supported employment programmes if they wish to return to work.

✓ Exercise programme – Patients suffering with psychosis, particularly those on antipsychotics, should be referred to a physical-activity programme.

✓ Talking therapies

› CBT – Consider CBT for all patients.

› Family intervention – This should be offered to families with members who live with them that are suffering from schizophrenia.

› Art therapies – Offer this to patients with negative symptoms.

*Medical*

✓ Antipsychotics – Do not initiate medication on first presentation unless this is done with advice from a consultant. Second-generation drugs (e.g. amisulpride, aripiprazole, clozapine [specialist], olanzapine, quetiapine, lurasidone and risperidone) are better at treating negative symptoms.

› Side effects – Weight gain (increased appetite), antimuscarinic (dry mouth, blurred vision, urinary retention and constipation), drowsiness, sexual dysfunction and DM.

› Extrapyramidal – Parkinsonism (tremor), dystonia (torticollis and oculogyric crisis), akathisia (severe restlessness) and tardive dyskinesia (rhythmic involuntary movement, such as chewing and the pouting of the jaw).

**Before initiating**

- Observation – Weight, BP, pulse, waist circumference, degree of physical activity and nutritional status.

- Investigation – HbA1c, lipid profile, LFTs, prolactin (hyperprolactinaemia), U&Es and ECG.

✓ Depot – Consider if the patient prefers this after an acute episodes or the patient attempts covertly to avoid adhering to taking the medication that is clinically essential.

## Referral

→ Early referral – Refer the patient urgently to the community team on first presentation of psychotic symptoms.

→ Re-referral – Re-refer them if they have a poor response to treatment, poor compliance, intolerable side effects, substance misuse, or pose a risk to themself and/or others.

## Safety Netting

» Suicide risk – Contact the crisis resolution and home treatment team for an urgent assessment.

» Sectioning – Try to persuade them to engage with services voluntarily; if they are not compliant, consider a referral for compulsory admission (if they pose a risk to themself or to others).

» Safeguarding – Follow the local safeguarding pathways for child protection or vulnerable adults.

» Follow-up – Offer a series of appointments in primary care, with short gaps in more serious cases.

*References*

National Institute for Health and Care Excellence (2014). *Psychosis and schizophrenia in adults: prevention and management.* https://www.nice.org.uk/guidance/cg178

Scottish Intercollegiate Guidelines Network (2013). *SIGN 131 Management of Schizophrenia.* https://www.sign.ac.uk/assets/sign131.pdf

# Eating Disorders

The term 'eating disorders' refers to the group of conditions that, as a result of a person's altered eating habits, puts their health and wellbeing at risk; this is usually out of a morbid fear that they will become obese or fat. The most common disorders are anorexia nervosa and bulimia nervosa, with bulimia being five times more common than anorexia. It is thought that well over 1.5 million people are affected by an eating disorder in the UK, with around 2% of women being affected at some point in their life. Although women are 10 times more likely to be diagnosed with an eating disorder than their male counterparts, its prevalence is beginning to increase in the male population as well.

## History

» Approach the topic sensitively in a non-threatening, non-judgemental manner. It can be quite difficult to broach the subject initially, so begin by designing your first few questions to put the patient at ease.

» Open questions

> *'Can you tell me more about the symptoms you have been experiencing? Could you tell me about what has been troubling you?'*

> Cues – If the patient appears embarrassed and is displaying little eye contact, reflect this non-verbal cue to them by saying something like *'You look upset. Is anything bothering you?'*

> Screening – In high risk patients (young women with a low BMI), ask screening questions such as *'Do you think you have an eating problem? Do you worry excessively about your weight?'*

» The SCOFF questionnaire (sick, control, one, fat, food)

This is used to screen for eating disorders. Two or more positive answers to these questions suggests a diagnosis of anorexia nervosa or bulimia.

> *'Do you make yourself sick because you feel uncomfortably full?'*

> *'Do you worry you have lost control over how much you eat?'*

> *'Have you recently lost more than one stone in a three month period?'*

> *'Do you believe yourself to be fat when others say you are too thin?'*

> *'Would you say that food dominates your life?'*

» Eating disorders

> Weight – Ask if they have had any problems with their weight. Ask about how much weight has been lost and over what time period. Ask if it was intentional.

> Diet – Ask about what they eat in typical day, if their eating pattern has changed recently, if they avoid certain foods and if they ever binge eat.

> Ask if they are eating more healthily at the present time (fruit and vegetables), and if they find themselves wanting to cook for others, but not wanting to eat themselves.

» Preventing weight gain

› Purging – Ask if they ever make themself throw up (self-induce) or use excessive laxatives.

› Medication – Ask if they use any medications to lose weight (diuretics or appetite suppressants).

› Exercise – Ask if they exercise, and if so, how much exercise they do.

» Psychological symptoms

› Fear of fatness – Ask if they worry about their weight, if they are scared of putting it on and if they enjoy losing it.

› Body image– Ask if they are happy with their body (have a desire to be thin).

› Denial– Ask if they believe that they may have a weight problem.

» Associated questions

› Depression – Ask if they have been feeling low recently, and if they feel disinterested in life or worthless inside

› Self-harm/suicide – Ask if they have ever harmed themself to feel better inside, or if they have ever felt so low that they wanted to end it all.

» Past history – Ask if they have ever had these symptoms before, or if they have any history of depression, anxiety or panic attacks. Ask if they have any medical conditions.

» Family history – Ask if there is a family history of any mental health issues, such as eating disorders, depression or substance misuse.

» Drug history – Ask if they are taking any medications, including laxatives, slimming pills and thyroxine.

» Social history – Ask if there is anything in their life that is causing much stress and anxiety; how their childhood was (abuse or neglect); if they smoke, drink alcohol or take recreational drugs; what their relationships are like; and what their support network is like (if their close friends or family have mentioned being worried about the patient's weight).

## RED FLAGS

Suicidal ideation, a BMI <14, electrolyte imbalance and bradycardia (<40bpm).

## Differential Diagnosis

| Anorexia nervosa | A BMI <17.5 or 15% below that expected for the person. The patient expresses that they avoid food that may increase their weight (fat), and may purge, use diuretics/laxatives, use appetite suppressants or do vigorous exercise. May have a body image misperception (believe they are fat). May have a reduced libido (men) or amenorrhoea (women). If it is before puberty, their growth and physical development can be affected. May also have acrocyanosis (hands/feet are red or purple), dry skin, hair loss, bradycardia, hypotension or lanugo hair (downy hair on the upper part of the body and face). |
|---|---|
| Bulimia nervosa | Patient is concerned about their body image, but has an uncontrollable desire to eat. Binge eating induces a feeling of relief followed by one of disgust, leading the patient to induce vomiting. Patient may suffer from low potassium (arrhythmias or renal impairment), eroded dental enamel, swollen parotid glands or calluses over their knuckles (from scraping against their incisors when inducing vomiting), but have a normal weight. |
| Binge-eating disorder | Characterised by a loss of control over the amount of food consumed. Patient eats more rapidly than normal until they are uncomfortably full, and they eat when not hungry. Patient eats alone (embarrassment), and feels guilty and distressed from overeating. Binging occurs more than once a week for at least three months. |

## Examination

» Vitals – Temperature, height, weight, BMI, BP and pulse (arrhythmia indicates hypokalaemia).

» Inspection – Inspect the teeth for erosion of the tooth enamel and the knuckles for calluses (Russell's sign from inducing vomiting). Check if they look pale, emaciated or have a bowed appearance, or if they have delayed puberty.

» Muscle power – Test their muscle power by asking them to sit up from lying down without using their hands (sit-up test). Ask them to stand from a squatting position without using their hands (squat test).

## Investigations

» Bloods – U&Es (hypokalaemia).

  › Others – FBCs, ferritin, LFTs, CK, bone profile, TFTs or ESR if indicated.

» ECG – The patient may have bradycardia, arrhythmias or a prolonged QT interval.

» X-ray – Only if there is concern about fractures.

» DEXA – When they are admitted as an inpatient.

## Management

*Conservative*

✓ Lifestyle measures

› Diary – Advise them to keep a food diary about what they eat and when they eat it. They should record their emotions at the time and see if there is any link.

› Eating – Advise them to only eat food at their regular mealtimes and not snack.

› Dietician – Refer them to an eating-disorder-trained dietician to discuss calories, food intake and a healthy diet.

› Weight – Advise them not to weigh themself more than once a week. They should try to avoid looking at themself in the mirror.

› Dental – If the patient is vomiting, advise them to avoid brushing their teeth after vomiting or rinsing with mouthwash, and to reduce their intake of acidic food. Refer them to a dentist for assessment of dentition.

✓ Self-help

› Material – Offer leaflets on understanding and managing eating disorders (*Overcoming* series).

› Group therapy – Suggest that they join group therapy.

✓ Talking therapies

› CBT – Consider referring them for CBT (individual or group).

› Family – For children and adolescents, consider helping the family implement a healthy diet, and also help resolve any family-based conflicts.

✓ Specialist

› Cognitive analytic therapy (CAT) – Consider referring them for CAT to help resolve unhealthy past events that are having an impact on current behaviours.

› Interpersonal psychotherapy (IPT) – Consider referring them for IPT to help them concentrate on their interactions with others and to deal with their emotional needs (reduced self-esteem or self-doubt).

*Medical*

✓ Laxatives – Advise them to stop taking or reduce the amount of laxatives they are taking.

✓ Vitamins – They may need oral multivitamins.

✓ Referral – Refer the patient to a specialist eating-disorder clinic. Consider inpatient admission if they pose a risk to themselves, have a very low BMI or have deranged electrolytes.

✓ Specialist

> Antidepressants – Consider SSRI (fluoxetine 60mg) for bulimia to reduce binging. Advise the patient that it may take two to three weeks before they feel any improvement. They can experience a worsening of anxiety in the first few weeks after medication has been started.

> Energy drinks – Fortisip/Complan may be prescribed by a dietician to aid weight gain.

> Antipsychotics – Olanzapine may be used in anorexia to reduce the anxiety and ruminations caused by the disorder. This is often initiated by a hospital.

## Safety Netting

» Suicide risk – Review the patient frequently. Consider contacting the crisis resolution and home treatment team for an urgent assessment. Give them the Samaritans' telephone number for emergencies.

» Sectioning – Try to persuade them to go voluntarily; if not, consider compulsory admission (if they pose a risk to themself or to others).

» Safeguarding – Follow the local safeguarding pathways for child protection or vulnerable adults.

» Follow-up – Offer a series of appointments in primary care, with short gaps in more serious cases.

---

### References

National Institute for Health and Care Excellence (2017). *Eating disorders: recognition and treatment.* https://www.nice.org.uk/guidance/ng69

# Suicidal Ideation

Patients suffering from mental health illnesses are at an increased risk of self-harming and attempting suicide. There were 19,000 deaths by suicide in in the period from 2011–2015 (about 4,800 per year in the UK), with many more self-harming and attempting suicide. It is important to screen for suicidal ideation in all patients who present with a low mood, anxiety, schizophrenia or self-harm, as evidence shows that almost 50% of patients who go on to die from suicide have visited their primary care physician within a month of their death, and of those who attempted suicide, over 90% have had suicidal thoughts or ideation in the past year.

## Risk Factors

➤ Gender – Men are three times than more likely to commit suicide than women

➤ Age – >30 years

➤ Depression – 70% of suicides suffered from a form depression

➤ Previous attempt – There is a 30–40 times increased risk of death in those who have attempted suicide before

➤ Alcohol abuse – Alcoholics have a lifetime risk of suicide of 3–4%

➤ Loss of rational thinking – Schizophrenics have a 10% lifetime risk of suicide

➤ Loss of support – Divorced or widowed women

➤ Organised plan – Patients who have planned their suicide, or left a note or will

➤ Unemployed – Those with a low socioeconomic status have a two to three times increased risk

➤ Chronic illness – Patients with chronic diseases (MS, epilepsy, pain, disability and cancer)

➤ Professions – Doctors, veterans, skilled and unskilled trade labourers

### *History*

Approach the topic sensitively in a non-threatening, non-judgemental manner. It can be quite difficult to broach the subject initially, so begin by designing your first few questions to put the patient at ease.

» Open questions

› Cues – If the patient appears withdrawn and is displaying little eye contact, reflect this non-verbal cue to them by saying something like *'You look upset. Is anything bothering you?'*

› Confidentially – Reassure the patient that everything they say is in confidence unless they or others are at risk.

» Focused questions

*Pre-attempt*

›   Trigger – Ask what they were thinking about before they made the attempt (bereavement or a significant life event).

›   Ask what their mood was like at the time.

›   Ask if there was any plan or if it was spontaneous.

›   Ask if they informed anyone.

›   Ask if they took any precautions (made sure no one was around).

›   Ask if they left a note or closed their bank accounts.

*Attempt*

›   Ask when it happened and where they were at the time.

›   Ask what method they used (using a weapon, taking an OD, trying to jump from a height, etc.).

›   If it was an OD, ask if they remember what medications they took and if they tried to mix different ones.

›   Ask what their intention was (if they actually wanted to end their life).

›   Ask if any alcohol or drugs were involved.

›   Ask how they were found, and if they sought help.

*Post-attempt*

›   Ask how they feel now that they are still alive, if they are happy that they are still with us, or if they are angry that they were not successful.

›   Ask what their intentions were, and what they were hoping to do when they did this (if they really wanted to die or it was more of a cry for help).

›   Ideation – Ask if they still have any thoughts or a desire not to be alive.

» Past history

›   Psychiatric – Ask if they have ever had similar issues in the past; if they have been treated for depression, anxiety or psychosis; if they have ever been admitted to a mental health ward; or if they have had any personality disorder (PD) or anorexia.

›   Self-harm – Ask if they have ever tried to commit suicide in the past or self-harmed before.

›   Ask if they have any chronic medical conditions such as CVA, DM, HIV, IHD, MS, epilepsy or chronic pain.

» Family history – Ask if there is a family history of depression or another mental illness.

» Drug history – Ask if they have taken SSRI, Champix or amitriptyline.

> » Social history – Ask about their current relationships (if they have any issues), what their support network is like (who lives with them, and if they have any close friends or family), what their occupation is (if they have any issues or financial worries), if they have suffered any abuse (physical, sexual or emotional), and if they smoke, drink alcohol or take recreational drugs.

## RED FLAGS

Ongoing suicidal ideation, meticulous planning, a violent method planned and past attempts.

## PROTECTIVE FACTORS FOR SUICIDE

There are factors that may decrease the risk of a patient attempting to commit suicide; some of these include having strong social support, having strong religious convictions, having children in the home or being pregnant, and having access to clinical interventions for mental and substance-misuse disorders.

## Examination

> » Vitals – BMI, BP and pulse.

> » Injuries – Assess and document any physical injuries.

> » Risk assessment – Determine whether the patient is a low, medium or high risk to themselves or to others.

## Investigations

Not routinely indicated in primary care.

> » Bloods – FBC, ESR, HbA1c, U&Es, LFTs, TFTs, calcium, paracetamol and salicylate levels.

> » Urine – For common recreational drugs (opiates, BDZs, barbiturates, amphetamines and methadone).

> » ECG – Look for comorbidities or cardiac arrhythmias post OD.

## Management

### Emergency

> ✓ In the case of acute injuries (for glue or stitches) or an OD, it is important to stabilise the patient and call 999 to take them to an emergency department.

*Prevention*

✓ Medication review – Offer regular medication reviews. Drugs such as aspirin, paracetamol, codeine, BDZs, sleeping tablets and amitriptyline should be rationalised.

✓ Weekly prescriptions – Consider giving weekly prescriptions for patients at a higher risk of suicide.

✓ Carer(s) – Advise them to have a carer or relative administer the medication from a locked cupboard or to observe them directly.

*Conservative*

✓ Lifestyle

  › Alcohol – Advise them to cut down their alcohol intake. Refer them to local detox programmes or alcohol advisors if indicated.

  › Drugs – Advise them to stop taking any recreational drugs (e.g. cannabis) and refer them to a drugs advisor. Consider referring them to dual diagnosis teams if they have concurrent mental illnesses.

✓ Benefits/job – Consider issuing a fit note if they are unable to work. Refer them to a benefits advisor, social services or local jobcentre if they need advice on housing and employment.

✓ Carer(s) – Refer them to social services for a care package if they are unable to cope (disability).

## Depression

✓ If the patient is depressed, then treat them via self-help, CBT or SSRIs.

## Bereavement

✓ If they have suffered a recent death, refer them to a bereavement counsellor first, instead of using SSRIs or CBT.

## Chronic disease

✓ Tighter control is required, so refer them to the appropriate secondary care specialist, rationalise their pain treatment or refer them to a pain team.

## Suicide

✓ Low risk – Consider offering telephone assessments or frequent follow-ups in primary care. Refer them to local psychotherapy services for the treatment of any anxiety or depression. Consider referring them to the local Primary Care Mental Health Team (PCMHT). Give them the telephone numbers for the Samaritans, the local 24-hour emergency crisis team and the emergency department.

✓ High risk – Refer them to the crisis resolution and home treatment team for an urgent assessment. Refer them for support from the local community mental health team (e.g. a community psychiatric nurse [CPN] or mental health key worker).

> › Sectioning – Try to persuade them to go voluntarily, but if they are not compliant, consider a compulsory admission (if they pose a risk to themselves or to others).

> › Safeguarding – Follow the local safeguarding pathways for child protection or vulnerable adults.

## Safety Netting

> » Offer a series of appointments in primary care, with short gaps in more serious cases. Give emergency details to the patient (e.g. the crisis team) in case they feel the need to self-harm again.

---

*References*

National Institute for Health and Care Excellence (2011). *Self-harm: longer-term management.* https://www.nice.org.uk/guidance/cg133/evidence/full-guideline-184901581

# Anxiety Disorder

The term 'anxiety disorders' refers to the range of mental disorders that present with symptoms of fear, anxiety, restlessness and irritability, and that may lead to physical symptoms, including palpitations, sweating and tremors. It may also present with physical ('somatic') symptoms, such as pain, tiredness or fits. There are a number of different conditions that come underneath the anxiety disorders umbrella, including social anxiety, generalised anxiety disorder (GAD), panic disorder and specific phobias. Although a specific trigger may be present, it is not necessary that one is for the diagnosis to be made.

GAD usually lasts for six months, causing social or occupational distress. Panic disorder is usually diagnosed if a patient has at least two attacks and at least a month of persistent worry around it. Social anxiety disorder is usually characterised with anxiety or fear in one or more social situations.

## History

Approach the topic sensitively in a non-threatening, non-judgemental manner. It can be quite difficult to broach the subject initially, so begin by designing your first few questions to put the patient at ease.

- » Open questions
    - › *'Can you tell me more about the symptoms you have been experiencing?'*
    - › *'Could you tell me about what has been troubling you?'*
    - › Cues – If the patient appears withdrawn and is displaying little eye contact, reflect this non-verbal cue to them by saying something like *'You look upset. Is anything bothering you?'*

- » Focused questions
    - › Anxiety – Ask when they started feeling like this, how long it has been going on for, and if it is always there (continuous) or it comes and goes (episodic).
    - › Ask what their triggers are, about avoidance, and if they have any palpitations or SOB.
    - › Ask if it affects their sleep.
    - › Others – Ask if they have any hot flushes, sweats, dizzy spells, pins and needles, tiredness, muscle aches or a sense of impending doom.

- » Associated questions – Perform a depression screen and a suicide-risk screen.

- » Past history – Ask if they have ever had similar symptoms before, or been treated for depression, anxiety or panic attacks; ask if they have an overactive thyroid or other medical condition.

- » Family history – Ask if there is a family history of any mental illnesses, including anxiety disorder or panic attacks.

- » Drug history – Ask if they have taken any medications, particularly salbutamol, thyroxine or diazepam.

» Social history – Ask what their occupation is (if they have any current stress at work); if they have any financial worries (losing their job, their mortgage, debt, etc.); if they smoke, drink alcohol or take recreational drugs; what their diet is like (coffee); and what their support network is like (who lives at home with them, and if they have any close friends or family).

## Differential Diagnosis

| GAD | Marked symptoms of generalised anxiety or excessive worry that impact most areas of their day-to-day functioning on most days for several months. Symptoms include stress, tension, restlessness and insomnia. |
|---|---|
| PTSD | Exposure to a traumatic life event. Impairing symptoms are re-experiencing the event as flashbacks or nightmares, avoiding thoughts or places, and emotional numbness with a hypervigilant state. Symptoms must be present six months after the event. |
| Acute stress reaction | Acute symptoms of anxiety, low mood, irritability and poor sleep, caused by a stressful event. Lasts minutes to hours. Physical symptoms include palpitations, headaches, SOB and nausea. |
| Adjustment disorder | Due to a change in a person's life or after a major life event (moving house / divorce). Symptoms are similar to an acute stress reaction or depression. Resolves once the stressor is removed. |
| Panic disorder | Unpredictable, recurrent panic attacks with a brief experience (five minutes to several hours) of severe anxiety, palpitations, tremors, SOB, chest pain or paraesthesia. These can occur anywhere, and may have multiple precipitants. |
| Obsessive-compulsive disorder (OCD) | Recurrent obsessions (unpleasant thoughts or ideas, or urges) and compulsions (mental or physical rituals). Often will believe that they would be responsible for something catastrophic if they don't attend to their rituals. Will experience anxiety if they resist, and only get temporary relief if they don't resist. |
| Phobia | Specific anxiety or fear of a particular thing (such as animals or travel) or a situation (social anxiety disorder or agoraphobia). Results in avoidance behaviour with an impact on daily function. |

## Examination

» Vitals – BMI, BP and pulse.

» Examination – Perform a cardiac or thyroid examination.

» Questionnaire – Complete the HADS and Generalised Anxiety Disorder Questionnaire.

## Investigations

» Bloods – Not routinely required. Consider FBC, ferritin, vitamin B12 and folate (deficiencies), and TFTs if indicated.

» ECG – Consider an ECG if they present with chest pain or palpitations to exclude arrhythmia.

## Management

*Conservative*

✓ Lifestyle measures

> Reassure – Explain the condition to the patient and attempt to reassure them by informing them that their symptoms are not due to a physical illness, but rather are anxiety related.

> Exercise – Advise them to take regular exercise (such as jogging, swimming or cycling), which helps to reduce stress and release tension. It is recommended that they do 2.5 hours weekly.

> Relaxation techniques – Recommend that they use relaxation techniques (e.g. deep-breathing exercises or yoga).

> Diet – Advise them to avoid consuming caffeine.

> Alcohol – Advise them to stop drinking alcohol or cut down their alcohol intake to under the safe limit (<=14 units/week).

> Drugs – Advise them to stop any recreational drug use (e.g. cannabis).

✓ Self-help

> Material – Offer books, audiobooks or leaflets on understanding anxiety and managing it (*Overcoming* series).

> Suggest that they try group therapy.

> Recommend that they try using online resources (FearFighter, Anxiety UK and Mind).

✓ Talking therapies

> Consider referring them for CBT (individual or group).

> Refer them to computerised or web-based CBT, supported by a practitioner.

> Exposure and Response Prevention (ERP) – This is a type of CBT that is used to confront repetitive thoughts and to reduce compulsive behaviour. Consider recommending this for OCD.

> Recommend group-based psychoeducational therapy.

> Applied relaxation – Refer them to speak to a trained CBT practitioner who offers training on a series of relaxation techniques (muscle and cue controlled), which may be applied in situations that trigger anxiety. Consider this for those with GAD.

> › Desensitisation – Systematic desensitisation is useful for treating phobias. This exposes the patient to the object of their phobia until their anxiety settles.

> › Hypnotherapy – There is little evidence on the effectiveness of this. Some suggest that it helps in social anxiety disorder and for phobias.

### Medical

✓ Antidepressants – Initiate an SSRI. Advise the patient it may take two to four weeks before they feel any improvement. Start with a very low dose and increase it slowly to reduce the worsening of the anxiety in the first two to four weeks after the medication is started. If there is no improvement after two months, consider increasing the dose or changing to an alternative SSRI or SNRI (venlafaxine).

✓ GAD – Sertraline is the first-line treatment; alternative SSRIs include escitalopram or paroxetine. If this is not tolerated, consider an SNRI or pregabalin (third-line treatment).

✓ BDZ – Diazepam can be considered for short-term (two to three weeks) use in cases of severe anxiety and irritability. Warn the patient about the risk of drug tolerance and dependency.

✓ B-blockers – Propranolol is useful in reducing the physical symptoms (sweating and palpitations).

✓ Insomnia – Advise them on good sleep hygiene. Consider offering a short course of hypnotics or sedative antidepressants (mirtazapine).

✓ Referral – Consider referring them to a psychiatrist if symptoms persist for more than a few weeks.

## Safety Netting

» Suicide risk – Review the patient frequently in primary care. Consider contacting the crisis resolution and home treatment team for an urgent assessment. Give them the Samaritans' telephone number for emergencies.

» Safeguarding – Follow the local safeguarding pathways for child protection or vulnerable adults.

» Follow-up – Offer a series of appointments in primary care, with short gaps in more serious cases.

---

### References

National Institute for Health and Care Excellence (2011). *Generalised anxiety disorder and panic disorder in adults: management.* https://www.nice.org.uk/guidance/cg113

# Post-Traumatic Stress Disorder

PTSD is a mental health condition that develops following exposure to an extremely stressful, distressing or frightening event. Common events that may induce PTSD include rape, robbery, military combat, severe natural disasters and serious RTAs. Sufferers usually present with recurrent memories, severe anxiety and flashbacks, whereby the patient may relive the event. It is thought that one in three people develop the symptoms of PTSD following an adverse event. However, the symptoms may not necessarily start immediately following it; rather, in most patients, symptoms develop many months afterwards.

## Professionals at Risk of Traumatic Events

➤ Armed forces (current/ex), police officers, prison guards, firefighters, paramedics, frontline nurses and doctors (casualty), and journalists.

## Screening for PTSD

➤ Consider screening for PTSD in patients who have experienced a major disaster (particularly less than one month previously), as well as for refugees and asylum seekers (particularly from conflict zones)

### History

Approach the topic sensitively in a non-threatening, non-judgemental manner. It can be quite difficult to approach the subject initially, so begin by designing your first few questions to put the patient at ease.

» Open questions

› *'Can you tell me more about the symptoms you have been experiencing?'*

› *'How long have they been going on for?'*

› Cues – If the patient appears withdrawn and is displaying little eye contact, reflect this non-verbal cue to them by saying something like *'You look upset. Is anything bothering you?'*

› Screening – For asylum seekers/refugees or any patients one month post a severe disaster, the patient should be asked if they have any PTSD symptoms.

» Focused questions

› Ask if they have ever experienced a traumatic event (abuse, torture, military combat, a natural disaster or serious RTA).

› Re-experiencing – Ask if they have had any flashbacks (repeated distressing memories or emotions of the event, or a sense of reliving it). Ask if they have had nightmares.

> › Avoidance – Ask if they have been avoiding people or situations that remind them of the event, or if they avoid talking about it.

> › Emotional numbness – Ask if they struggle to experience feelings or feel detached.

> › Hyperarousal – Ask if they often get irritable for no reason or feel they are always on edge (hypervigilance).

» Associated questions

> › Ask if they have any anxiety.

> › Conduct a depression screen.

> › Ask if they have had any suicide ideation.

» Past history – Ask if they have had any previous psychiatric issues, or a medical issue such as cancer or HIV.

» Family history – Ask if there is a family history of any mental health issues.

» Drug history – Ask if they have taken any salbutamol, Ritalin, thyroxine, L-dopa or b-blockers.

» Social history – Ask what their occupation is; if they smoke, drink alcohol or take recreational drugs; how their relationships are (if they have any issues); and what their support network is like.

## Differential Diagnosis

| PTSD | Exposure to a traumatic life event. Impairing symptoms are re-experiencing the event as flashbacks or nightmares, avoiding thoughts or places, and emotional numbness with a hypervigilant state. Symptoms must be present six months after the event. |
| --- | --- |
| Depression | Persistent low mood and effects – with cognitive and biological symptoms, including delusions (worthlessness) and hallucinations (derogatory auditory) – for at least two weeks. |
| Abnormal bereavement reaction | Abnormal reaction to a bereavement (more than two months). Feelings of guilt, a preoccupation with worthlessness, and psychomotor retardation. Can have thoughts of death. May have dreams about their deceased partner. |
| Acute stress reaction | Acute symptoms of anxiety, low mood, irritability, flashbacks and avoidance. Physical symptoms such as palpitations, headaches, SOB and nausea may be present. Starts suddenly, almost immediately after a stressful event, and usually does not last for more than a few months. |
| Adjustment disorder | Occurs due to a change in a person's life or after a major life event. Symptoms include anhedonia, hopelessness, anxiety and crying. The condition usually resolves once the stressor is removed. |

| GAD | Marked symptoms of generalised anxiety or excessive worry that impact most areas of day-to-day functioning on most days for several months. Symptoms include distress, tension, restlessness, fatigability and insomnia. |
|---|---|

## Examination

» Vitals – BMI.

» Questionnaire – Conduct a Trauma Screening Questionnaire (TSQ). Do this one month or more after they were exposed to the trauma. Ask which symptoms they have experienced. If they have experienced five or more in the past week, consider an intervention.

## Management

*Conservative*

✓ Lifestyle measures

> Alcohol – This is a known risk factor. Advise them to stop drinking alcohol or refer them to an alcohol programme.

> Drugs – Advise them to stop taking any recreational drugs (e.g. cannabis).

> Sleep – Advise them to relax in a dark room with minimal distractions, and to go to sleep at the same time every night.

✓ Advice

> Dos – Advise them to return to a normal routine, talk to friends/family about what happened, return to work, eat and exercise regularly, return to where the traumatic event occurred, make time to be with family and friends, and be careful about driving if their concentration is poor.

> Don'ts – Advise them not to beat themself up or bottle up their feelings, avoid discussing it, miss meals, or drink excessive coffee/alcohol.

✓ Watchful waiting – Where there are mild symptoms for less than four weeks, consider monitoring the patient to see if it resolves without treatment.

✓ Self-help

> Material – Offer books or leaflets on understanding PTSD and how to manage it.

> Group therapy – Suggest that they join group therapy. Consider signposting members of their family to a support group.

> Online – Suggest that they try using online resources (UK Psychological Trauma Society, Veterans UK or Anxiety UK).

✓ Talking therapies

> CBT – Consider recommending trauma-focused CBT (8–12 sessions). This tries to change the cognitive process for interpreting traumatic events (e.g. rape victims often blame themselves not the perpetrator, and war survivors blame themselves for not saving a comrade/friend).

> Exposure treatment – Expose the patient to the traumatic memories (e.g. by asking them to recount the event). Repeat their exposure to situations that elicit fear and avoidance behaviour.

> Eye movement desensitisation and reprocessing (EMDR) – Consider referring them for EMDR. This helps the brain reprocess flashbacks and understand the traumatic event.

### Medical

Note that the evidence base for drug treatments in PTSD is very limited (NICE, 2005).

✓ Antidepressants – Consider medications such as paroxetine, mirtazapine or, alternatively, amitriptyline if the patient has declined a referral to specialist services. Consider this if they have a poor response to other forms of therapy.

✓ Anxiety – Diazepam can be considered in the short term (up to two weeks) to improve anxiety and irritability. Propranolol may be helpful for panic-attack-like symptoms.

✓ Insomnia – Consider a short course of hypnotics or sedative antidepressants (mirtazapine).

✓ Referral – Consider referring them to community psychological therapy if their symptoms persist for more than a few weeks.

## Safety Netting

» Suicide risk – Review the patient frequently in primary care. Consider contacting the crisis resolution and home treatment team for an urgent assessment.

» Safeguarding – Follow the local safeguarding pathways for child protection or vulnerable adults.

» Follow-up – Offer a series of appointments in primary care, with short gaps in more serious cases.

### References

Royal College of Psychiatrists (2013). *Post-traumatic stress disorder.* https://www.rcpsych.ac.uk/mental-health/problems-disorders/post-traumatic-stress-disorder

National Institute for Health and Care Excellence (2005). *Post-traumatic stress disorder. The management of PTSD in adults and children in primary and secondary care.* https://www.nice.org.uk/guidance/ng116/evidence/march-2005-full-guideline-pdf-6602623598

# Alcoholism

Alcohol dependence syndrome is due to the excessive consumption of alcohol such that one finds it difficult to cut down, despite being at risk of significant mental or physical harm. It is thought that 9% of men and 4% of women suffer from alcohol dependence syndrome at some point in their lifetimes. Excessive alcohol consumption can cause a number of physical ailments, including gastritis, hepatitis, cirrhosis, erectile dysfunction and pancreatitis, as well as mental problems such as depression, insomnia and anxiety. Excessive alcohol consumption also causes numerous social problems, including relationship breakdowns, loss of employment and criminality. It is now recommended that men and women should not drink >14 units a week, along with having two or more drink-free days per week to minimise harmful consequences. However, the advice for pregnant women is abstinence to prevent foetal-alcohol spectrum disorders.

## History

- » Open questions
  - › *'Can you tell me more about the symptoms you have been experiencing? Could you tell me about what has been troubling you?'*
  - › Cues – If the patient appears embarrassed and is displaying little eye contact, reflect this non-verbal cue to them by saying something like *'You look upset. Is anything bothering you?'*

- » Focused questions
  - › Alcohol – Ask how long they have been drinking for, and how much they drink in a typical day (convert this to units).
  - › Ask about the pattern of their drinking (on a typical day).
  - › Ask what types of alcohol they drink (spirits, beer or wine).
  - › Ask if they binge drink.
  - › Ask if there are any reasons/triggers for the drinking.

- » Associated questions
  - › Neurology – Ask if they have had LOC, dizzy spells, poor coordination, or pins and needles.
  - › Liver – Ask if they have had any jaundice or abdominal pain.
  - › Depression – Ask if they have been feeling low, and do a self-harm / suicidal ideation risk assessment.
  - › Psychosis – Ask if they have experienced any formication or hallucinations.
  - › Injuries – Ask if they have sustained any injuries from drinking.

- » Past history – Ask if they have had any previous psychiatric issues, any past drinking issues (if they have been to any local groups), or if they have had any medical issues such as PUs, pancreatitis or liver disease.

» Family history – Ask if there is a family history of mental health issues, or alcohol or substance misuse.

» Drug history – Ask if they have taken any OTC preparations, warfarin, COCP or anti-epileptics.

» Social history – Ask if they have suffered any stress (any childhood issues, abuse, neglect or parental alcoholism), ask what their occupation is, if they drive, if they smoke or take recreational drugs, how their relationships are (if the drinking has had any impact on them or there are any issues), if they have children (if there is any involvement from social services), and about any criminality.

## RED FLAGS

Depression, liver disease (jaundice), encephalopathy and neuropathy.

## Differential Diagnosis

| Alcohol dependence | Patient experiences cravings and a preoccupation with drinking alcohol (despite knowing it is harmful). Alcohol is drunk to reduce the withdrawal symptoms (tremors, insomnia, sweating and hallucinations), and it overtakes life to the point of neglect and tolerance (volume drunk would cause LOC for normal drinkers). The Severity of Alcohol Dependence Questionnaire (SADQ) can be used. |
|---|---|
| Delirium tremens | Often develops two to three days after the cessation of heavy alcohol consumption. Patient experiences delirium (disorientation towards time and place), drowsiness, agitation, tremors of the hands, sweating and hallucinations (formication). |
| Pancreatitis | Inflammation of the pancreas presenting with acute upper abdominal pain, radiating to the back, and nausea and vomiting. Can cause peritonitis (shoulder-tip pain and abdominal tenderness). |
| Wernicke encephalopathy | Caused by thiamine deficiency and is reversible. Wernicke encephalopathy symptoms include acute confusion, ataxia (broad-based gait), ophthalmoplegia (fixed pupil, nystagmus and bilateral lateral rectus palsies) and peripheral neuropathies (legs). |
| Korsakoff psychosis | A lack of thiamine that causes irreversible damage. Patient presents with retrograde amnesia (before the onset of the condition), anterograde amnesia (the inability to memorise new information), confabulation (invented memories where there are gaps in the memory) and lack of insight. |

| Liver cirrhosis | End-stage liver disease. Patient presents with lethargy, pruritus, fever, weight loss and swelling of the abdomen (ascites). Signs include jaundice, clubbing, palmar erythema, leukonychia, spider naevi and gynaecomastia. |
| --- | --- |

## Units and Measures of Alcohol

➤ Beer – Half a pint is one unit, half a pint of strong beer is two units, and a large bottle is three units.

➤ Wine – A small (125ml) glass is 1.5 unit, a medium (175ml) glass is two units, a large (250ml) glass is two units, and a bottle of wine (750ml) is nine units.

➤ Spirits – A single shot (25ml) is one unit, and a bottle (750ml) is 30 units.

## CAGE Questionnaire

» Cut down – Ask if they have tried to cut down how much alcohol they drink.

» Angry – Ask if they have felt angry if people comment on their drinking.

» Guilty – Ask if they have felt guilty about how much they drink.

» Eye opener – Ask if they ever drink first thing in the morning.

## Dependence Syndrome

» Check if they have the following symptoms:

› Cravings (desire to drink)

› Primacy (alcohol is a priority over other aspects of life)

› Tolerance (they need to drink more alcohol to get the same effect)

› Neglect (neglecting other responsibilities because of drinking)

› Withdrawal symptoms (tremors, shakes, nausea, fits and hallucinations)

» Ask if the above symptoms are relieved by drinking more alcohol.

## Examination

» Vitals – BMI, BP and pulse (AF).

» Inspection – Inspect for signs of liver disease (ascites and spider naevi), tremors and jaundice.

» Abdomen – Check for an enlarged liver, ascites and signs of chronic liver disease.

» Neurology – Check for a wide-based gait (ataxia), confusion and peripheral neuropathy.

## Investigations

» Bloods – FBC (macrocytosis), vitamin B12, LFTs, GGT, ALT, AST, albumin, clotting and lipids.

» Questionnaires – Offer a brief alcohol screening to newly registered patients. Screen using the Fast Alcohol Screening Test (FAST) or the alcohol use disorders identification test for consumption (AUDIT-C). If these are positive, offer a full alcohol use disorders identification test (AUDIT) questionnaire.

## Management

### Conservative

✓ Brief intervention – Provide a brief five-minute intervention. Discuss the patient's drinking habits and the costs verses benefits of drinking. Also explore the health risks and the impact it is having on their life. Explain the maximum number of units that may be consumed per week. Consider using the FRAMES model: feedback (discuss the risk), responsibility (take charge), advice (give clear advice), menu (give options for change), empathy and self-efficacy (encourage).

✓ Lifestyle changes

› Advise them to try to avoid places that have alcohol readily available, such as pubs, clubs and supermarkets. They should throw out from the house any reminders of alcohol (alcoholic beverages and empty bottles).

› Advise them that if they are drinking in a group, they should ensure they are the slowest drinker and sip their drink instead of gulping. They should buy less-concentrated forms of alcohol as they attempt to wean themself off it.

› Advise them to try having days off alcohol to reduce their tolerance. They should replace alcohol with other types of drinks.

› Advise them that anyone with alcohol dependence must inform the DVLA. They cannot drive until they have been free of the alcohol dependence problem for one year and free of alcohol misuse for six months. This may require licence revocation and normalisation of blood tests.

✓ Self-help

› Material – Offer books or leaflets on understanding alcoholism and managing it (*Overcoming* series).

› Group therapy – Suggest that they join Alcoholics Anonymous.

✓ Talking therapies – Consider referring them for CBT to help alter unrealistic thoughts and beliefs.

### Detoxification

✓ Community – Consider daily monitoring and treatment to ensure compliance for patients who drink >15 units per week.

✓ Inpatient – Consider inpatient treatment for those who drink more than 30 units a day; have delirium tremens, epilepsy or Wernicke's encephalopathy; or who drink 15–20 units a day, but have severe depression or psychosis. A patient who is homeless or has an increased risk of suicide should be considered for an inpatient detox.

*Medical*

✓ Acute withdrawal

› BDZ – Chlordiazepoxide is classically used to help reduce tremors and agitation. An alternative may be diazepam. Give short courses to reduce the chances of dependency.

› Oral vitamin B complex or as multivitamins – This is to reduce neurological symptoms.

› Relapse prevention (specialist led) – This includes acamprosate, naltrexone or disulfiram.

## Safety Netting

» Offer a series of appointments in primary care, with short gaps in more serious cases.

» Advise them that if they develop symptoms of delirium tremens, they are to come for review as soon as possible.

» Equally, advise them that if they develop signs of jaundice, haematemesis, abdominal pain (pancreatitis) or drowsiness, they are to come for urgent review.

*References*

National Institute for Health and Care Excellence (2010). *Alcohol-use disorders: diagnosis and management of physical complications*. https://www.nice.org.uk/guidance/CG100

# Drug Dependency

Substance misuse or drug dependency is an increasingly common phenomenon whereby a person has a compulsive need to use drugs in order to function. Failure to obtain drugs leads to uncomfortable withdrawal symptoms, such as anxiety, shaking, excessive sweating and a lack of concentration. A person can become addicted to a large number of substances, including glue, nicotine, alcohol and caffeine; however, in this chapter, we will focus on illegal substances such as heroin, 3,4-methylenedioxymethamphetami (MDMA), LSD and cocaine.

Patients presenting with drug dependence or substance abuse may not disclose their behaviour unless you provide them with reassurance that everything they tell you will be confidential and will not be shared with any outside agencies unless there is a risk of harm to others or to themselves.

## History

- » Open questions
    - › Expectations – *'How were you hoping I could help you today?'* (Detoxification or maintenance therapy, methadone for withdrawal symptoms, letter for court, housing, etc.)
    - › Cues – If the patient appears embarrassed and is displaying little eye contact, reflect this non-verbal cue to them by saying something like *'You look upset. Is anything bothering you?'*

- » Focused questions
    - › Confidentiality – Reassure them that everything they say will be in confidence unless it puts themselves or others at risk.
    - › Screening – Screen for substance abuse if they have or suffer from mental health disorders or alcoholism, or have been in prison.
    - › Drugs – Ask what they are currently taking, how long they have been taking it for, when they started taking it, how much they are using and if the amount has changed recently.
    - › Method – Ask how they are taking it (orally, injection, snorting or smoking), and if they use any needles or share any needles.
    - › Costs – Ask how much they are spending.
    - › OD – Ask if they have ever ODed before.
    - › Detoxification – Assess the patient's motivation to change. Ask if they have any reason why they want to stop now and if they have tried to stop before.

- » Dependence syndrome – Ask about cravings, control, tolerance and withdrawal symptoms, and ask if they have neglected any other responsibilities.

- » Associated questions
    - › Liver – Ask if they have any jaundice or abdominal pain.

> › Depression – Ask if they have a low mood or are disinterested in life. Conduct a suicide-risk screen.

> › Anxiety – Ask if they have any anxiety.

> › Insomnia – Ask if they have any insomnia.

» Past history – Ask if they have hep B or C, HIV, depression, anxiety, panic attacks, schizophrenia or any other medical conditions.

» Family history – Ask if there is a family history of mental health issues, problems with alcohol or substance misuse.

» Social history – Ask if they smoke or drink alcohol, what their housing situation is (where they live or if they are homelessness), what their occupation is, what their finances are like (how they finance their drug habit), about any criminality, what their support network is like (who lives at home with them, and if they have any close friends or family), what their relationships are like, and if they have any children (if so, if there is any social services involvement).

## RED FLAGS

If they are a risk to themselves and/or others, vulnerable children/adults (pregnancy), liver disease and low weight.

## Differential Diagnosis

| Drug dependence | Patient experiences cravings and a preoccupation with the drug (despite knowing it is harmful). Drugs are taken to reduce withdrawal symptoms (tremors, insomnia, sweating and hallucinations), and it overtakes their life to the point of neglect and tolerance. |
|---|---|
| Cocaine | Patient with excessive use presents with dilated pupils, increased energy levels and excitability, insomnia, hallucinations, paranoia and palpitations. |
| Ecstasy | Patient with excessive use may present with headaches, chest pain, blurred vision, nausea and vomiting, fainting, raised BP and hyperthermia. An OD may cause LOC, seizures and paranoia. |
| Heroin | OD presents with depressed breathing, a dry mouth, pinpoint pupils, low BP and constipation. May cause drowsiness, delirium and, eventually, a coma. |
| LSD | Overuse may lead to hallucinations, panic attacks, despair, and feelings of death, fear and synaesthesia (sensory crossover). |

## Examination

» Vitals – BP, pulse and temperature.

» Inspection

  › Inspect for signs of liver disease if indicated.

  › Inspect for poor dental caries and poor nutrition.

  › Skin – Look for any puncture marks on the elbows or legs.

  › Look for signs of infections (sepsis, thrombophlebitis, cellulitis and abscesses).

» Auscultation – If clinically indicated, listen to the chest to exclude chest infections and TB.

» Palpation – Feel the liver for signs of hepatomegaly (hepatitis).

## Investigations

» Bloods – LFTs, GGT, hep B and C, HIV and FBC (anaemia and infections).

» Urine – Urine drug screen (usually done by drug-addiction centres) prior to initiating opioid-substitution treatment.

» ECG – Check for bradycardia (opiates) or arrhythmias. Methadone can cause long-QT syndrome.

## Management

*Conservative*

✓ Brief intervention – Discuss their drug habits and the cost verses benefits of using drugs. Also explore the health risks and the impact it is having on their life. Do not recommend that they go 'cold turkey'.

  › Withdrawal – Explain to the patient the possible withdrawal symptoms they may experience. If they suffer from depression, anxiety or insomnia, these symptoms may worsen from drug withdrawal (opiate dependency).

  › Care plans – Offer the patient information leaflets.

✓ Harm reduction

  › Sharing needles – Inform them of the risks of sharing needles (hep B and HIV) and recommend testing. Offer a needle exchange programme for safe disposal.

  › Immunisation – Recommend immunisation for tetanus, and hep A and B.

✓ Self-help

  › Citizens Advice (CA) – Refer them to CA if they are having financial problems.

> Social services – Refer them to social services for assistance with housing or social issues.

> Group therapy – Suggest they join Narcotics Anonymous, Cocaine Anonymous, or Self-Management and Recovery Training (SMART).

✓ Other

> Social – Support the patient's access to welfare benefits and offer a housing letter from their GP.

> Driving/DVLA – It is illegal to drive whilst under the influence of drugs. Drug users must inform the DVLA if they have used in the past three years. The patient must not drive a car or ride a motorcycle if they are suffering from persistent drug misuse or dependence (cannabis, amphetamines, ecstasy, LSD, etc.). They may drive if they have been free of misuse for six months. Patients on heroin, morphine, methadone, cocaine or BDZ must not drive if they are still misusing, and they can apply for relicensing one year (Group 1) after being assessed and having a clear urine drug screen, or less if they are on a consultant-led maintenance programme.

*Medical*

✓ Prescriptions – Prescriptions for these patients are done by a local drug-dependence unit. Involve a drug worker / key worker to support the patient.

> Opioids – Consider withdrawal through a slow dose reduction of BDZ or z-drug, or switch to an equivalent diazepam dose with tapering doses. Consider changing to diazepam if they are on a short-acting BDZ (lorazepam or alprazolam).

> Methadone – This is often the first choice. If their alcohol intake is significant, methadone may not be appropriate. Often initiated on a low dose (10mg), and only liquid methadone is licensed. Side effects are GI effects, dry mouth, headaches, reduced libido and amenorrhoea.

> Buprenorphine can be considered if they have suffered side effects from methadone, they wish to detoxify from heroin, or are on a liver-enzyme inducer/inhibitor drug (rifampicin anticonvulsants). However, they will be more likely to develop withdrawal symptoms.

   - Both methadone and buprenorphine can be offered under supervised consumption (i.e. via a pharmacist).

✓ Travelling abroad – This requires a letter from the prescribing doctor. Advise them to keep their medication in their hand luggage. If they are travelling for more than three months, this requires a special licence to travel with a controlled drug.

✓ Pregnancy – Involve social services and child protection if appropriate. Maintenance therapy of methadone is recommended. Vomiting from morning sickness can reduce their methadone intake, so offer antiemetics or a quick prescription replacement.

✓ Pain – For acute pain, continue a maintenance dose of opioid medication. Offer paracetamol or NSAIDs. If the pain is severe and they are on methadone, speak with a GP, who may offer morphine sulphate with the dose titrated for pain.

## Safety Netting

» Child protection – If there are any concerns for the welfare of any children, refer as per local guidance. Have a low threshold for discussing issues with the local authority and assessment-duty social workers.

» Offer an appointment within the week to establish if they are coping, achieving shared targets or are tied in with the local services. Offer daily appointments if initiating detoxification or maintenance treatment.

---

### References

National Institute for Health and Care Excellence (2007). *Drug misuse – psychosocial interventions*. https://www.nice.org.uk/guidance/cg51/evidence/drug-misuse-psychosocial-interventions-full-guideline-195261805

National Collaborating Centre for Mental Health (UK) (2011). *Psychosis with coexisting substance misuse, assessment and management in adults and young people*. British Psychological Society.

# Obsessive-Compulsive Disorder

OCD is a mental health condition that is characterised by repetitive, unpleasant, intrusive thoughts that create feelings of fear and unease in the sufferer, which are sometimes made to subside by undertaking repetitive behaviours. Approximately 2% of adults suffer from it. Sufferers usually recognise their actions as being excessive or irrational, but are compelled to repeat them to reduce anxiety levels. They recognise that the thoughts originate from themselves and not someone else. Common symptoms include excessive hand washing, repeated checking of whether doors are locked, being obsessively meticulous and making sure that everything is in a specific order.

## Definition of OCD

➤ Obsession – An unwanted intrusive thought, urge or image that intrudes into one's mind repeatedly, causing distress and anxiety; e.g. contamination (dirt, fluids or chemicals), a need for order/symmetry, or a fear of harm.

➤ Compulsions – Repetitive actions the patient feels obliged to perform, which are driven by their obsession; e.g. handwashing, checking doors/plugs/gas, or arranging items.

## History

» Open questions

> *'Could you tell me about what has been troubling you?'*

> If the patient appears withdrawn and is displaying little eye contact, reflect this non-verbal cue to them by saying something like *'You look upset. Is anything bothering you?'*

» Focused questions

> OCD – Ask when they first started feeling like this, how long it has been going on for, if anything has made it worse or triggered their symptoms (life events or stressors).

> Obsessions – Ask if they have any unpleasant thoughts or ideas, how these thoughts make them feel (disgusted or anxious), how often they have these thoughts, if they are intrusive (entering their mind against their will), what the content of the thoughts is, if they are able to resist or ignore the thoughts, and what happens if they do resist.

> Compulsions – Ask what type of compulsions they have (cleaning, checking things repeatedly, putting things in order or hoarding) and if they get relief when they give in to compulsions.

» Associated questions – Conduct a depression screen and a suicide-risk assessment.

» Past history – Ask if they have had any other psychiatric issues or if they have any medical issues.

» Family history – Ask if there is a family history of psychiatric problems (anxiety, panic attacks or OCD).

» Drug history – Ask if they have taken any medications, particularly Ritalin.

» Social history – Ask about their occupation, if the symptoms make it hard or impossible to work, or if anyone has commented on their behaviour; ask if they smoke, drink alcohol or take recreational drugs; and ask what their support network is like.

## RED FLAGS

If they are a risk to themself and/or others.

## Differentials

➤ Depression

➤ Schizophrenia

## Examination

» Vitals – BMI, BP and pulse.

» Examination – Perform a cardiac or thyroid examination if indicated.

» Questionnaire

› Obsessive-Compulsive Inventory (OCI) – The OCI consists of 42 questions covering a range of repetitive behaviours and thoughts that may have distressed or bothered a patient over the past month. Each question is rated using a frequency score from 0 (never) to 4 (almost always) and a similar 0–4 score for a distress scale. It is scored out of a total of 168, with an OCI score >40 suggesting OCD.

› Yale Brown Obsessive Compulsive Scale (Y-BOCS) – This is an alternative tool consisting of 10 items, with each question scored from 0–4 with a maximum score of 40.

## Investigations

Not routinely required.

## Management

*Conservative*

✓ Reassure – Explain the condition to the patient and attempt to reassure them by informing them that their symptoms are not due to a physical illness, but are anxiety related.

✓ Self-help – Offer material such as books and leaflets on OCD and managing it (*Overcoming* series). Suggest that they join group therapy.

✓ Talking therapies

› ERP – Consider referring them for ERP, which is the gold-standard treatment, and is a modified form of CBT, usually comprising weekly sessions for 12–14 weeks (individual or group).

› CBT – Consider referring them for CBT.

› Cognitive therapy (CT) – CT can be used in addition to ERP. Consider referring a patient who suffers from obsessions but not compulsions, for whom it is helpful. This can be individual or group based.

› Hypnotherapy – There is little good evidence around the effectiveness of this. Some suggest it provides short-term help in cases of OCD.

*Medical*

✓ Antidepressants – Consider initiating an SSRI. Advise the patient that it may take 12 weeks before they feel an improvement. They can experience a worsening of anxiety in the first two to four weeks after the medication has been started.

› If they are <30 years, review in one week, with their risk of suicide monitored weekly for the first month.

✓ TCA – If they have a poor response to two SSRIs, you may consider clomipramine 25mg od, increasing to 100–150mg od after two weeks. Continue the treatment for 12 months (this is sometimes initiated by a specialist).

› Baseline – Check BP and perform an ECG if CVD is indicated.

› Side effects – Dry mouth, drowsiness, blurred vision, constipation and urinary retention.

› Contraindications – Immediately after an MI or for arrhythmia (block).

✓ Antipsychotics – These may be used in addition to an SSRI to augment the patient's response.

# Referral

→ Refer them to a psychiatrist if the patient has a marked impairment to daily function, is at risk of self-harm/neglect or has significant comorbidity (drugs, severe depression or schizophrenia)

## Safety Netting

» Review the patient frequently in primary care. Consider contacting the crisis resolution and home treatment team for an urgent assessment. Give them the Samaritans, telephone number for emergencies.

» Follow-up – Offer a series of appointments in primary care, with short gaps in more serious cases.

## References

Seibell, P.J, Pallanti, S., Bernardi, S., Hughes-Feltenberger, M. and Hollander, E. (2018). *Obsessive-compulsive disorder.* https://bestpractice.bmj.com/topics/en-gb/362

National Institute for Health and Care Excellence (2005). *Obsessive-compulsive disorder and body dysmorphic disorder: treatment.* https://www.nice.org.uk/guidance/cg31

# Bipolar Disorder

Bipolar disorder is an affective mood disorder that causes the patient to alternate between the extremes of low and high (mania) moods. In between these fluctuations, the patient has a normal mood. The causes could be multifactorial, such as childhood experiences. Risk factors may include a family history of bipolar disorder or traumatic experiences. In addition, the disorder may be medication induced (phencyclidine, amphetamine, cocaine, BDZs and dexamethasone).

The pathophysiology of bipolar disorder has not been determined. Twin studies have revealed that environmental factors / traumatic life events increase the risk of developing the disorder.

## Subtypes of Bipolar Disorder

➤ Bipolar I disorder – The disorder includes episodes of depression, mania or mixed states, separated by periods of normal mood. A state of depression is not usually required for a diagnosis.

➤ Bipolar II disorder – The patient does not experience mania, but does have periods of hypomania, depression or mixed states.

## *History*

» The features are those of depression or hypomania, which usually occur with months between them.

» Focused questions

  › Ask a depressed patient about any high-mood episodes.

» Family history – Ask if there is a family history of bipolar disorder (5–10 times increased chance of bipolar disorder).

» Depression – Perform a depression screen. They must have at least five of the following symptoms, and one symptom must be either a depressed mood or anhedonia:

  › Low mood that is present for most of the day, almost everyday

  › Sleep disturbance (insomnia or hypersomnia)

  › Anhedonia

  › Feelings of worthlessness or guilt

  › Fatigue

  › A lack of concentration

  › A change in appetite that has resulted in a weight change

  › Suicidal ideation

» Mania or hypomania – Conduct a screening for mania or hypomania. They must have at least three of the following:

> › Increased goal-directed activity (sexually, at work, socially, etc., or psychomotor agitation)

> › Pressure of speech causing increased talkativeness

> › Flights of ideas

> › A loss of social inhibitions (e.g. inappropriate behaviour, recklessness, aggression or hostility)

> › A decreased need for sleep

> › Heightened self-esteem or grandiosity

» Remember DIGFAST (distractibility, irresponsibility, grandiosity, flights of ideas, activity increase, sleep deficit and talkativeness).

## Examination

» Perform a general assessment of the patient to determine if they are well kempt and if there are any signs of drug use (remember that an organic cause must be ruled out).

» Determine if they require hospitalisation; that is, if there is significant dysfunction to life, risk to themselves or others, or psychotic symptoms.

## Differentials

➤ Depression

➤ Schizophrenia

➤ Caused by a drug (e.g. amphetamines or cocaine)

➤ Hyperthyroidism

## Investigation

» The diagnosis is clinical.

» Bloods – Routine bloods, such as TFTs, to rule out an organic cause of the symptoms.

» Urine – Conduct a urine drug screen, especially in patients with mania.

» Questionnaire

> › Conduct a mood-disorder questionnaire for manic disorders.

> › Conduct a PHQ-9 for depressive episodes.

## Management

*Medical*

✓ Do not start medications in primary care!

✓ Within secondary care/specialist areas

> During a manic episode – Commence an antipsychotic such as haloperidol, olanzapine, quetiapine or risperidone can be commenced – if this is not effective, lithium can be added.

> The patient should be reviewed four weeks after the resolution of the mania symptoms.

> In patients who suffer with a moderate–severe bipolar depression, fluoxetine can be used in combination with the antipsychotic.

## Referral

→ If a new diagnosis of bipolar disorder is suspected within a primary care setting, refer the patient to a mental health team (note that the symptoms must have been present for at least four days).

→ An urgent referral to mental health is required in patients who are at risk of harm to themselves or others, or for patients who have had an escalation of symptoms.

→ If a patient is being managed in primary care, a routine mental health referral is required in the following cases:

> They have only had a partial response to treatment.

> Their adherence to treatment is poor.

> Morbid alcohol use is suspected.

> They are considering stopping taking the medication.

> They are or are trying to become pregnant.

*References*

National Institute for Health and Care Excellence (2014). *Bipolar disorder: assessment and management.* https://www.nice.org.uk/guidance/cg185

# Personality Disorders

Personality traits reflect people's characteristic patterns of thought, feelings and behaviours. A PD arises when a patient's personality traits are inflexible and maladaptive across a wide range of situations, such that they cause significant distress and the impairment of social and occupational functioning. Usually, the person is not aware of the problem. The American Psychiatric Association (2013) defines PD as 'An enduring pattern of inner experience and behaviour that deviates markedly from the expectations of the individual's culture.' Causes of PD may be genetic factors or traumatic events (bullying, neglect, or sexual, emotional or physical abuse).

Individuals with PD often pose a challenge for clinicians, as features of their behaviour may compromise care.

## *Often patients may have the following:*

➤ Frequent mood swings

➤ Angry outbursts

➤ Anxiety that is sufficient to cause difficulty making friends

➤ A need to be the centre of attention

➤ A feeling of being widely cheated or taken advantage of

➤ Not feeling there is anything wrong with their behaviour

➤ Externalising and blaming the world for their behaviours and feelings

## PD Clusters

PD can be characterised into three 'Clusters':

### *Cluster A – 'Weird'*

Those falling into this cluster are known as odd or eccentric. The patients in this group usually have an inability to develop social relationships. There is no psychosis, but some genetic association with schizophrenia.

» Paranoid

› They usually suffer intense paranoia and tend to be highly suspicious.

› They typically suspect, without sufficient basis, that others are exploiting or deceiving them.

› They may be preoccupied with unjustified doubts about the loyalty or trustworthiness of friends and colleagues.

› They can be reluctant to confide in others due to fearing that information will be used against them, and they persistently bear grudges.

› In addition, there could be recurrent suspicions about the fidelity of a spouse, without justification.

» Schizoid

› It is important to remember that there is no psychosis, such as hallucinations.

› They are detached from social relationships.

› They have a restricted range of expression of emotions in interpersonal settings, due to not desiring or enjoying close relationships.

› They have a lack of close friends, other than immediate family.

› They appear indifferent to praise or criticism by others.

» Schizotypal

› They have odd beliefs or magical thinking.

› They have unusual perceptions, including bodily illusions.

› They have odd thinking and speech.

› They exhibit behaviour or an appearance that is eccentric or peculiar.

## Cluster B – 'Wild'

Those falling into this cluster are known to be dramatic, emotional and erratic in their emotions/behaviour.

» Histrionic

› They display excessive emotions and attention-seeking behaviour.

› They display inappropriate sexual or seductive behaviour.

› They have shallow expressions of emotion.

› They use their physical appearance to draw attention to themself.

› They are easily influenced by others and by circumstances.

» Narcissistic

› They have a grandiose sense of self-importance, a need for admiration and a lack of empathy.

› They exaggerate their achievements and talents.

› They have a sense of entitlement.

› They only wish to be associated with high-status people or institutions.

› They are unwilling to recognise or identify with the feelings of others.

» Borderline

› They have a pervasive pattern of instability in interpersonal relationships, alternating between extremes of idealisation and devaluation.

› They have an unstable self-image.

› They have a chronic sense of emptiness and fear of abandonment.

› They have affective instability, including difficulty controlling anger.

› They display recurrent suicidal behaviour (gestures or threats).

» Antisocial

› They have a pervasive pattern of disregard for and violating the rights of others.

› They lie, steal and default on debts.

› They neglect their children or other dependents.

› They demonstrate impulsivity and a failure to plan ahead.

› They show aggressiveness.

› They display a lack of remorse.

## Cluster C – 'Worried'

Those in this cluster are known to be anxious or fearful. There is some genetic association with anxiety disorders.

» Avoidant

› They have a pervasive pattern of social inhibition, feelings of inadequacy and hypersensitivity to negative evaluation.

› They fear criticism and disapproval by others.

› They avoid interpersonal closeness because of a fear of being shamed.

› They are preoccupied with being criticised or rejected in social situations.

› They view themselves as socially inept or inferior.

» Dependent

› Their excessive need to be taken care of leads to submissive and clingy behaviour.

› They have feelings of being inadequate.

› They cannot make their own decisions.

› They avoid confrontation for fear of losing a source of support.

› They urgently seek other relationships for care.

› They have a fear of being alone.

» Obsessive compulsive

› They have a pervasive pattern of preoccupation with perfectionism, mental and interpersonal control, and orderliness, at the expense of flexibility and efficiency.

› They are preoccupied with details, order and organisation.

› They want perfectionism at the expense of task completion.

› They show rigidity and stubbornness.

## Management

### Conservative

✓ Studies suggest that it is more useful to target specific behavioural difficulties through psychodynamic, CBT, IPT or group therapy.

### Medical

✓ Low dose antipsychotics have been shown to be of some benefit in schizotypal PD.

✓ SSRIs are often used as first-line treatment for some PDs.

✓ Mood stabilisers may help with moods and aggression.

## Referral

→ Patients with suspected PD may benefit from an early referral to the appropriate mental health team, as such patients who have an increased risk of adverse outcomes related to physical trauma, suicide, substance abuse and concurrent psychiatric disorders.

### References

American Psychiatric Association (2013). Personality disorders. In *Diagnostic and statistical manual of mental disorders, fifth* ed. https://dsm.psychiatryonline.org/doi/10.1176/appi.books.9780890425596.dsm18

American Psychiatric Association (2013). *Diagnostic and Statistical Manual of Mental Disorders, Fifth Edition.* American Psychiatric Association Publishing.

National Health Service (2020). *Personality disorders.* https://www.nhs.uk/conditions/personality-disorder/

# 16

# Care of the Elderly

## Dementia

Dementia is an irreversible and progressive condition that usually affects the elderly, causing impairment of cognitive function and personality, but without affecting consciousness. In the UK, there are just over 800,000 people with dementia, and the prevalence increases with age. Patients may suffer from amnesia (memory loss), anomia (the inability to recall names), apraxia (the inability to coordinate), aphasia (a communication disorder that makes it difficult to read, write or speak) and agnosia (loss of the ability to recognise objects and persons). The diagnosis is made once two cognitive domains are impaired enough to affect the patient's ADLs. In addition, the symptoms should be present for more than six months. As symptoms progress, patients may wander, suffer hallucinations, become doubly incontinent and, eventually, need 24-hour care. Over 50% of dementias are caused by Alzheimer's disease, 25% are due to vascular dementia and 15% due to Lewy bodies. Although there are no treatments to cure dementia, there are medications that might delay cognitive deterioration.

### History

It is important to approach the topic sensitively in a non-threatening manner. It may be difficult to approach the subject as the patient may lack insight, so begin by designing your first few questions to put the patient at ease. If any carers are present, seek permission from the patient to take a collateral history.

» The history can be given by a relative, carer or neighbour.

» Open questions

> *'Can you tell me more about your memory difficulties?'*

» Focused questions

*Cognitive symptoms*

> Memory – Ask when they first noticed problems with their memory and how long it has been going on for.

> Pattern – Ask if it developed suddenly (delirium), over a period of time (Alzheimer's disease) or in a step-like fashion (vascular dementia)?

> Types – Ask if they forget immediate things (appointments, names or where their keys are), recent things (their phone numbers or what they cooked for dinner last night) or past things (birthday / important dates, or recognising family and friends).

> › Orientation – Ask if they have ever been disorientated with respect to what day or what time it is.

> › Communication – Ask if they have had problems with speaking or writing, if they have misunderstood people at times, or if they are finding themself repeating questions more often than before.

> › Tasks – Ask if they feel it has become more difficult to make decisions, if they are making more decisions now that they regret later on, or if they are finding it difficult to complete everyday tasks that they could do previously (paying bills or following recipes).

*Behaviour / emotional symptoms*

> › Low mood – Ask if they have been feeling low recently, and if so, which came first: the low mood or the forgetfulness (pseudodementia).

> › Anhedonia – Ask if they have lost interest in doing things they used to do.

> › Withdrawal – Ask if they are no longer interacting with people, or if they feel withdrawn from life.

> › Sleep – Ask how their sleep has been recently.

> › Delusions – Ask if they have felt that someone was out to harm them in any way.

> › Hallucinations – Ask if they have seen or heard anything that others have not noticed.

> › Disinhibition – Ask if they have ever done something that they feel embarrassed about (going outside undressed).

*Neurological symptoms*

> › Walking – Ask if there are any problems with mobility, such as any shuffling when walking or falling more often.

> › Apraxia – Ask if there are any problems with dressing or grooming themself, or with cooking.

» Associated history

> › ADLs – Ask if there are any problems with looking after themself, being able to cook and feed themself, or washing themself regularly.

> › Suicide – Ask if they have felt so low that they wanted to end it all, if they have ever acted upon these thoughts, and how they feel today.

» Past history – Ask if they have had any depression, anxiety or psychosis, or if they have / have had CVA, DM, IHD, high cholesterol, HIV, syphilis, Parkinson's disease, a head injury, or a recent infection such as a UTI or chest infection.

» Family history – Ask if there is a family history of Alzheimer's or any other mental health illnesses.

» Drug history – Ask if they have taken anticholinergics, TCAs, opiates, BDZs or phenytoin.

» Social history – Ask what their support network is like; if they have any carers, and if so, how often they visit and what they help with; what their occupation is; if they drive; and if they smoke or drink alcohol.

## RED FLAGS

Suicidal ideation, severe memory loss, risky or aggressive behaviour, abuse or neglect, risk to themself (leaving the gas cooker on), or wandering (getting lost when going out and being unable to find their way back home).

## Differential Diagnosis

| | |
|---|---|
| Alzheimer's disease | Progressive memory loss (often short term). Behavioural changes such as wandering and withdrawal. Dyspraxia (difficulty dressing) and problems communicating (dysphasia). Can result in personality changes. A family history of the condition. |
| Vascular dementia | Stepwise deterioration with evidence of vascular disease (IHD, PVD or BP issues). Often starts more acutely, with gait problems, personality changes with insight intact until late. |
| Lewy body | Fluctuant, with Parkinsonian symptoms (rigidity, gait problems and tremors). May have delirium-like periods and visual hallucinations. |
| Frontotemporal degeneration | Found in younger patients <65 years. Patient mainly suffers from disinhibitions, early loss of insight and personality changes with the preservation of memory. |
| Delirium | Clinical diagnosis. Sudden onset and fluctuating consciousness that is usually worse at night. May have confusion and disorientation with fear and aggression. Delusions and hallucinations may be present. Common causes include infections (UTI / chest infection), drugs (sedatives or analgesics), constipation and poor nutrition. |

## Examination

» Vitals – BMI, BP and temperature.

» Inspection – Inspect for signs of increased CVD risk factors, carotid bruit and reduced peripheral pulses.

» Screening – Conduct a dementia identification direct enhanced service (DES) to screen all at-risk patients for memory loss. Those at risk include patients >60 years with CVD, CVA, PVD or DM; patients >40 with Down's syndrome; and patients >50 years with LD or neurodegenerative conditions (PD).

» Mini-Cog test

> Memorise (score 0–3) – Ask them to recall three unrelated words (e.g. 'banana', 'sunrise' and 'chair') and repeat them to ensure they are able to learn.

> Clock (score 0 or 2) – Request that they draw a clock and show the time 11.10.

> Recall (score 0–3) – Ask them to recall the three words used previously.

> Interpretation – A score <3 suggests possible dementia.

» MMSE

> A detailed memory test for checking orientation (time and place), registration (name three objects), recall (address), calculation (count backwards from seven), language (reading and writing), drawing (pentagon). It is scored out of 30.

» Other – Conduct an abbreviated mental test score (AMTS) and screen for depression (PHQ-9).

## Investigations

» Bloods – FBC, serum vitamin B12 and folate, ESR, CRP, HbA1c, U&Es, LFTs, TFT and calcium.

» Non-routine investigations

> Bloods – Syphilis, and HIV if risk factors are present.

> Urine – MSU for infection, to exclude delirium.

> CXR – To exclude chest infection and bronchial carcinoma.

> ECG – If CVD is suspected.

> CT/MRI – For evidence of vascular dementia (subcortical vascular changes).

## Management

*Conservative*

✓ Advice – Discuss sensitively with the patient and their family/carer the possibility of dementia.

✓ Lifestyle

> Diet – Advise them to cut down their alcohol intake (it exacerbates forgetfulness), eat well and regularly, stop taking any recreational drugs and stop smoking.

> Exercise – Advise them to take regular exercise to reduce their weight. Recommend structured exercise programmes (when done over six months, this improves cognition) or dancing.

> Mind – Offer cognitive stimulation programmes (problem-solving and memory provoking), multisensory stimulation (being exposed to light effects, tactile sensations and sound), music or art therapy, massage, aromatherapy or animal-assisted therapy (interacting with a trained pet or animal).

✓ Memory – Advise them to develop a routine to help compensate for poor memory (having a fixed place for leaving keys), use memory aids such as writing things down, populating to-do lists (daily planner), and using a diary for important dates or events.

✓ Disorientation – Advise them to fit higher door handles or locks to prevent them wandering and getting lost, fit alarms to the door to contact carers when the main door is opened, and consider a pendant alarm.

✓ Hazards – Advise them to declutter the house (by removing excess clothes, and pots and pans), remove trip hazards, and label drawers with their contents.

✓ Support for carers

> Peer group – Give them details about peer-support groups for carers of dementia sufferers (Alzheimer's Society, Carers UK and dementia support groups).

> CBT – Consider offering CBT or group psycho-education.

> Respite – Offer short-break care (day care, adult replacement, or short-term or overnight residential care) to allow their carer some respite.

✓ End-of-life care – Discuss with the patient, while they still have the capacity, end-of-life strategies, including a place-of-care plan to enable them to die with dignity. Consider palliative care measures, including the Liverpool care pathway or Gold Standards Framework.

✓ Do Not Attempt Resuscitation (DNAR) order – Discuss the resuscitation decisions with the GP and/or patient.

*Medical*

✓ Medication – This must be initiated by a specialist (psychiatrist or neurologist); for example, acetylcholinesterase inhibitors (donepezil and galantamine) are often prescribed for moderate Alzheimer's disease (MMSE of 10–20) or mild to moderate Lewy body dementia (rivastigmine). It is not given for vascular dementia or mild cognitive impairment. Memantine is given in severe Alzheimer's disease or to those with moderate Alzheimer's disease who are intolerant of other treatments.

✓ Antipsychotics – These should not be prescribed routinely (e.g. haloperidol, olanzapine and risperidone). There is an increased risk of CVA and increased mortality rates. This is considered only for those with severe symptoms (psychosis and anxiety-causing distress), as a last resort.

✓ Antidepressants – These can be offered for a major depressive disorder. Care must be taken due to interaction with anticholinergics (it affects cognition). This is often specialist-led. Instead, consider CBT.

✓ Safety

› Housing – Consider sheltered accommodation or a change in residence.

› Driving – They should inform the DVLA. Their licence is to be reviewed annually and a formal driving assessment may be necessary (Group 1). A Group 2 licence will be refused or revoked.

✓ Capacity – Advise them to assess their capacity to make decisions (Mental Capacity Act 2005).

› Mental Capacity Act (2005)

- Principles – Patients are assumed to have capacity. People have the right to have support when making decisions and are permitted to make unwise ones. If a patient lacks capacity, then the decision should be made in their best interests, with the least restrictive intervention regarding their rights and freedom.

- Lack of capacity – Patients lack capacity if they have an impairment to their mental function, and if they do not understand the information related to the decision, are unable to retain it, unable to utilise it, unable to make a decision or unable to communicate their decision to others.

› Power of attorney – While they still have capacity, the patient can nominate (in a legal written document called a health and welfare lasting power of attorney[LPA]) an individual to act on their behalf to make healthcare decisions if they were to lose capacity in the future.

› Advance decisions – This is similar to a living will and legally binding. It permits the decision to refuse treatment even if it results in their death (e.g. antibiotics for pneumonia).

› Advance statements – These can recommend treatment and request that their beliefs are respected. These must be considered by doctors, but it is not legally binding.

› Place-of-care plan – Patients can request their preferred place of care (i.e. where they would like to die).

› Will – They should write a will while they still have the capacity to direct their financial matters after their death.

› Independent mental capacity advocate (IMCA) – An IMCA is for patients who lack capacity and who do not have someone (a friend, family member or carer) to act as an advocate. They can challenge serious medical treatments, a change of residence or provide support in vulnerable adult cases (abuse).

## Referral

→ Memory clinic – Refer them for a diagnosis of dementia or if they are a known sufferer of significant depression/psychosis, risky behaviour or medico-legal issues (capacity or driving).

→ MDT – Refer them to an MDT (OT, physiotherapy, neuropsychiatry and social services) to assess their functional capacity (continence, safety at home, self-care, etc.).

› OT – This is to evaluate performance and need, and to identify and facilitate environmental modifications to help them complete tasks independently such as cooking, cleaning and washing.

› Social services – Consider referring them to have their needs at home assessed.

## Safety Netting

» Suicide risk – Review the patient frequently in primary care. Consider contacting the crisis resolution and home treatment team for an urgent assessment.

» Sectioning – Try to persuade them to go voluntarily, but if not, consider a compulsory admission (if they are a risk to themself or others).

» Safeguarding – Follow the local safeguarding pathways for child protection or vulnerable adults.

» Follow-up – Offer a series of appointments in primary care, with short gaps in more serious cases.

---

## References

National Institute for Health and Care Excellence (2018). *Dementia: assessment, management and support for people living with dementia*. https://www.nice.org.uk/guidance/ng97

# Falls

A fall is the unintentional loss of balance that results in the individual coming to a rest on the ground. These are very common in the elderly, with 30% of those >65 years having a fall in the last year, and one in two people who have suffered a fall have had a history of two or more previous falls in the last year.

Falls predispose patients to serious injuries, such as fractures (wrist or femur), particularly in patients with osteoporosis. They can have a significant impact upon the patient, creating a fear of having another fall, which results in the patient failing to mobilise or exercise. This in turn causes muscle weakness, which puts them at risk of further falls.

## History

» Focused questions
  › Ask when they last had a fall, and what happened exactly (e.g. a trip).
  › Ask about the frequency of their falls.
  › Ask if there were any witnesses and what they said happened.
  › Ask if there were any injuries (fractures or head injuries).
  › Ask if this has happened before, and if so, when exactly.
  › Ask if they have had any dizziness or vertigo, and if it happened after looking up (benign paroxysmal positional vertigo [BPPV]).
  › Ask if they had any LOC.

» Associated history – Ask if there were any hazards (loose rugs anywhere, they tripped over a cable, or there was a footwear issue), if they have arthritis (joint pains that mean they can't exercise), or if they have vision issues (cataracts, partial sight or macular degeneration), incontinence, a UTI (dysuria or an increase in frequency) or dementia (memory problems).

» Past history – Ask if they have ischaemic problems (AF, DM, HTN or CVD), osteoporosis, or CNS issues (dementia, strokes, epilepsy or Parkinson's disease).

» Drug history – Ask if they have taken polypharmacy, antihypertensives (postural hypotension), hypoglycaemics, antiarrhythmics or psychoactives (BDZ anticonvulsants).

» Family history – Ask if there is a family history of osteoporosis.

» Social history – Ask if they have any mobility issues (e.g. with stairs), what their support network is like (who lives with them at home, if they have any close friends or family, if they have any carers, and how they are coping), what their occupation is (working or retired), and if they smoke or drink alcohol.

## RED FLAGS

Sudden onset, recent head injury, exercise-induced LOC, or focal neurology.

## Differentials

➤ Cardiac issues

➤ Epilepsy

➤ TIA

➤ Postural hypotension

➤ Situational syncope

## Examination

»	Vitals – Lying and standing BP (hypotension), pulse (AF and bradycardia) and BMI.

»	Inspect – Look at their general appearance (anxious or pale), and check for any muscle wastage or tremors.

»	Cardiovascular – Listen for heart murmurs (AS), an enlarged heart (HOCM) or carotid bruits.

»	Neurological – Perform a focused examination based on clinical findings:

	›	Gait – Check for a broad-based, ataxic, scissoring gait.

	›	Do a turn-180° test – Ask them to stand up and turn around 180°. If this requires more than four steps, a further assessment is required.

	›	Timed 'get up and go' test – Time the patient getting up from a chair without using their arms, walking 3m, turning around, returning to the chair and sitting down in it. They can use their own walking aid.

	›	Tone – Check for hypertonia.

	›	Reflexes – Consider checking their reflexes in their biceps, triceps, supinator, knee or ankle.

	›	CNs – Perform a CN examination (e.g. Snellen chart, nystagmus and visual fields).

## Investigations

»	Urine – MSU or dipstick to exclude a UTI.

»	Bloods – Hb (anaemia), glucose (DM), U&Es (dehydration), LFTs, TFTs and vitamin B12.

»	Imaging – CXR (enlarged heart) and DEXA (osteoporosis).

»	Cardiac – ECG (arrhythmia and bradycardia), 24-hour ECG, echo (heart murmurs) and 24-hr BP.

»	CT/MRI – Consider for subdural/subarachnoid bleeds, carotid doppler (TIA), tilt-table and carotid sinus massage.

## Management

### Conservative

✓ Polypharmacy – Rationalise their medications if they are on multiple ones.

✓ Exercise – Recommend that they do muscle strengthening and balance training. Recommend exercises (e.g. tai chi).

✓ Support groups – Suggest that they contact Age Concern and Age UK.

✓ Adaption – Recommend that they use non-slip mats in the bathroom, mop up wet floors, declutter the house (move furniture and wires), and insert bright lightbulbs.

✓ Feet – Advise them to only wear well-fitting shoes and to trim their toenails.

✓ Housing – Advise them to consider wearing a pendant alarm, or moving into sheltered accommodation / a warden-controlled flat.

✓ Alcohol – Advise them to cut down or avoid drinking alcohol.

### Medical

✓ Osteoporosis – Consider offering vitamin D and calcium, including bisphosphonates if they have a history of fractures/osteoporosis.

## Referral

→ Physiotherapy – Refer them to physiotherapy for structured exercise programmes.

→ OT – Refer them for a home-hazards assessment (loose rugs, cables, furniture, wet surfaces and dim light), to determine if equipment needs to be installed (handholds or rails) or if they require walking aids (a walking stick or a Zimmer frame).

→ Chiropodist or podiatry – Refer them if they require foot care or a footwear assessment.

→ Vision – Refer them to an optician for a vision assessment, or to an ophthalmologist if they have cataracts.

→ Endocrinologist – Refer them to an endocrinologist if you suspect autonomic neuropathy.

→ Falls clinic – If it is a multifactorial, complex case or there is an unknown cause, refer them to the falls clinic.

## Safety Netting

» Review them annually to check for risk factors, or sooner if they have recurrent falls.

### References

National Institute for Health and Care Excellence (2013). *Falls in older people: assessing risk and prevention.* https://www.nice.org.uk/guidance/cg161

# End-of-Life/Palliative Care

Patients suffering from life-threatening illnesses should expect care and support in the periods during the last days of their life. Palliative care relates to the branch of medicine that deals with a patient's symptom management once there are no curative treatment options and the illness becomes terminal. The ultimate aim is to improve the quality of life for both the patient and their family, and to make the patient's life comfortable in the final stages of their illness. Palliative care usually involves a multidisciplinary approach, with hospital specialists, GPs, community nurses, matrons, Macmillan nurses and pain specialists involved in delivering the care.

Common symptoms that present in patients under palliative care include chronic pain, SOB, nausea, vomiting and constipation. Such symptoms may be extreme or constant, affecting the patient's quality of life and causing distress. Good care planning and multidisciplinary working can help patients and carers be prepared throughout this turbulent time.

## History

- » Open questions
  - › *'Can you tell me more about the symptoms you have been experiencing? Can you tell me what has been troubling you?'*

- » Focused questions
  - › Pain – Ask when it started and how long it has been going on for. Ask about the frequency, site, severity (pain score), character, radiation and triggers.
  - › Dyspnoea – Ask when it started, how long it has been going on for, and if it has worsened recently. Ask about the frequency, triggers, increased noisy secretions, and the impact on their QOL (if it is affecting their sleep, if they are able to talk, and how far they are able to walk).
  - › Cough – Ask when it started, how long it has been going on for and if it has worsened recently. Ask about the frequency and character (dry, barking or harsh). Ask if there is any phlegm (if so, what colour it is and if there is any blood), any noisy secretions, any chest pain or any SOB.
  - › Constipation – Ask how often they are opening their bowels, if it has changed, if they are able to pass wind, if there has been any vomiting, if they have any abdominal pain, if there is any blood in their stools, or if they have had any dark stools.
  - › Nausea and vomiting – Ask when it started, how long it has been going on for, if it has worsened recently, what colour it is, what the frequency is, if there are any triggers (medications), if there is any haematemesis, and if they have heartburn.
  - › Mental health – Ask if they have a low mood, are feeling disinterested in life, or have any thoughts of self-harm or suicidal ideation.

- » Associated history – Ask how their appetite is, if they have lost any weight or if they have fatigue.

» Past history – Ask if they have had any medical conditions, particularly cancer (if so, which treatment they had), and if they have any advanced directives and a care co-ordinator.

» Drug history – Ask if they take / have taken any medications and what the delivery route for them was, if they have taken anything OTC or herbal remedies, and if they have taken any analgesia and how often it is used (opioids may cause constipation).

» Social history – Ask if they follow a religion (if so, if they have spoken to a priest, chaplain, etc.), who lives at home with them, if they have any current relationships, if they have any carers (if so, how often they attend), if they are coping, what things they can do independently (cooking, bathing, dressing, feeding themselves and continence), and if they smoke or drink alcohol.

## RED FLAGS

Dyspnoea at rest, intractable pain or a bowel obstruction.

## Examination

» Vitals – BP, pulse, temperature and oxygen saturations.

» Inspection – Inspect the appropriate system.

## Investigations

» Bloods – FBC, ferritin, calcium and U&Es.

» X-ray – An AXR if an obstruction is suspected, or a CXR if they have SOB.

» CT/MRI – Brain/spine scan if pathology is suspected (raised ICP or spinal compression).

## Management

✓ Finances – If they are terminally ill (there is an expectation that they will not live for longer than six months) request their named GP to issue a DS1500 form. This will mean that disability living allowance and attendance allowance can be fast tracked. Discuss them having a living will.

✓ Dying – Check if the patient knows about the DNAR status, advanced directive and LPA. *See Dementia section, page 597.*

### Pain

✓ Utilise the analgesic ladder (adapted from WHO) as follows:

› Mild – Use a non-opioid, such as paracetamol with or without NSAIDs.

> › Moderate – Use a weak opioid (e.g. codeine, dihydrocodeine or tramadol) in addition to a non-opioid if necessary (co-codamol). Also offer a stimulant laxative (senna or bisacodyl) or a stool softener (sodium docusate).

> › Severe – Consider a strong opioid (e.g. morphine). Discuss with the GP to start immediate release (rapid onset in 20 minutes) oramorph 5mg four-hourly (2mg in the elderly). Titrate the dose in 30–50% increments until they are pain free. Offer a laxative.

> Offer modified release morphine (onset in one to two hours with a slow peak at four hours) for continuous pain or once the pain is controlled on immediate release.

> The side effects are drowsiness (this often settles), nausea and vomiting (metoclopramide), constipation (senna, bisacodyl or docusate) and a dry mouth (sip cold water, ice cubes or lollies, and have unsweetened drinks).

## Other pain

✓ Intestinal colic – Try hyoscine hydrobromide.

✓ Muscle spasms – Suggest a heat pad, massage or TENS, or consider offering diazepam.

✓ Neuropathic – Try amitriptyline/nortriptyline, pregabalin/gabapentin, or carbamazepine.

## Nausea and vomiting

*Treat the underlying cause.*

✓ Conservative – Eat small meals/snacks with cool fizzy drinks, and consider acupuncture.

✓ Medical – Treat with cyclizine (most instances), metoclopramide (gastric stasis), domperidone (gastric distension), ondansetron (post radiotherapy) or haloperidol (opioid induced).

## Cough

*Treat the underlying cause*

✓ Conservative – Recommend that they sit upright, do breathing exercises, inhale steam and open the windows.

✓ Medical – Try a simple linctus or codeine linctus. If persistent, try codeine phosphate or MST.

## Constipation

*Treat the underlying cause*

✓ Medical – Offer a stimulant laxative (senna or bisacodyl), a stool softener (sodium docusate) or suppositories (glycerol) for hard stools.

### Hiccups

*Treat the underlying cause*

- ✓ Conservative – Recommend that they breathe into a paper bag or undergo vagal stimulation.
- ✓ Medical – Offer haloperidol or chlorpromazine. For intractable hiccups, consider carbamazepine or gabapentin.

### QOF

- » There should be a register of palliative-care patients, with three-monthly MDT discussions with allied health professionals regarding all the patients on the register.

## Referral

- → Macmillan nurse – Refer them to a Macmillan nurse for support and advice regarding medication or symptom control (pain, and nausea and vomiting).
- → Marie Curie nurse – Refer them to a Marie Curie nurse for care for the terminally ill, including hands-on care at home.
- → Pain clinic – Refer them to a pain clinic if they have ongoing pain despite maximal doses of painkillers.
- → Dietician – Consider referring them for advice on feeding and thickeners if they have problems swallowing.
- → Chaplain – Consider referring them for advice around spiritual needs.

## Safety Netting

- » Review in one to two days if their symptoms are not improving. Offer home visits if they are deteriorating or bed bound.

# 17

# Paediatrics

## Approach to Taking a Paediatric History

Taking a history from a parent and child is a key skill that all PAs in primary care have to master. You may have to deal with two (or possibly more) participants in the consultation, which will definitely impact the dynamics of the conversation. When dealing with parents of young children, be aware that they may be tired, anxious or fearful. In the case of teenage children, the parents may be intrusive and over-controlling. In all situations, it is important that you establish and maintain a rapport, and try to be empathic to their plight.

### Principles

> Listen to the mum – Listen carefully and acknowledge what they say. The mother should be considered correct until proven otherwise.

> Address them by name – When talking to the parents about the child, avoid addressing them as 'he' or 'she'; rather, call them by their first name, especially if they are in the room (e.g. *'Does Johnny have any tummy pain?'*)

> Rapport – Greet the child as well as the parents when they come into the room. Maintain good eye contact with them when talking to them.

> Interaction – Observe the interaction between the child and the parent(s). Is it positive or negative?

> Use open questions and avoid too many closed questions to allow the child to use their own vocabulary.

> When questioning the child, avoid using medical jargon.

> If the child is very young, try using props (toys or teddy bears); e.g. when trying to locate pain.

> Verify and correlate their history with their parents if necessary. Avoid being dismissive of what the child says.

### *History*

» Establish, in a chronological order, how their symptoms have developed.

› Ask when the onset was, when the child was last well, if there were any triggers, if they have had any similar episodes, if they have had any unwell contacts at home, and if they have they been off school or nursery.

» Cough
  › Ask if it is worse during the day, at night or is bad during both.
  › Ask if it is made worse by exercise.
  › Ask what it sounds like (barking, a whoop, wet or dry).
  › Ask if there is an associated wheeze, and any sputum or catarrh.

» Fever
  › Ask how high the temperature went.
  › Ask if they have a swinging fever.
  › Ask if there has been any shaking (rigors) or fits (seizures).
  › Ask if they have had any headaches or intolerance to light (photophobia).
  › Ask if they have had any rashes (face/trunk/nappy area), and if so, ask what it looks like and if it changes colour when pressed (blanching/non-blanching).

» Diarrhoea
  › Ask how many times they have passed stools (for neonates, ask about dirty nappies).
  › Ask if the stools are loose, watery or fully formed.
  › Ask if there has been any blood, mucus or tummy pain.
  › Ask if there has been any pain associated with feeding.
  › Ask if they are passing urine every day.

» Vomiting
  › Ask how many times they have vomited.
  › Ask if it is related to meals.
  › Ask if there has been any projectile vomiting (pyloric stenosis).
  › Ask what colour the vomit is, and if there is any blood.

» Seizures
  › Ask if they had any fever before the fit and how long it lasted for.
  › Ask if there was any tongue biting or if they wet themself.
  › Ask if there was any LOC.
  › Ask if the limbs were jerking, and if they felt sleepy or drowsy afterwards.

» Infant – If taking a history about an infant, ensure that you ask questions pertinent to their age.
  › Bowels – Ask how their bowel movements are and if they have had any dirty nappies.
  › Weight – Ask if they have lost or gained any weight recently.
  › Feeds – Ask how often they feed and if it has changed.
  › Type of feeding – Ask if they are breastfed, bottle fed or it is mixed.

» Behaviour – Ask what the child's usual mood or demeanour is like, if there has been any change, if they have temper tantrums, if they hit themself or carry out any repetitive behaviours (autism), if they are hyperactive (ADHD), and how their sleep is.

» Past history

> Medical – Ask whether the child suffers from any medical conditions (asthma, DM, epilepsy or atopy) and if they have a learning disability.

> Hospital – Ask if they have had any operations, any A&E attendances, any hospital admissions or any special care baby unit (SCBU) admissions.

> Immunisations – Check if they are up to date with their childhood immunisations and if they have had any travel vaccinations.

» Birth history

> Pregnancy - Ask whether the mother had any problems during pregnancy (epilepsy, DM, BP, or viral illnesses such as hep B, HIV and varicella).

> Delivery – Ask how the child was delivered (via a c-section or naturally), if there were any problems in childbirth (prolonged labour), if forceps or ventouse was required, if the child was breech (developmental dysplasia of the hip [DDH]), if the child was born prematurely or at term, and if there was any shoulder dystocia.

> Treatment – Ask if they were admitted to the SCBU, and if they had jaundiced and require light treatment.

> Feeding – Ask if they have been breastfed or bottle fed, and if there have been any problems with weaning.

> Development – Ask if there have been any problems with the child's development or achieving milestones (walking, eating, speaking and potty training).

» Family history

> Genetic – Establish if there are any genetic conditions that run in the family (CF or sickle cell disease).

> Medical – Ask if there are any medical conditions that affect other family members (asthma or allergies).

» Drug history – Ask if they have taken any medications.

» Social history

> Ask who lives with them at home, and if the parents are consanguineous.

> Ask if they have brothers or sisters, what the relationship between them is like, and if their siblings have any illnesses.

> Ask if anyone smokes at home, and if they have any pets at home.

> Ask if they are known to social services.

> Ask about school, particularly if there is any bullying, how they are performing and if they have any unauthorised days off.

> Ask if they eat a balanced diet, if they avoid any foods (dairy or meat), and if they have any allergies to foods (seafood or peanuts).

## RED FLAGS

Poor growth on centiles, child-protection concerns or a developmental delay.

# Examination

» Vitals – Check the centiles (compare them to the red book). If they are under two years, check their head circumference.

» Inspection – Inspect the system that is appropriate to the physical complaint.

# Management

✓ Explanation – In your explanation, incorporate vocabulary that the parent used to describe their child's illness; e.g. saying something like *'You mentioned Johnny was "wheezy" and "croupy".'*

✓ Prognosis – Explain the natural course of the illness and what they should expect within a timeline.

## Safety Netting

» Red flags – Be sure to explain to the parents what red-flag symptoms they need to look out for and that they must seek medical advice if they encounter those symptoms.

» Follow-up – Offer the patient a convenient follow-up appointment if relevant. If a complaint is being made, explain when the patient can expect to get a response.

# Asthma

Asthma is a chronic inflammatory disorder of the airways that is characterised by a variable airway obstruction and hyperreactivity. The exposure of the airway to environmental allergens causes bronchospasm, excessive mucus secretions and oedema. Over time, continued exposure leads to the airway narrowing, which gives rise to symptoms including a wheeze, breathlessness, chest tightness and coughing. Its severity can be assessed using a peak flow meter, which also helps to confirm the diagnosis. There is reversibility and improvement in peak expiratory flow rate (PEFR) following admission for a short course of a bronchodilator (salbutamol).

## History

» Focused questions

  › Cough – Ask if they have had a cough, when it started and how long it has lasted for.

  › Diurnal variation – Ask if it is worse at night or in the morning.

  › Triggers – Ask if anything makes their symptoms better (inhalers or seasons) or worse (exercise, pets, going to the park or cold weather).

  › Breathing – Ask if they have had SOB, any noisy breathing or a wheeze.

  › Chest tightness – Ask if they experience any chest pain in the morning.

» Associated history

  › Exacerbation – Ask if they have had a fever, brought up any phlegm or had a runny nose.

  › Vomiting – Ask if they vomit after coughing.

» Past history – Ask if they have had any atopy (hay fever, eczema or urticaria), any bronchiolitis or a wheeze as an infant (if so, how old they were), any asthma attacks (if so, how many), and if they have ever attended A&E or been admitted due to asthma.

» Birth history – Ask if their mother had any issues in pregnancy, or the child was born prematurely.

» Drug history – Ask if they have taken/used any medications, inhalers or spacers, particularly if they have used oral steroids in the last year (if so, how many times).

» Immunisations – Ask if their immunisations are up to date.

» Social history – Ask who lives at home with them, if they have any siblings, if anyone in the family smokes at home, if they have any pets (cats or dogs), if they have any fluffy toys (allergens), if they go to school or if they have missed school because of this issue, if they play sports, and if so, whether it has interfered with their ability to do so.

## RED FLAGS

Severe SOB, speaking in incomplete sentences, exhaustion, fast breathing and confusion.

## Examination

» Vitals – Pulse (tachycardia), respiratory rate (tachypnoea), temperature, height, weight (growth charts) and oxygen saturations.

» Respiratory

  › Inspection – Inspect for signs of respiratory distress, accessory muscles, barrel chest, Harrison's sulcus or being unable to complete sentences.

  › Auscultation – Listen to the chest for a prolonged expiratory phase, a wheeze or a silent chest.

## Investigations

» CXR – This is needed for an overinflated chest or unclear diagnosis.

» Peak flow – This is unreliable in young children (under five years) due to poor technique. It is used to determine reversibility with B-agonist/inhaled steroids.

» Specialist – Perform spirometry if they are over five years and the diagnosis is uncertain. Do not routinely use fractional nitric oxide (FeNO) to monitor asthma control. Skin-prick tests for aeroallergens or specific IgE can be considered to identify any triggers after the diagnosis.

## Diagnosis

The diagnosis is based on the history and examination. If they are under five years, treat their symptoms based upon judgement, and review regularly. If possible, perform objective tests once they reach five years. Refer them to a primary care diagnostic hub where the diagnosis can be made using a combination of spirometry and variable peak flow readings:

➤ Significant – Obstructive spirometry of FEV1/FVC <70%, and a bronchodilator reversibility (BDR) test with improvement >=FEV1 or 12%, and a peak flow variability of >20%.

➤ Avoid using skin-prick tests for aeroallergens, total serum IgE, FBC (eosinophil) and the exercise challenge for diagnosis.

### Increased probability of a diagnosis of asthma

» Symptoms – A wheeze, SOB, chest tightness and a cough (at night, early morning, after exercise, when cold and in the presence of allergens).

»      Past history – Atopy.

»      Family history – Atopy or asthma.

»      Examination – A widespread wheeze (expiratory and bilateral), prolonged expiration and an increased respiratory rate.

## Management

### Conservative

✓      Lifestyle changes

>      Advise them to avoid potential allergens.

>      Dust mites – Advise them to remove (from the child's room) carpets, curtains and soft toys; cover pillows and their mattress; and do regular hoovering (advise that the child does not return to their room within 20 minutes).

>      Advise them to avoid pets (cats or dogs).

>      Explain that breastfeeding is protective against asthma.

>      Advise them to stop exposing the child to passive smoking where possible.

>      Advise them to lose weight, and exercise programmes can be recommended.

✓      Refer them for self-management programmes and offer a personalised care plan.

✓      Give advice on the patient's inhaler technique.

### Medical

✓      NICE (2017) guidelines recommend reviewing their response four to eight weeks after a change in treatment.

**Under five years old**

✓      SABA – Offer an inhaled SABA (salbutamol) as required if asthma is suspected.

✓      ICS – If the child's asthma is uncontrolled using a salbutamol inhaler, they have asthma symptoms more than three times a week or they have nocturnal symptoms, do an eight-week trial of paediatric moderate-dose ICS therapy at presentation.

>      After eight weeks, stop the ICS and monitor their symptoms.

>      If it is not resolved during the trial period, consider an alternative diagnosis.

>      If it is resolved in less than four weeks after stopping the ICS, restart it, but use a paediatric low-dose ICS.

>      If is resolved in more than four weeks after stopping the ICS, repeat the eight-week trial of a paediatric moderate-dose ICS.

✓      LRTA – If it is uncontrolled on low-dose ICS maintenance therapy, add an LTRA.

✓      If it is uncontrolled on a low-dose ICS plus LTRA, stop the LTRA and refer them to a consultant.

**5–16 years old**

✓ SABA – Offer an inhaled SABA (salbutamol) as required.

✓ ICS – If the patient is uncontrolled on salbutamol, their asthma symptoms are occurring more than three times a week or they have nocturnal symptoms, start them on a paediatric low-dose ICS.

✓ LTRA – Add an LTRA (montelukast).

✓ LABA – Consider stopping the LTRA and adding a LABA (salmeterol).

✓ If the asthma is uncontrolled, discuss the following recommendations with their GP:

› Maintenance and reliever therapy (MART) – Consider changing the LABA and low-dose ICS to a MART such as Symbicort or Fostair, with a paediatric low-maintenance dose of ICS.

› If the asthma is uncontrolled, consider increasing the ICS to a paediatric moderate-maintenance dose (either as MART or via a fixed-dose regimen, such as ICS plus LABA plus SABA).

**Over 16 years old (NICE, 2017)**

✓ Low dose of ICS is <=200mcg of budesonide or equivalent.

✓ Moderate dose of ICS is 200–400mcg of budesonide or equivalent.

✓ High dose of ICS is >400mcg of budesonide or equivalent.

## Safety Netting

» If patients have acute SOB, chest tightness, wheezing, or are unable to complete sentences, exhausted, confused or drowsy, they should seek medical advice

» Follow-up – Follow up every three months to consider stepping down or changing to the lowest inhaled steroid dose if symptoms are controlled.

---

## References

National Institute for Health and Care Excellence (2017). *Asthma: diagnosis, monitoring and chronic asthma management.* https://www.nice.org.uk/guidance/ng80

# Autism

Autism spectrum disorder is a complex and lifelong neurological and developmental problem that appears during childhood. It affects the sufferer in a number of ways, including impairing their ability to interact socially with others, as well as their ability to communicate verbally and nonverbally. It is often noticed by parents as the child reaches three years of age and begins to display odd, repetitive behaviours or has problems interacting with them. The causes of autism are not known, but it is thought that there is a complex interplay between genetic, environmental and neurological factors that affect brain development. In the UK, it is believed that one in 100 people has autism or autistic traits, amounting to almost 700,000 sufferers.

## History

Approach the topic sensitively in a non-threatening, non-judgemental manner. Adopt a relaxed, open posture that is calm and inviting. Try not to appear patronising nor paternalistic towards the parent(s). Do not be dismissive, but try to engage with and explore the patient's ideas and concerns.

- » Focused questions
  - › Ask when they noticed a change in their child.
  - › Communication – Ask how their child communicates, if their child speaks and when they started to speak (on time), if the child repeats themself or says a single phrase a lot (echolalia), and if the child is able to understand if they are being joked with.
  - › Social interaction – Ask if their child has many friends, if they enjoy playing with others or are more happy being alone, if they avoid eye contact with their parents or others, and if they do not like it when others enter their personal space.
  - › Playing – Ask if their child plays with different toys or concentrates on one, and if they play with the whole toy or just with a small part of it.
  - › Routine – Ask if they have to have a clear routine, such as when dressing or eating.
  - › Emotion – Ask if they smile much and if they like cuddling.
  - › Skills – Ask if their child has any exceptional talents (memorising lists, drawing or music related).
  - › Behaviour – Ask what their child's usual mood or demeanour is, if there has been any change, if they have temper tantrums or demonstrate challenging behaviour, if they do not like change, if they hit themself or carry out any repetitive behaviours (such as rocking their body or flapping their hands), and if they display the same behaviour whether they are at home, in social situations or at school.

- » Associated history
  - › Ask if they have any sleeping problems.
  - › Feeding – Ask what their appetite is like, if they eat well, if they refuse any foods, and if so, why they refuse them.

> › GI – Ask if they have any problems with their bowels (constipation, diarrhoea or pain).

> › Development – Ask if there have been any problems with the child's development or achieving milestones (walking, eating or potty training), and if they had any delay in using language (<10 words by two years of age).

» Past history – Ask if they have Down's syndrome, tuberous sclerosis, epilepsy, ADHD or a learning disorder (LD), and if they are up to date with immunisations.

» Birth history – Ask if there were any problems during pregnancy, if any medications were taken during it (sodium valproate) and about the gestation period.

» Drug history – Ask if they are taking / have taken any medications.

» Family history – Ask if there is a family history of autism or schizophrenia.

» Social history – Ask who lives at home with them, if they have any siblings, and if there are any issues at school or nursery.

## RED FLAGS

If a child under three years regresses on language or developmental milestones, or there is suspicion of child abuse.

## Differentials

➤ ADHD

➤ Anxiety/depression

➤ Psychosis

➤ Hearing/visual problems

## Measles, Mumps and Rubella (MMR) Vaccine and Autism

» The consensus of the medical and scientific community states that there is no scientific evidence for a credible link between the MMR vaccine and autism, and that the lack of confidence in MMR has damaged public health. Single separate vaccines instead of the MMR vaccine would not reduce the chance of adverse effects, but would increase the risk of children catching the disease due to the increased time waiting for full immunisation cover. In 2010, both Dr Wakefiels and *The Lancet* published a public retraction around the findings and conclusions of the paper.

## Examination

»     Vitals – Not routinely required unless there are worries about autism.

## Investigations

»     Bloods – Not routinely required. Genetic tests are usually undertaken by a genetic centre.

»     EEG – Done by specialists if there is a suspicion of epilepsy.

## Management

✓     Explanation – Explain the likely diagnosis and what will happen next.

## Referral

→     Refer them to a local autism clinic, child development centre or child psychiatrist to confirm the diagnosis.

→     Social services – Consider referring them to social services for an assessment for benefits or an assignment of a key worker. Consider referring them for a carer's assessment.

→     Education – Consider referring them for extra help or an educational needs assessment for school performance.

→     Psychological – Refer them for early intensive behavioural intervention therapy to reduce challenging behaviours, and for CBT to reduce anxiety.

→     SALT – Refer them for speech therapy to improve communication.

→     OT – Refer them to OT, which can help with sensory integration therapy or adapting their environment.

→     Neurologist – Refer them to a paediatrician or neurologist if the child has a regression of motor skills or is over three years with a regression in language.

### Safety Netting

»     Offer the patient a convenient follow-up appointment that is relevant to their needs.

---

### References

National Institute for Health and Care Excellence (2011). *Autism spectrum disorder in under 19s: recognition, referral and diagnosis.* https://www.nice.org.uk/guidance/cg128

# Attention Deficit Hyperactivity Disorder

ADHD is a behavioural disorder that is characterised by inattention, hyperactivity or acting in impulsive ways that are not appropriate for their age. It often presents in childhood (three to seven years) with impairment to their daily function (at home, in social activities and at school), and it is seen more often in boys than girls. Often, the child is easily distracted, forgets things, and has difficulty following instructions or completing tasks. They also can get bored after only a few minutes of doing an activity before switching swiftly to another.

For a formal diagnosis, symptoms must be present for at least six months, other causes (such as learning difficulties) must have been excluded, and there must be an impact upon at least two settings (e.g. their home, school or social situations). The diagnosis should be made by a specialist.

## History

Approach the topic sensitively in a non-threatening, non-judgemental manner. Adopt a relaxed, open posture that is calm and inviting. Try not to appear patronising nor paternalistic towards the parent(s). Do not be dismissive, but try to engage with and explore the patient's ideas and concerns.

- » Focused questions
    - › Ask when they first noticed a change in their child's behaviour, and if they display the same behaviour whether they are at home, in social situations or at school.
    - › Inattention – Ask if they have difficulty concentrating on a task or play activity, if they make careless mistakes in their school work or other activities, if they are easily distracted, and if they struggle to complete tasks or follow instructions.
    - › Hyperactivity – Ask if they are more restless than other children, if they can remain seated throughout a class lesson, if they are always fidgeting, and if they run or climb during times when it is not appropriate.
    - › Impulsive – Ask if their child is generally impatient (e.g. when waiting their turn in games), if they blurt out things without thinking or worrying about the consequences, or if they interrupt others a lot (in conversation or playing).

- » Associated history
    - › Developmental delay – Ask if there have been any problems with the child's development or achieving milestones (walking, eating, speaking and potty training).
    - › School – Ask if there have been any problems with school, how they are performing and what their relationships with their friends are like.
    - › For an adolescent, ask if they have had any problems with the police and if they use drugs.

» Past history – Ask if they have Down's syndrome, tuberous sclerosis, epilepsy, any LD, any psychiatric issues (low mood or anxiety), and if they are up to date on their immunisations.

» Birth history – Ask if there were any issues during pregnancy or delivery (low birth weight or born prematurely).

» Drug history – Ask if they are taking / have taken any medications.

» Family history – Ask if there is a family history of autism or ADHD.

» Social history – Ask who lives with them at home; how things are at home; if they have any brothers or sisters, and what the relationship between them is like; if they are known to social services; and if they have had any brushes with the law or the youth justice system.

## RED FLAGS

Any child-protection issues or abnormal development.

## Differential Diagnosis

| Autism | Changes in social interaction, playing and communication. |
|---|---|
| Anxiety/depression | Ask about their mood, if there is any stress at school or if there is any bullying. |

## Examination

» Vitals – Height, weight and growth charts. If they are on medication, take a baseline pulse and BP.

## Management

✓ Explanation – When explaining the condition to the family, incorporate vocabulary that the parent used to describe their child's problems. Try to involve the whole family in the management of the condition. The diagnosis should be made by a specialist and not in primary care.

✓ Talking therapies

› Family therapy – Consider offering this to the family.

› Group CBT – Consider offering this to the child or offer individual psychological treatment for older children.

› Education programme – This teaches the parents behaviour therapy techniques to use with their child, such as offering structure to child's daily routine/day, rewarding positive interactions and implementing clear rules for behaviour.

*Specialist*

✓ Medication may be initiated (methylphenidate is the first-line treatment) if talking therapies fail. Side effects include abdominal pain, nausea and indigestion. Growth is not usually affected, but it is recommended to monitor growth during treatment. Lisdexamfetamine and dexamphetamine can be considered if the side effects render methylphenidate unsuitable. If there is no response after six weeks, atomoxetine or guanfacine may be considered.

✓ Shared care – Medication is usually prescribed under the shared-care protocol. Height and weight should be measured every six months and after every dose change.

## Referral

→ Moderate – Consider watchful waiting for up to 10 weeks. Refer them for educational programmes.

→ Education – Consider referring them for extra help, an educational needs assessment for school performance, or the assignment of a special educational needs coordinator (SENCO).

→ Severe – Refer them to the Community Adolescent Mental Health Service (CAMHS) or a specialist paediatrician.

## Safety Netting

» Offer the patient a convenient follow-up appointment as is relevant to their needs.

*References*

National Institute for Health and Care Excellence (2018). *Attention deficit hyperactivity disorder: diagnosis and management.* https://www.nice.org.uk/guidance/ng87

# Meningitis

Meningitis relates to the infection or inflammation of the protective surface layer of the brain and spinal cord, which is known as the meninges. It can become infected via bacteria, viruses or even due to TB. The most common cause is viral meningitis, which usually presents as a mild disease; however, all suspected meningitis cases should be considered bacterial unless proven otherwise, since bacterial meningitis is a life-threatening condition that is particularly serious in children and young people. Due to the introduction of child immunisation with meningitis C (MenC), meningitis B (MenB) and *Haemophilus influenzae* type B (Hib) vaccines, the demographics of the causes of meningitis is changing, with *Streptococcus pneumoniae* (pneumococcal disease) and *Neisseria meningitidis* (meningococcal) being the most common causes.

## History

Principles

» Listen to the mum – If the child is of a young age and attends with a parent (e.g. the mother), listen carefully and acknowledge what the mother is saying. Acknowledge the level of concern of the parent/carer in making your diagnosis.

» Focused questions

 › Ask when the symptoms began, how long it has been going on for, and if it is getting worse or better.

 › Ask if there is a rash, and if so, ask if it goes away when you press on it.

 › Ask if they have any neck stiffness or headaches, if they are irritable or drowsy, what their mental state is like (confused or semi-conscious), if they have any photophobia, and if they have had any seizures.

 › Screen for septicaemia – Ask if they have any joint pains, cold limbs despite having a fever or rigors.

» Associated history – Ask if they have had any nausea and vomiting, fever, lethargy or headaches (if so, what the location is), if they are feeding and taking fluids, and if they are passing urine okay (or ask how many wet nappies they have had).

» Past history – Ask if they were born prematurely or had a low birth weight, if they have had a shunt or hydrocephalus, and if they are up to date on their immunisations.

» Drug history – Ask if the child is taking any medications.

» Social history – Ask who lives at home with them; if they have any siblings, and if so, if their siblings have any illnesses; if they are studying; if they have attended any crowded events (boarding school or youth camps); and if they have travelled abroad recently.

» Family history – Ask if there is a family history of any medical conditions.

## RED FLAGS

An evolving, non-blanching rash, delirium, focal neurological signs or if they are deteriorating rapidly.

## Examination

»   Vitals – BP (hypotension), pulse (tachycardia), temperature, respiratory rate, CPT (more than two seconds) and oxygen saturations.

*Normal Heart and Breathing Rates for Healthy Children*

| Age | Normal (Beats per Minute) | Normal (Breaths per Minute) |
|---|---|---|
| Birth – 1 year | 100–160 | 30–60 |
| 1–3 years | 90–150 | 24–40 |
| 3–6 years | 80–140 | 22–34 |
| 6–12 years | 70–120 | 18–30 |
| 12–18 years | 60–100 | 12–16 |

»   Inspection

  ›   General – Inspect the child generally. Check if they are tired, withdrawn, limp or confused. Check if they look pale, have a high-pitched cry or look dehydrated (sunken eyes and reduced skin turgor).

  ›   Rash – Look for a rash anywhere on the body. Check if it blanches and if each spot is >2mm in diameter.

»   Palpate – Feel the peripheries for evidence of being cold. In infants, check if the fontanelle is bulging.

»   Neurological – Perform a general screening using AVPU (check if they are **a**lert, if they respond to **v**oice, if they are in **p**ain or if they are totally **u**nresponsive). Perform a generalised CN examination (abnormal pupils) and a neurological assessment. Check if they flinch when a bright light is shone into their eyes.

»   Special tests

  ›   Kernig's sign – Determine whether the child complains of pain when the knee is passively extended, while keeping the hips flexed.

  ›   Brudzinski's sign – Check if the hips flex when the head is bent forwards.

## Investigations

Initiated in secondary care:

- » Bloods – FBC (infection), CRP, glucose, U&Es, coagulation screen (disseminated intravascular coagulation [DIC]), blood cultures (bacterial infection) and PCR (*Neisseria meningitidis*).

- » Urine – To exclude alternative causes.

- » CXR – To exclude alternative causes of fever.

- » Lumbar puncture – CSF sent for gram stain, TB, cytology, and glucose protein and culture.

- » CT/MRI – To exclude brain abscess and herniation.

## Management

### Conservative

- ✓ General – Advise them to wash their hands and practice good hygiene. They should not share drinks, straws or utensils. Advise them to stay healthy, and cover their mouth when coughing or wheezing.

- ✓ Travel – If they are travelling to the Hajj or sub-Saharan Africa, they should consider having a meningococcal groups A, C, W-135 and Y conjugate (MenACWY) injection.

- ✓ Gatherings – Advise them to avoid large social gatherings.

- ✓ Immunisations – Ensure they are immunised in line with the DoH schedule (MenC/Hib vaccine [pre-university] and pneumococcal vaccine).

- ✓ Health Protection Agency – Inform the Health Protection Agency / consultant in communicable disease control (CCDC) about the diagnosis.

### Medical

- ✓ Admission – Call 999 and request an ambulance to attend urgently.

  - › Bacterial (rash) – If bacterial meningitis is suspected, then give stat IM benzylpenicillin. If they are under one year old, give 300mg; if they are one to nine years old, give 600mg; and if they are >10 years old, give 1,200mg.

  - › Allergy – If they have a penicillin allergy, withhold the aforementioned and consider cefotaxime as an alternative.

  - › Viral – Refer them to a hospital for supportive therapy and possible initiation of acyclovir.

- ✓ Prophylaxis – Identify possible close contacts in the week before the onset of the illness (household contacts, partners, pupils in the same dormitory, etc.). Offer prophylaxis for meningococcal disease in the form of ciprofloxacin stat (azithromycin stat in pregnancy).

## Safety Netting

> » Red flags – Ensure it is explained to the parents what the red-flag symptoms are (non-blanching rash and photophobia), and that they are to seek medical advice should those symptoms occur.

> » Follow-up – Review the patient after discharge from hospital.

> » Audiology – Ensure that the patient is booked for an audiological assessment four weeks after discharge.

*References*

National Institute for Health and Care Excellence (2010). *Meningitis (bacterial) and meningococcal septicaemia in under 16s: recognition, diagnosis and management.* https://www.nice.org.uk/guidance/cg102

# Urinary Tract Infections

A UTI is defined as any infection that affects the urinary tract from the kidneys to the urethra. It is fairly rare in children, with girls being more prone to it than boys. It is estimated that around 8% of girls and 2% of boys will have a UTI by the age of seven. Structural abnormalities such as abnormal kidneys, vesicoureteric reflux or genital malformations may increase the risk of developing a UTI; however, in most cases, there is no evidence of an underlying problem. More commonly, functional problems such as holding the urine or constipation may be found and should be corrected. The most common bug implicated is *E. coli* (>75%) then *Klebsiella*.

## History

- » Focused questions
  - › Ask when the urinary problems began, how long it has been going on for, and if it is getting worse or better.
  - › Ask if they have any dysuria (any burning or stinging when passing urine), any tummy pain or any pain in the kidney area.
  - › Frequency – Ask if they are passing urine more often and how many times they are going a day (or how many wet nappies there are when appropriate).
  - › Nocturia – Ask if the child is passing urine at night, how many times they are going and if they are wetting the bed.
  - › Ask if there is any offensive smell or if there is blood in the urine.
  - › Ask if they have any constipation, and how often are they opening their bowels.
  - › Holding – Ask if their child voluntarily holds their wee to not to go to the toilet, if they urinate fewer than three times a day, and if they feel that their bladder is full even after they have been to the toilet.

- » Associated history – Ask if they have had any nausea and vomiting, fever or lethargy, and if they are feeding and taking fluids.

- » Past history – Ask if they were born prematurely, have any abnormalities (kidney or spinal problems from birth), or have had any UTIs in the past.

- » Birth history – Ask about the pregnancy, and if there was any renal malformation on the scans.

- » Drug history – Ask if they are taking / have taken any medications and if their immunisations are up to date.

- » Social history – Ask who lives at home with them.

- » Family history – Ask if there is a family history of any renal disorders.

- » Consider the presence of child abuse in a child who presents with recurrent UTI symptoms in the absence of a medical cause or in the presence of other factors (excessive genital itching, bruising or inappropriate sexual play).

## RED FLAGS

Dehydrated, lethargic or if there is suspected child abuse.

## Differentials

➤ DM – Ask if they feel thirsty all the time, and if they have lost any weight.

## Examination

» Vitals – BP, pulse, temperature, height and weight (growth charts).

» General – Inspect the child generally to check if they are tired, withdrawn or limp; or if they look pale or dehydrated (sunken eyes and decreased skin turgor).

» ENT – Examine the ears and throat to exclude other causes of fever. Examine for swollen cervical chain LNs.

» Abdomen – Examine the abdomen for swelling (bladder), masses (kidney) or pain. Palpate for constipation and loin pain.

» Genitals – Examine for any evidence of vulval adhesions or phimosis in boys, and check if there is any evidence of superficial irritation.

### Distinguishing Between Lower and Upper UTIs

» Upper UTI – Affects the kidneys (and ureter), with signs of loin pain, high swinging fever and rigors.

» Lower UTI – Affects the bladder (and urethra), with signs of dysuria, frequency and urgency.

## Investigations

» Bloods – Not routinely indicated. If necessary, consider FBC (infection), CRP, HbA1c and U&Es.

» Urine – Urine dipstick (leucocytes, nitrates and blood) and send for MC&S (even if the dipstick test is negative) to confirm the diagnosis.
**When to treat based on the dipstick results for children three years old and over**
> Positive leucocytes and negative nitrates – Do not give antibiotics and do not send for MSU.

> Negative leucocytes and positive nitrates – Start antibiotics and send for MSU.

> Positive leucocytes and negative nitrates – Do not start antibiotics (unless clear history), but send for MSU.

> › Positive leucocytes and positive nitrates – Start antibiotics, and only send for MSU if there has been a previous UTI or a risk of serious illness.

» USS – If there are recurrent UTIs, do a USS to look for a structural deformity or a thickening bladder.

» Specialist – Micturating cystography (urethral defects) if a UTI is suspected in a child under three months old. DMSA scintigraphy (renal defects) if a UTI is suspected in a child under three years old, or for a recurrent UTI in a child over three years old.

## Management

### Conservative

✓ Fluids – Advise them to ensure that the child is drinking plenty of water in small amounts regularly.

✓ Hygiene – Advise them to ensure the child washes their hands after going to the toilet, and avoid bubble baths.

✓ Toileting – Advise the parents on correct techniques, such as wiping from front to back for girls and not to repeat using the same piece of tissue. They should ensure the child has good access to a potty or toilet, and encourage to go when they feel the need.

✓ Clothing – Advise them to avoid the child wearing tight-fitting clothes and that they should wear cotton underwear.

✓ Constipation – Advise them to increase the child's fibre intake (brown bread, cereal, fruit and vegetables) and ensure they exercise regularly.

✓ Dysfunctional voiding – Advise them to take the child to urinate every two to three hours, even if they do not feel the need. They should increase the child's water consumption and treat constipation.

### Medical

✓ Aged under three months – If a UTI is suspected, then admit them under a paediatrician.

✓ Aged three months or over – If this is their first UTI, treat it with trimethoprim (lower UTI) or augmentin (upper UTI).

✓ Urgent – If there are any high-risk factors (poor urine output, a dilated bladder, poor growth or a genetic abnormality), then refer them urgently to hospital.

✓ Recurrent UTI – If the child has had three lower UTIs, two upper UTIs, or one lower and one upper UTI, then refer them to a paediatrician for assessment.

✓ Prophylaxis – Initiated in secondary care. Consider long-term antibiotics in patients with severe, recurrent UTIs or structural abnormalities (first-line treatment is trimethoprim or nitrofurantoin, and second-line treatment is cephalexin or amoxicillin).

✓ Culture – If the culture shows that the organism is resistant to the initial antibiotic, check if the symptoms have improved. If they have, complete the course and recheck the culture to ensure that the infection has cleared. If the symptoms have not improved, then change the antibiotic to one to which the organism is sensitive.

## Safety Netting

> » Ensure the parents have an appropriate follow-up appointment to return in two to four weeks if there is no improvement. Ensure they know to return as an emergency if the child is dehydrated or lethargic.

---

### References

National Institute for Health and Care Excellence (2007). *Urinary tract infection in under 16s: diagnosis and management.* https://www.nice.org.uk/guidance/cg54

National Institute for Health and Care Excellence (2018). *Urinary tract infection (recurrent): antimicrobial prescribing.* https://www.nice.org.uk/guidance/ng112

# Nocturnal Enuresis

Nocturnal enuresis relates to the problem of bedwetting in a child who is of an age where control is expected. It is defined as involuntary wetting during sleep in the absence of congenital or acquired defects. It occurs more commonly in boys and in those of lower social classes. It can be quite a distressing and embarrassing disorder for parents and child alike, and it is important to broach the subject in an emphatic and non-judgemental way. Any underlying illness or side effects of medication need to be reliably excluded if the child had been previously dry at night for more than six months.

Most children with enuresis do not suffer from psychological disorders, other illnesses or conditions associated with urinary symptoms (e.g. UTI or DM), which rarely present with enuresis. Daytime enuresis is more common in girls and is usually due to urge incontinence as a result of bladder instability.

Medical management for nocturnal enuresis is often considered after the child is over five years old. Most children are continent during both night and day by the age of three to four years. However, approximately 20% of five-year-olds wet the bed twice a week, which falls to 9% of nine-year-olds. Primary nocturnal enuresis is when the child has never stopped bedwetting, while secondary is when the child had been dry for the previous six months.

## Causes of Enuresis

*Primary*

➤ Without daytime symptoms – Sleep-arousal challenges (inability to sense a full bladder, contraction or waking due to noise), polyuria and an overactive bladder.

➤ With daytime symptoms – Overactive bladder (daytime wetting, urgency, frequency and a poor stream), chronic constipation, UTI, structural abnormalities or neurogenic bladder.

*Secondary*

➤ DM, constipation, UTI, psychological (stress) and child maltreatment.

## History

» Focused questions
› Ask when they first noticed the bed wetting.
› Ask about the onset (sudden or over a period of time).
› Pattern – Ask how long it has been going on for, how many nights a week, how many times a night and at what time of night it occurs.
› Ask about the amount of urine passed.
› Primary/secondary – Ask if they are wet during the day and if they have ever been dry.
› Daytime – Ask how often they pass urine during the day, and if they have any accidents or a feeling of urgency.

» Associated history – Ask if there are any issues with the child's development or achieving milestones (walking, eating, speaking and potty training).

» Past history – Ask if they have DM or ADHD.

» Family history – Ask if they have enuresis or DM.

» Drug history – Ask if they are taking / have taken any medications.

» Social history – Ask who lives with them at home and how things are at home; if they have brothers or sisters, what the relationship between them is like, and if any of them have any illnesses; if they are known to social services; and if they go to nursery or school, how they are performing and if they have any unauthorised days off.

## RED FLAGS

Painless jaundice or weight loss.

## Differential Diagnosis

| Nocturnal enuresis | More common in boys. Associated with FH, ADHD and obesity (30% of obese children have nocturnal enuresis). Often caused by sleep-arousal difficulties (inability to sense a full bladder), polyuria or bladder dysfunction (overactive). Exclude other causes such as UTI, constipation and psychological issues. |
|---|---|
| UTI | Common (8% of girls at five years). Nocturia, frequency and urgency. May have smelly and dark urine. OE: suprapubic pain. Dipstick test for leukocytes and nitrates, and if both are positive, MSU if they are under five years, which needs a referral. |
| Type 1 DM | Rare. Causes weight loss, severe thirst, hunger, tiredness, frequency and nocturia. If it is very high, it may lead to ketoacidosis. O/E: thin, unwell child, with raised BMs. Dipstick for ketones and glucose. Needs an urgent referral to hospital. |

## Examination

» Vitals – Temperature (fever), BMI and monitor growth.

» Abdominal – Examine the abdomen (constipation) and genitalia if appropriate.

» Neurological

› Spine – Inspect the back for sacral simple, naevus or hair (meningomyelocele).

> Lower limbs – Perform a neurological assessment of the lower limbs, including ankle reflexes.

## Investigations

» Urine – Urine dipstick and MC&S (DM and UTI).

» Specialist – USS of bladder and kidneys.

## Management

*Conservative*

✓ Reassure

> Child under five years – Reassure that nocturnal enuresis is common (5% of 10-year-olds) and often resolves spontaneously without treatment. Advise them to consider placing a potty by the bed and ensure easy access to the toilet. If they have been trained for more than six months, consider one or more nights in a row without nappies/pull-ups (with a waterproof mattress / mattress cover).

> Child over five years – If it has been happening less than two times per week, consider monitoring only. If it is more than this, consider offering treatments (alarms).

✓ Diary – Offer a bladder diary, including recording fluid intake and urine output over two weeks.

✓ Toilet – Encourage toilet training. Advise them to take the child to the toilet if the child wakes up in the night. They should trial several nights (at least two) in a row without nappies/pull-ups. They should always get the child to empty their bladder before going to sleep.

✓ Voiding – Advise them that, during day, the child should void their bladder every two to three hours and they should avoid holding it when they have the urge to urinate.

✓ Mattress – Advise using a waterproof cover for their mattress, and absorbent quilted sheets or pads.

✓ Excess fluid – Advise them to avoid the child having an excessive fluid intake, particularly one hour before bed, or having abnormal toileting patterns. The daily intake for four- to eight-year-olds is 1–1.4l, and for 9–13-year-olds it is 1.2–2.3l.

✓ Behaviour

> Rewards – Suggest using star charts for agreed behaviour rather than simply a dry night (e.g. drinking the correct volume of fluid, going to the toilet before sleeping and having clean sheets).

> Advise them to stress that it is not the child's fault. They should not use penalty systems if the child fails (taking stars away). Punitive measures and blame should be avoided.

*Medical*

✓ Enuresis alarm – Consider an enuresis alarm if they have not responded to lifestyle advice (often in those >10 years old). It wakes the child when they start urinating. They can be worn in the trousers or be a sensor pad that is placed under the child. This conditions the child to wake up and go to the toilet once they start passing urine. Eventually, the child learns to wake up and hold their bladder before wetting the bed. This can be trialled for four months until two weeks of continuous dry nights have been achieved. The treatment may last for three to five months. Alarms are not recommended for children under five years, as it requires cooperation.

✓ Desmopressin – Usually started by a specialist. Offer desmopressin (200mcg po or 120mcg sublingual) for those over seven years old if a rapid or short-term improvement is sought (e.g. for a social occasion), or if the alarm is unsuccessful or inappropriate. It is taken at night as a tablet. Only sips of drink are allowed one hour before taking the medicine and up to eight hours after. It is effective for short-term use or one off measures (short holiday trips). Review within four weeks.

✓ TCAs (imipramine) – These have antimuscarinic effects, and are prescribed by specialists. They should be considered when all other options have been explored. Alternatives include antimuscarinics (e.g. oxybutynin).

## Referral

→ Refer them to the enuresis clinic if a primary cause is identified or there are daytime symptoms.

→ Refer them if treatment has failed despite two courses (alarm, desmopressin or both).

*References*

National Institute for Health and Care Excellence (2010). *Nocturnal enuresis – the management of bedwetting in children and young people.* https://www.nice.org.uk/guidance/cg111/evidence/cg111-nocturnal-enuresis-the-management-of-bedwetting-in-children-and-young-people-full-guideline3

Caldwell, P.H.Y., Deshpande, A.V., Von Gontard, A. (2013). Management of nocturnal enuresis (clinical review). *BMJ, 347,* f6259. doi: https://doi.org/10.1136/bmj.f6259

# Functional Constipation

Constipation is a common problem in children, with some estimates claiming that up to 30% of children suffer from it. In both the primary and secondary care settings, it is one of the most common attendances with around 25% of a paediatric gastroenterologist's workload being due to it. It is defined as the decrease in the frequency of bowel movements with the passage of hard stools, which may give rise to pain. Normal bowel movements vary depending on the age of the child.

For the vast majority of sufferers, this is due to functional problems, with only 5% being due to an underlying medical condition. There is no single agreed definition as to when a patient is constipated. However, Rome IV (Drossman, Chang, Chey, Kellow, Tack and Whitehead, 2017) has created some diagnostic criteria for functional constipation. Chronic constipation is defined as when the problem persists for more than two months, and it is found in around 33% of cases.

## Rome IV Diagnostic Criteria for Functional Constipation (Drossman et al., 2017)

In children over four years, it must include two or more of the following, occurring at least once a week for the past month:

➤ Two defecations or fewer per week

➤ At least one episode per week of incontinence after the acquisition of toileting skills

➤ A history of retentive posturing or excessive volitional stool retention

➤ A history of painful or hard bowel movements

➤ The presence of a large faecal mass in the rectum

➤ A history of large diameter stools that may obstruct the toilet

## *History*

» Focused questions

› Ask when the problems began, how long it has been going on for, and if it is getting worse or better.

› Frequency – Ask if their child opens their bowels regularly and how often they go.

› Ask if there is any straining (struggling to pass a motion).

› Ask about the appearance of the stools (rabbit droppings), and use the Bristol stool chart to identify the stool type.

› Ask if there is any pain when going to pass stools.

› Incontinence – Ask if they soil their undergarments or overflow.

› Posture – Ask how the child sits when they go to the toilet.

› Ask if there have been any triggers, such as moving house, starting school, after potty training, new stress in the family (including new additions) or their parents arguing.

» Associated history – Ask if they have had any nausea and vomiting, how they are feeding (what milk is being used and if there has been any weaning onto solids), what their fluid intake is like (if they are passing urine okay and how many wet nappies they have), and if there is any blood on the toilet paper after wiping.

» Past history – Ask if they were born prematurely, have any disability (Down's syndrome, cerebral palsy [CP] or autism), or have any anal problems or a UTI.

» Birth history – Ask about the pregnancy and the birth; ask if the child passed stools within 48 hours of the birth.

» Drug history – Ask if they are taking / have taken any medications (particularly opiates or antihistamines), and if they are up to date with their immunisations.

» Social history – Ask who lives at home with them; if they have moved recently; if they have any siblings and what the current relationships between them are like; and if they have any issues at nursery/school.

» Family history – Ask if there is a family history of Hirschsprung's disease.

## RED FLAGS

Constipation from birth, abdominal distention, vomiting, suspected child abuse or blood in the stools.

## Differential Diagnosis

| Anal fissures | A tear to the anal mucosa that is often posterior to the anal canal. Pain on defecation with blood on the toilet paper after wiping. Associated with constipation. On examination, a fissure is visible. Very tender on PR exam. |
|---|---|
| Obstruction | Colicky abdominal pain, distension and absolute constipation, including wind. Bowels not opened. Tinkling bowel sounds. |
| Hirschsprung's disease | Constipation present from the first week of birth. A delay in passing meconium of >48 hours after delivery at full term. May vomit when fed. OE: abdominal distension. Failure to thrive. |

## Examination

» Vitals – BP, pulse, temperature, weight and height (growth charts).

» General – Inspect the child generally. Check if they are well, silent and listless, or have signs of Down's syndrome. Look for signs of bruising.

» Abdomen – Inspect for distention. Palpate for swelling (impacted faeces), pain and constipation. Auscultate for bowel sounds.

» PR – Not routinely required. If only one Rome IV criterion is present and there is diagnostic uncertainty, a PR may be helpful. If you suspect congenital abnormalities, inspect the anus. Look for anal fissures.

## Investigations

» Bloods – Not routinely indicated. If indicated, FBC (infection), U&Es (dehydration), TFTs (hypothyroid) and TTGA antibodies (coeliac).

» AXR/USS – Not usually needed in primary care. May help if faecal impaction is suspected.

» Specialist – Transit studies or a rectal biopsy (Hirschsprung's disease).

## Management

### Conservative

✓ Reassure – Reassure them of the diagnosis of functional constipation and that no underlying serious medical condition has been found. Explain that it is very common (30% of children) and treatable.

✓ Diary – Offer a bowel diary, including daytime fluid intake and dietary intake.

✓ Fluids – Advise them to ensure that the child drinks plenty of water in small amounts regularly.

✓ Toileting – Advise the parents on correct techniques. They should try scheduled toileting where the child is taken to the toilet at regular intervals. They should use warm water or Vaseline around the anus to soothe it and help pass the stools. Consider a simple massage of the abdomen prior to going to the toilet, starting from the right hip area (RIF) up and across, then down towards the left hip (LIF).

✓ Diet

> Fruit – Advise them to increase their intake of fruit and vegetables (particularly apples, pears, prunes and apricots). This can be via fresh fruit juice. Dry fruits have a higher concentration of sorbitol.

> Fibre – Advise them to increase their fibre consumption by eating coarse bran, wholegrain bread, wholemeal flour, brown rice and wholemeal spaghetti.

✓ Exercise – Encourage them to exercise for 30–60 minutes daily.

✓ Behaviour

> Rewards – Use star charts for agreed behaviour (e.g. drinking the correct volume of fluid and going to toilet at regular intervals).

> Advise them to stress that it is not the child's fault. They should not use penalty systems if the child fails (taking stars away). Punitive measures and blame should be avoided.

### Medical

✓ Oral – Use Movicol Paediatric Plain as the first-line treatment. If there is no improvement after two weeks, then add a stimulant laxative (bisacodyl or senna). Consider lactulose instead of Movicol if the patient is intolerant.

✓ PR – Do not use unless PO treatment has failed. Consider a sodium citrate enema. Do not use a phosphate enema except in a hospital setting.

✓ Maintenance – Commence maintenance treatment and continue until several weeks after regular bowel motion is established. Titrate down the doses over a period of months, depending on stool consistency and frequency.

## Safety Netting

» Follow-up – Ensure the parents have an appropriate follow-up appointment to return in one to two weeks to adjust the response.

## Referral

→ Consider referring them to a specialist if there are any red flags or a poor response to treatment (if they are under one year old and there is no response to treatment after one month, or they are over one year old and there is no response to treatment after three months).

→ Specialist – They may manually evacuate, offer enemas or employ psychological therapies.

---

### References

National Institute for Health and Care Excellence (2010). *Constipation in children and young people: diagnosis and management*. https://www.nice.org.uk/guidance/cg99

Drossman, D. A, (Author, Ed.), Chang, L. (Ed.), Chey, W.D. (Ed.), Kellow, J. (Ed.), Tack, J. (Ed.) and Whitehead, W.E. (2017). *Rome IV Functional Gastrointestinal Disorders: Disorders of Gut-Brain Interaction Volume 1*. Rome Foundation, Inc.

# Upper Respiratory Tract Infections

URTIs are illnesses that are caused by an infection affecting the throat (pharyngitis or tonsillitis), sinuses (sinusitis), nose (rhinitis), ears (otitis), trachea (tracheitis) or larynx (laryngitis). They are extremely common, with children experiencing an average of six colds per year. They all usually present as self-limiting conditions, most commonly triggered by viruses (rhinoviruses or coronaviruses), and give symptoms such as lethargy, myalgia and fever. Symptoms worsen for the first three days before gradually clearing on their own, usually within two weeks. Occasionally, bacteria may be implicated in the infection process and may require clearing with a course of antibiotics.

Despite being extremely common, URTIs still cause much angst and worry for parents and carers alike. Looking after a hot, feverish and miserable child is not an easy task, and parents frequently attend the GP for a magical panacea that will make everything better overnight; it is still incorrectly believed that this is in the form of antibiotics. When dealing with a tired and stressed carer, it is important to remain empathetic and show your concern about the child's health. You will have to educate them and explain the natural course of the illness before safety netting and advising if and when they may have to return.

## History

» Principles

  › Listen to the mum – If the child is of a young age and attends with a parent, listen carefully and acknowledge what they are saying. Acknowledge the level of concern of the parent or carer in making your diagnosis.

» Open questions – *'Can you tell me more about your child's problems? Could you tell me about what has been troubling them?'*

» Focused questions

  › Otitis media – Ask if they have any otalgia (ear pain) and if they are tugging at their ears; ask if there has been any otorrhoea (discharge from the ear), and if so, what colour it was and if the ear pain settled afterwards; and ask if there are any problems with hearing, any delay in speech or language, or any concentration issues at school.

  › Tonsillitis – Ask if they have had a sore throat, dysphagia (affecting swallowing), otalgia or stridor (noisy breathing).

  › Croup – Ask if they have had a cough (barking in nature and worse at night), hoarseness of their voice or stridor (noise when breathing in), and if there are any triggers.

  › Sinusitis – Ask if they have any nasal symptoms, such as a discharge (and if so, what colour it was); any facial pain (headache or pain on the face); a cough; or any problems with their sense of smell.

» Associated history – Ask if they have any fever, nausea and vomiting, lethargy or headaches; ask how they are feeding and what their fluid intake is like (are they passing urine or have wet nappies); and ask how their bowels are functioning.

» Past history – Ask if they have had otitis media, and if their immunisations are up to date.

» Birth history – Ask if they were born prematurely, and how they are being fed (breastfed or bottle fed).

» Drug history – Ask if they are taking / have taken any medications or have any allergies.

» Social history – Ask if they have experienced passive smoking, who lives at home with them, if they go to nursery and if they have any unwell contacts.

## RED FLAGS

Evolving, non-blanching rash; delirium; focal neurological signs; a rapidly deteriorating child; stridor or a breathing difficulty.

## Differential Diagnosis

| Otitis media | A common condition with a peak age of 6–15 months; it is rare in children of school age. Risk factors include passive smoking, going to a nursery, bottle feeding, craniofacial abnormalities and winter dummy use. Can be viral (respiratory syncytial virus [RSV] or rhinovirus) or bacterial (*Streptococcus pneumoniae* or *Haemophilus influenzae*). Child reports ear pain (older child), pulling or rubbing their ears, a cough, poor feeding and a high fever (>40°C). OE: red, cloudy, bulging tympanic membrane with or without fluid level. Occasional perforation with discharge. |
|---|---|
| Otitis media with effusion | Known as 'glue ear'; a collection of fluid within the middle ear with signs of inflammation. Seen in one- to six-year-olds. Can cause hearing loss (resolves in weeks to months), which can sometimes cause language delays. Similar risk factors to otitis media. OE: often no signs of inflammation of the tympanic membrane, effusion (blood, mucoid or purulent) with loss of light reflex, yellow or blue retracted drum, and a fluid level with air bubbles. |
| Tonsillitis | Common illness in children. May present with sore throat, painful swallowing, headache and loss of voice. Pain may radiate to the ears. OE: red tonsils with exudate, and tender anterior cervical LNs. |
| Sinusitis | Bacterial or viral infection of the sinuses (frontal, maxillary or ethmoid). Presents with cold- or flu-like illness, and symptoms include fever, tenderness over the sinuses, halitosis, nasal congestion with rhinitis, and pressure/throbbing over the head that worsens when bending forwards. |

| Croup | Viral infection (e.g. parainfluenza) that affects infants aged from 6–36 months, particularly in the autumn and spring seasons. Starts with coryzal symptoms of a sore throat and mild fever, progressing to a barking cough, hoarseness or inspiratory stridor with a high fever (>40°C). The cough often occurs at night or when a child is agitated. |
|---|---|
| Bronchiolitis | Caused by RSV. Often seen in winter months. Typically affects those under one year old, and presents with a fever and a runny nose. Worsening symptoms include an irritable cough, worsening SOB and feeding difficulties. OE: widespread fine crepes with a high-pitched wheeze. |
| Scarlet fever | Produces a characteristic red-blush blanching rash, which starts on day two and fades slowly over three weeks. Can start from the upper chest or neck, spreading to the abdomen and extremities, and skin creases that can peel off (toes and fingers). Has a sandpaper-like texture. Associated with exudative tonsillitis (red spots on the palate, a flushed face and a strawberry tongue). |
| Glandular fever | Infectious disease spread by saliva and is caused by EBV. Presents with a fever and acute fatigue with a worsening sore throat, lymphadenopathy and a macular rash. Can last for two to three weeks. Check for splenomegaly. Complications includes a splenic rupture. |

## Examination

Perform a focused examination based on the clinical findings.

- » Vitals – Pulse, temperature, respiratory rate, CPT and oxygen saturations.

- » General – Inspect the child to see if they are tired, withdrawn or pale. Look for signs of dehydration (sunken eyes and decreased skin turgor).

  - › Check for a rash on the body (if found, check for blanching and size), skin texture (a sandpaper-like texture indicates scarlet fever) and peeling of the skin.

- » Throat – Use a tongue depressor, and inspect for enlarged, red tonsils or exudate (tonsilitis). Inspect the tongue for colour (strawberry indicates scarlet fever). Check for halitosis (sinusitis).

- » Ears – Inspect the ears and check they are not displaced. Look at the tympanic membrane and determine the colour (red or cloudy), the shape (bulging or retracted) and the presence of a fluid level. Check for any perforations or discharge, and for loss of the light reflex. Check for any redness or tenderness of the mastoid area.

- » Sinuses – Palpate the frontal, maxillary and ethmoid sinuses.

- » Chest – Inspect for tachypnoea, intercostal recession and stridor. Listen for a wheeze or crepitations.

- » LNs – Consider palpating the cervical LNs (tonsils, anterior, posterior, pre- and post-auricular, and occipital).

» Other – Palpate for splenomegaly if glandular fever is suspected.

## Investigations

*Investigate the underlying cause*

» Bloods – Not routinely required. If indicated, FBC, CRP and antistreptolysin O (ASO) titres.

> Others – LFTs, blood film (mononuclear leukocytosis) and the monospot test for glandular fever.

» Swab – Not routinely required. If indicated, ear discharge swab and throat swab.

» Urine – Consider checking this if their fever >38°C and there is no source of infection.

» Specialist – Audiometry (persistent hearing loss) or pneumatic otoscope for otitis media with effusion.

## Management

*Treat the underlying cause*

### Conservative

✓ General – Advise them to wash their hands and practise good hygiene. They should not share drinks, straws or utensils. Advise them to stay healthy, and cover their mouth when they cough or sneeze.

✓ OTC – Advise that steam inhalation may help to relieve congestion. Vapour rubs may soothe respiratory symptoms (apply to the chest and back, and avoid using in the nose area). Gargling with salt water or sucking menthol sweets may help relieve the symptoms of a sore throat or nasal congestion.

✓ Avoidances (for those under six years old) – Advise them to avoid giving cough syrups and antihistamines to young children.

### Otitis media

✓ Advice – Reassure the parents that this often resolves within four days without antibiotics. Advise the parents not to smoke, to avoid giving the child dummies, and to consider breastfeeding.

✓ Analgesia – Offer paracetamol with or without NSAIDs.

✓ Antibiotics – Avoid prescribing these unless the condition is severe. Recommend five days oral (not drops) amoxicillin or clarithromycin/erythromycin.

> When considering giving antibiotics for otitis media, only prescribe them for one of the following:

- Bilateral, acute otitis media in a child under two years old.

- If the child is systemically very unwell.

- Acute otitis media in children with otorrea.

- If the child has signs of complications (if mastoiditis is suspected, refer them).

- If there is a high risk of comorbidity (immunosuppressed, premature, or has CF or organ disease).

✓ Admission – Admit the child if they are under three months old, have mastoiditis or are systemically very unwell.

✓ Referral – Refer them to ENT if they have persistent symptoms that are irresponsive to antibiotics, a discharge or perforation after two to three weeks, or impaired hearing.

## Otitis media with effusion

✓ Advice – Reassure the parents that it often resolves in 6–12 weeks (90%) with monitoring. Advise the parents not to smoke around the child.

✓ Antibiotics – Not recommended.

✓ Referral – If there is hearing loss, refer them to audiology. If there is significant hearing loss (including bilateral), they have Down's syndrome or a development delay, refer them to ENT.

✓ Surgery – Consider for surgery if they have persistent bilateral otitis media with effusion for more than three months and with hearing loss. Treatment is with grommets or an adenoidectomy. Alternatively, hearing aids or autoinflation may be offered.

## Tonsillitis / sore throat

✓ Advice – Reassure the parents that a sore throat, pharyngitis and acute tonsillitis often resolves within one week. Advise them to avoid hot drinks, but have an adequate fluid intake. For older children, recommend salt-water gargles, lozenges, hard-boiled sweets and ice cream for symptomatic treatment.

✓ Analgesia – Offer paracetamol or NSAIDs.

✓ Antibiotics – Use the Centor criteria to support the decision. If antibiotics are indicated, give 10 days of penicillin V, or if they have a penicillin allergy, give erythromycin for five days. Avoid prescribing broad-spectrum antibiotics (amoxicillin is more appropriate for maculopapular rashes). Give a delayed prescription that may be used if symptoms are worsening or they have not improved in three days.

## Centor Criteria for Diagnosing Group A Beta-Haemolytic Streptococcus

A patient with a sore throat and three or more of the following features may benefit from antibiotic use:

› Tonsillar exudate

› Absence of a cough

› Tender anterior cervical LNs

› Fever

✓ Admission – Admit them if there are signs of peritonsillar abscess.

✓ Referral

› Refer them if they have had a sore throat or painful swallowing for more than three weeks.

› Refer them for a tonsillectomy if they have had five or more infections a year, it is severe enough to impact daily function or causes sleep apnoea.

✓ Follow-up – Review as soon as possible if they have SOB, stridor, drooling, dysphagia, severe pain, cannot keep fluids down or they become systemically unwell.

## Croup

✓ Advice – Reassure the parents that it is often a self-limiting illness, which often resolves within two days, but it can persist for one week. Advise them to get the child upright if they are crying or they have stridor, and to ensure they have an adequate fluid intake. Do not recommend steam inhalation, but rather breathing cool air by taking a stroll outside.

✓ Antipyrexia – Offer paracetamol or NSAIDs for a high fever.

✓ Antibiotics – Not recommended.

✓ Steroids – Give stat oral dexamethasone (0.15mg/kg) or prednisolone (1mg/kg).

✓ Admission – Admit them if they have severe croup, persistent stridor, respiratory distress, intercostal recession or cyanosis.

✓ Follow-up - Review them as soon as possible if they have worsening SOB, a high fever, or are restless or pale. Call 999 if they become cyanotic, become drowsy or unusually sleepy, struggle to breathe, or start drooling.

## Acute sinusitis

✓ Advice – Reassure the parents that this is a self-limiting illness that often lasts for two and a half weeks. Advise that they ensure the child has an adequate fluid intake. They should apply warm face packs.

✓ Analgesia – Offer paracetamol or NSAIDs for the pain. Sodium chloride nasal drops can be considered.

✓ Nasal steroids – Consider these in children >12 years old, but only for prolonged symptoms (two weeks or more).

✓ Antibiotics – Only give antibiotics if there is evidence of a bacterial infection, such as a purulent discharge (often unilateral), severe local pain (often unilateral), a high fever >38°C or a marked worsening of symptoms. Offer a prescription of penicillin V or co-amoxiclav, but if they are allergic to penicillin, offer doxycycline, or offer clarithromycin if they are >12.

✓ Admission – Admit them if they are systemically unwell, or there is intracranial (meningitis) or orbital spread (cellulitis).

✓ Referral – Refer them to ENT if it is recurrent (more than three instances requiring antibiotics in a year).

✓ Follow-up – A follow-up is required if the symptoms worsen, or they have a high fever or severe pain that is mainly unilateral.

## Natural Average Length of Conditions

| Condition | Length of time |
|---|---|
| Acute otitis media | Four days |
| Acute tonsillitis | Seven days |
| Acute pharyngitis | Seven days |
| Common cold | 10 days |
| Acute rhinosinusitis | 16–18 days |
| Acute cough/bronchitis | 21 days |

## References

National Institute for Health and Care Excellence (2008). *Respiratory tract infections (self-limiting): prescribing antibiotics.* https://www.nice.org.uk/guidance/CG69

National Institute for Health and Care Excellence (2018). *Sore throat (acute): antimicrobial prescribing.* https://www.nice.org.uk/guidance/ng84

National Institute for Health and Care Excellence (2019). *Fever in under 5s: assessment and initial management.* https://www.nice.org.uk/guidance/ng143

# Limping

Children are often active, mobile beings who are difficult to keep still. When a child presents with a limp, it can be quite a worrying sight for the parents. A limp is often caused by a simple sprain, a minor injury or even a splinter in the foot. However, if there is no obvious cause of the limp, then further evaluation is required. The most common cause of a limp is an irritable hip triggered by a URTI, but other more serious causes – such as septic arthritis or Perthe's disease – should be excluded.

## *Common causes of limping in a child by age*

| | |
|---|---|
| <3 years | Fracture or soft-tissue injury (child abuse or a toddler fracture – a twisting injury), DDH, or an infection (septic arthritis / osteomyelitis). |
| 3–10 years | Fracture or soft-tissue injury (child abuse or stress fracture), transient synovitis, an infection (septic arthritis / osteomyelitis), or Perthe's disease. |
| 10–18 years | Fracture or soft-tissue injury (child abuse or stress fracture), slipped upper femoral epiphysis (SUFE), an infection (septic arthritis / osteomyelitis), Perthe's disease, Osgood-Schlatter disease, Sever's disease, osteochondritis dissecans, or chondromalacia patellae. |
| Rarer causes | Cancer (sarcoma, leukaemia or lymphoma), rickets, sickle cell disease, muscular dystrophy or juvenile idiopathic arthritis. |

## *History*

» Focused questions

› Ask when they first noticed the limp and how long it has been going on for.

› Site – Ask if the limp is with one or both legs.

› Onset – Ask if the onset was sudden or gradual.

› Trauma – Ask if they had any fall or injury.

› Ask if there is any pain anywhere (hip, knee or bone), when the pain is worse, and if it is on one or both sides.

› Infants – Ask if there is any pain when changing the child's nappy (back flexion indicates discitis).

› Ask if there is any swelling of the joints.

› Movements – Ask if they have any difficulty walking or if they refuse to stand.

› Ask if the limp has changed over time.

» Associated history – Ask if they have any fever, sweats or shivers; a recent URTI; any weight loss; or any skin or nail changes.

» Past history – Ask if they have sickle cell disease, rickets or SLE; what the delivery at birth was like (breech); and if they have had any delay in reaching milestones (walking, eating, speaking and potty training).

» Family history – Ask if there is a family history of any hip problems (RA, juvenile idiopathic arthritis or muscular dystrophy).

» Drug history – Ask if they are taking / have taken any medications, particularly steroids.

» Social history – Ask how things are at home, if they go to nursery or school, and if they have had any days off because of their symptoms.

## RED FLAGS

» Fever or sweats (septic arthritis), trauma (fracture), weight loss or night pain (malignancy), or child maltreatment (e.g. bruising in a child who is not independently mobile – particularly in clusters).

## Examination

*See Hip Pain section, page 431.*

## Differential Diagnosis

| Irritable hip (transient synovitis) | Common in boys from two to twelve years old (the mean is six years), and associated with a viral infection (mild fever) or mild trauma. Presents with acute hip pain and a limp that improves gradually over 10 days. Both hips are often affected. The child is systemically well. OE: hip held in flexion, abduction and moderate external rotation. Limited ROM, particularly in adduction and extension (it increases the intracapsular pressure). Often a diagnosis of exclusion. |
|---|---|
| Perthe's disease | Avascular necrosis to the femoral head resulting in abnormal growth. Seen in children from three to eleven years (with the peak age of four to seven years), and more common in boys. Around 10% is bilateral. Presents with insidious onset (over one month) of hip pain, knee pain (synovitis) or groin pain, which causes a limp. OE: short stature, reduced abduction, internal rotation, leg length inequality and positive Thomas test. |
| Malignancy | For example, neuroblastomas, leukaemias (all) and osteosarcomas. Presents with pain at night and/or bone pain that is distant from the joint. |

| Juvenile idiopathic arthritis | Arthritis developing in those <16 years for more than three months. Varies in presentation, but often affects the large joints. May present with a painless limp. Associated features include fever (swinging), maculopapular rash and arthralgia. Similar features to RA. |
|---|---|
| Septic arthritis / osteomyelitis | Bacterial infection of the joint space that often spreads from the blood, a penetrating wound or a local infection (chronic osteomyelitis). Often seen in those who are immunosuppressed, those who have DM or RA, or as a result of steroid use or recent joint surgery. Presents with a high fever and an unwell child with a swollen, tender, red hip joint. Often absent movements due to pain, with point tenderness. Signs of tachycardia and swinging pyrexia. |
| SUFE | The upper femoral epiphysis slips across the femur and is displaced posteroinferiorly. Believed to be caused by rapid pubertal growth. Rare cause of a limp. More common in boys than girls, with the peak age in early adolescence (10–15 years). More often in the left hip than the right, but it can be bilateral. The child is often overweight and with hypothyroidism. Presents with pain in the hip, groin, medial thigh or referred to the knee. Made worse by walking or running. OE: reduced ROM of the hip (resists internal rotation), and the leg is rotated externally and shortened. |
| DDH | Otherwise known as the congenital dislocation of the hip. If it is not identified at birth through screening, it may present with hip pain, a limp or OA when older. More common in girls, those who are first born, those with a family history of DDH, those born from a breech presentation and those with a heavy birth weight. |
| Osgood-Schlatter disease | Presents with anterior knee pain during the teenage years. Occurs during a pubertal growth spurt when the quadriceps has grown and enlarged before the apophysis has fused to the tibia, causing several small avulsion fractures within the apophysis. Caused by excessive physical exertion (repeated knee flexion and forced extension) before skeletal maturity, and seen in young athletes. Often unilateral, and it affects males more than females. |

## Investigations

*Depends on the cause*

> » Infection screen – Hb, WCC, CRP and ESR.

> » Others – MSU, throat swab, aspiration of synovial fluid (septic arthritis), and blood C&S.

» X-ray – This is to exclude a fracture or the avascular necrosis of the femoral head (Perthe's disease). Consider an AP/lateral hip x-ray for SUFE.

» Other imaging – USS (irritable hip), MRI and bone scan.

## Management

*Treat the underlying cause*

### Irritable hip

✓ Reassure the parents, as it often resolves within two weeks. Recommend rest and analgesia. Advise that they keep the leg flexed and rotated externally.

✓ If there is effusion, consider aspiration.

✓ Once the pain settles, recommend mobilisation (e.g. swimming).

✓ Consider a follow-up x-ray after six weeks to exclude Perthe's disease.

✓ Referral – Refer them if the otherwise well child has not improved within one week of onset or has multiple presentations with a limp.

### Perthes' disease

✓ Advise that they rest, and that this generally heals over two to three years.

✓ Referral – Refer them to orthopaedics for bracing or surgery.

### SUFE

✓ Advise that they rest and avoid walking.

✓ Offer analgesia.

✓ Referral – Refer them to orthopaedics for a screw insertion or reconstructive surgery.

### Septic arthritis

✓ If this is suspected, admit them to hospital for surgical drainage and antibiotics.

### Juvenile arthritis

✓ Referral – Refer them to a rheumatologist. The treatment is similar to RA (e.g. NSAIDs, steroids [intra-articular or oral] and methotrexate.

## Referral

» Organise an urgent assessment if the child is under three years old with a limp, unable to bear weight or in severe pain.

» Also refer them if there are any red flags (fever, pain waking the child at night, weight loss, night sweats or signs of maltreatment).

» Refer them if SUFE is suspected and they are over nine years old with pain or restricted internal rotation.

## Safety Netting

» Review in one to two weeks to ensure the limp is improving.

---

### *References*

Partners in Paediatrics (2013). *Paediatric guidelines 2013–14*. https://www.networks.nhs.uk/nhs-networks/partners-in-paediatrics/documents/Paediatric%20guidelines%202013-14%20with%20links.pdf

# Glossary

| Acronym/Initialism | Meaning |
| --- | --- |
| 2WW | Two-week wait |
| A&E | Accident and Emergency |
| AAA | Abdominal aortic aneurysm |
| ABCT | Active cycle of breathing techniques |
| ABG | Arterial blood gas |
| a-blocker | Alpha blocker |
| ABPI | Ankle-brachial pressure index |
| ABPM | Ambulatory blood pressure monitoring |
| ACEI | Angiotensin-converting enzyme inhibitors |
| ACJ | Acromioclavicular joint |
| ACL | Anterior cruciate ligament |
| ACR | Albumin to creatinine ratio |
| ACS | Acute coronary syndrome |
| ADHD | Attention deficit hyperactivity disorder |
| ADLs | Activities of daily living |
| AF | Atrial flutter |
| AFP | Alpha-fetoprotein |
| AION | Anterior ischaemic optic neuropathy |
| AKI | Acute kidney injury |
| ALP | Alkaline phosphatase |
| ALT | Alanine transaminase |

| Acronym/Initialism | Meaning |
| --- | --- |
| AMH | Anti-mullerian hormone |
| AMTS | Abbreviated mental test score |
| ANA | Antinuclear antibody |
| anti-D | Antibody against D antigen |
| anti-dsDNA | Anti-double stranded deoxyribonucleic acid |
| anti-Sm | Anti-Smith |
| ARB | Angiotensin II receptor blocker |
| AS | Aortic stenosis |
| ASIS | Anterior superior iliac spine |
| ASO | Antistreptolysin O |
| AST | Aspartate aminotransferase test |
| AUDIT | Alcohol use disorders identification test |
| AUDIT-C | Alcohol use disorders identification test for consumption |
| AV | Arterio-venous |
| AVM | Arteriovenous malformation |
| AVN | Avascular necrosis |
| AXR | Abdominal x-ray |
| BASHH | British Association for Sexual Health and HIV |
| b-blocker | Beta blocker |
| BCC | Basal cell carcinoma |
| BCG | Bacillus Calmette-Guerin |
| bd | Twice a day |
| BDZ | Benzodiazepine |
| BHCG | Beta human chorionic gonadotropin |
| BM | Blood-sugar measurement |
| BMA | British Medical Association |
| BMI | Body mass index |
| BP | Blood pressure |
| BPAS | British Pregnancy Advisory Service |
| BPPV | Benign paroxysmal positional vertigo |
| BTS | British Thoracic Society |
| C&S | Culture and sensitivity |

| Acronym/Initialism | Meaning |
|---|---|
| C. diff | Clostridium difficile |
| CA | Citizens Advice |
| CA125 | Cancer antigen 125 |
| CABG | Coronary artery bypass graft |
| CAH | Congenital adrenal hyperplasia |
| CAMHS | Community Adolescent Mental Health Service |
| CAT | Cognitive analytic therapy |
| CCB | Calcium channel blocker |
| CCF | Congestive cardiac failure |
| CCG | Clinical Commissioning Group |
| CEA | Carcinoembryonic antigen |
| CF | Cystic fibrosis |
| CFS | Chronic fatigue syndrome |
| CHD | Coronary heart disease |
| CK | Creatine kinase |
| CKD | Chronic kidney disease |
| CMV | Cytomegalovirus |
| CN | Cranial nerve |
| CNS | Central nervous system |
| COCP | Combined oral contraceptive pill |
| COPD | Chronic obstructive pulmonary disease |
| CP | Cerebral palsy |
| CPN | Community psychiatric nurse |
| CREST | Calcinosis, Raynaud phenomenon, oesophageal dysmotility, sclerodactyly, and telangiectasia. |
| CRP | C-reactive protein |
| CSA | Clinical Skills Assessment |
| CSF | Cerebrospinal fluid |
| CT | Computerised tomography |
| CT | Cognitive therapy |
| CVA | Cerebrovascular accident |
| CVD | Cardiovascular disease |
| CVI | Certificate of visual impairment |
| DAFNE | Dose Adjustment For Normal Eating |

| Acronym/Initialism | Meaning |
|---|---|
| DDH | Developmental dysplasia of the hip |
| DES | Direct enhanced service |
| DESMOND | Diabetes Education and Self-Management for Ongoing and Newly Diagnosed |
| DEXA | Dual energy x-ray absorptiometry |
| DHEA | Dehydroepiandrosterone |
| DIC | Disseminated intravascular coagulation |
| DIP | Distal interphalangeal joint |
| DKA | Diabetic ketoacidosis |
| DLA | Disability Living Allowance |
| DM | Diabetes mellitus |
| DMARDs | Disease-modifying anti-rheumatic drugs |
| DN | District nurse |
| DNA | Deoxyribonucleic acid |
| DNAR | Do Not Attempt Resuscitation |
| DoH | Department of Health |
| DPP-4 | Dipeptidyl peptidase 4 |
| DRE | Digital rectal exam |
| DRSP | Daily Record of Severity of Problems |
| DTP | Diphtheria, tetanus and pertussis |
| DU | Duodenal ulcer |
| DUB | Dysfunctional uterine bleeding |
| DVLA | Driver and Vehicle Licensing Agency |
| DVT | Deep vein thrombosis |
| E. coli | Escherichia coli |
| EBV | Epstein-Barr virus |
| EC | Emergency contraception |
| ECG | Electrocardiogram |
| echo | Echocardiogram |
| ECT | Electroconvulsive therapy |
| EDD | Estimated date of delivery |
| EEG | Electroencephalogram |
| eGFR | Estimated glomerular filtration rate |
| ELISA | Enzyme-linked immunoassay |

| Acronym/Initialism | Meaning |
|---|---|
| EMA | Endomysium antibodies |
| EMDR | Eye movement desensitisation and reprocessing |
| EMG | Electromyography |
| ENT | Ear, nose and throat |
| ERCP | Endoscopic retrograde cholangiopancreatography |
| ESA | Employment and support allowance |
| ESR | Erythrocyte sedimentation |
| ESS | Epworth Sleepiness Scale |
| FAP | Familial adenomatous polyposis |
| FAST | Fast Alcohol Screening Test |
| FB | Foreign body |
| FBC | Full blood count |
| FGM | Female genital mutilation |
| FIT | Faecal immunochemical test |
| FOB | Faecal occult blood |
| FSH | Follicle stimulating hormone |
| G6PD | Glucose-6-phosphate dehydrogenase |
| GA | General anaesthetic |
| GAD | Generalised anxiety disorder |
| GCS | Glasgow coma scale |
| GET | Graded exercise therapies |
| GGT | Gamma-glutamyl transferase |
| GHD | Growth hormone deficiency |
| GI | Gastrointestinal |
| GP | General practice or general practitioner |
| GPPAQ | General Practice Physical Activity Questionnaire |
| GPwSI | General practitioner with special interest |
| GTN | Glyceryl trinitrate |
| GUM | Genitourinary medicine |
| H. pylori | Helicobacter pylori |
| HADS | Hospital Anxiety and Depression Scale |
| Hb | Haemoglobin |
| HbA1c | Haemoglobin A1c |

| Acronym/Initialism | Meaning |
| --- | --- |
| HBPM | Home blood pressure monitoring |
| hCG | Human chorionic gonadotropin |
| HDL | High-density lipoproteins |
| hep A | Hepatitis A |
| hep B | Hepatitis B |
| hep C | Hepatitis C |
| HF | Heart failure |
| Hib | Haemophilus influenzae type B |
| HIV | Human immunodeficiency virus |
| HLA | Human leukocyte antigen |
| HNPCC | Hereditary nonpolyposis colorectal cancer |
| HOCM | Hypertrophic obstructive cardiomyopathy |
| HONK | Hyperglycaemic hyperosmolar non-ketotic coma |
| HPA | Hypothalamic pituitary adrenal |
| HPV | Human papilloma virus |
| HR | Heart rate |
| HRT | Hormone replacement therapy |
| HSG | Hysterosalpingogram |
| HSV | Herpes simplex virus |
| HTLV | Human T-cell lymphotropic virus |
| HTN | Hypertension |
| HUS | Haemolytic uraemic syndrome |
| HVS | High vaginal swab |
| HZV | Herpes zoster virus |
| IBD | Inflammatory bowel disease |
| IBS-C | Constipation-predominant irritable bowel syndrome |
| IBS-D | Diarrhoea-predominant irritable bowel syndrome |
| IBS-M | Mixed type irritable bowel syndrome |
| ICAS | Independent Complaints Advocacy Service |
| ICD | Implantable cardioverter-defibrillator |
| ICS | Inhaled corticosteroid |
| IgA | Immunoglobulin A |
| IGF | Insulin-like growth factor |

| Acronym/Initialism | Meaning |
| --- | --- |
| IHD | Ischaemic heart disease |
| II | Integrase inhibitors |
| IIDB | Industrial Injuries Disablement Benefit |
| IM | Intramuscular |
| IMB | Intermenstrual bleeding |
| INR | International normalised ratio |
| IOP | Intraocular pressure |
| IP | Interphalangeal |
| IPSS | International Prostate Symptom Score |
| IPT | Interpersonal psychotherapy |
| IT | Information technology |
| ITU | Intensive Therapy Unit |
| IUCD | Intrauterine contraceptive device |
| IUI | Intrauterine insemination |
| IUS | Intrauterine system |
| IVF | In vitro fertilisation |
| IVU | Intravenous urography |
| JVP | Jugular venous pulse |
| LA | Local anaesthetic |
| LABA | Long-acting beta-antagonist |
| LAMA | Long-acting muscarinic antagonist |
| LARC | Long-acting reversible contraception |
| LBBB | Left bundle branch block |
| LD | Learning disorder |
| LDH | Lactate dehydrogenase |
| LDL | Low-density lipoprotein |
| L-dopa | Levodopa |
| LFT | Liver function test |
| LH | Luteinizing hormone |
| LIF | Left iliac fossa |
| LMP | Last menstrual period |
| LMWH | Low molecular weight heparin |
| LN | Lymph node |

| Acronym/Initialism | Meaning |
| --- | --- |
| LOC | Loss of consciousness |
| LOS | Lower oesophageal sphincter |
| LP | Lumbar puncture |
| LPA | Lasting power of attorney |
| LRINEC | Laboratory risk indicator for necrotising fasciitis |
| LTRA | Leukotriene receptor antagonists |
| LUQ | Left upper quadrant |
| LUTS | Lower urinary tract symptoms |
| LV | Left ventricular |
| LVH | Left ventricular hypertrophy |
| MAOI | Monoamine oxidase inhibitors |
| Max fax | Maxillofacial |
| MC&S | Microscopy, culture and sensitivity |
| MCP | Metacarpophalangeal |
| MCV | Mean corpuscular volume |
| MDMA | 3,4-methylenedioxymethamphetamine |
| MDT | Multidisciplinary team |
| ME | Myalgic encephalomyelitis |
| MenB | Meningitis B |
| MenC | Meningitis C |
| MFQ | Mood and Feelings Questionnaire |
| MI | Myocardial infarction |
| MMR | Measles, mumps and rubella |
| MMSE | Mini mental-state examination |
| MND | Motor neurone disease |
| MRC | Medical Research Council |
| MRCGP | Membership of the Royal College of General Practitioners |
| MRI | Magnetic resonance imaging |
| MRSA | Methicillin-resistant *Staphylococcus aureus* |
| MS | Multiple sclerosis |
| MSK | Musculoskeletal |
| MSU | Midstream specimen of urine |
| MTP | Metatarsophalangeal |

| Acronym/Initialism | Meaning |
| --- | --- |
| MTP | Metatarsophalangeal |
| NAFLD | Non-alcoholic fatty liver disease |
| NBM | Nil by mouth |
| NHS | National Health Service |
| NICE | National Institute for Health and Care Excellence |
| NNRTIs | Non-nucleoside reverse transcriptase inhibitors |
| NOAC | Non-Vitamin K antagonist oral anticoagulant |
| NRT | Nicotine replacement therapy |
| NRTIs | Nucleoside/nucleotide reverse transcriptase inhibitors |
| NSAIDs | Nonsteroidal anti-inflammatory drugs |
| NSPCC | National Society for the Prevention of Cruelty to Children |
| NTD | Neural tube defect |
| NYHA | New York Heart Association |
| OA | Osteoarthritis |
| OAB | Overactive bladder |
| OCI | Obsessive-Compulsive Inventory |
| OCP | Oral contraceptive pill |
| od | Once per day |
| OD | Overdose |
| OE | On examination |
| OGD | Oesophago-gastro-duodenoscopy |
| on | Once per night |
| OSA | Obstructive sleep apnoea |
| OSAHS | Obstructive sleep apnoea-hypopnoea syndrome |
| OSCE | Objective structured clinical examination |
| OT | Occupational therapy |
| OTC | Over the counter |
| PA | Physician associate |
| PAD | Peripheral arterial disease |
| PALS | Patient and Advice Liaison Service |
| PCB | Postcoital bleeding |
| PCMHT | Primary Care Mental Health Team |
| PCOS | Polycystic ovarian syndrome |

| Acronym/Initialism | Meaning |
| --- | --- |
| PCR | Protein-creatinine ratio |
| PD | Parkinson's disease |
| PD | Personality disorder |
| PDE5 | Phosphodiesterase type 5 inhibitor |
| PE | Pulmonary embolism |
| PEFR | Peak expiratory flow rate |
| PEG | Percutaneous endoscopic gastrostomy |
| PET | Positron emission tomography |
| PGL | Persistent generalised lymphadenopathy |
| PHQ 9 | Patient Health Questionnaire 9 |
| PI | Protease inhibitors |
| PID | Pelvic inflammatory disease |
| PIP | Personal independence payment |
| PMB | Post-menopausal bleeding |
| PMR | Polymyalgia rheumatica |
| PND | Paroxysmal nocturnal dyspnoea |
| PO | By mouth |
| pO2 | Partial pressure of oxygen |
| PO4 | Phosphate |
| POM | Practice of Medicine |
| POP | Progestogen-only pills |
| Post-op | Post-operative |
| PPI | Proton pump inhibitor |
| PR | Per rectum |
| PRN | *Pro re nata* (as needed) |
| proBNP | Pro b-type natriuretic peptide |
| PSA | Prostate-specific antigen |
| PTH | Parathyroid hormone |
| PTSD | Post-traumatic stress disorder |
| PU | Peptic ulcer |
| PUVA | Psoralen and ultraviolet A |
| PV bleeding | Per vaginal bleeding |
| PVD | Peripheral vascular disease |

| Acronym/Initialism | Meaning |
|---|---|
| PVPS | Post-vasectomy pain syndrome |
| qds | Four times a day |
| QFit | Quantitative faecal immunochemical test |
| QOF | Quality and Outcomes Framework |
| RA | Rheumatoid arthritis |
| RAST | Radioallergosorbent test |
| RBBB | Right bundle branch block |
| RCGP | Royal College of General Practitioners |
| RCPsych | Royal College of Psychiatry |
| REM | Rapid eye movement |
| RF | Radio frequency |
| Rh | Rhesus |
| RIF | Right iliac fossa |
| RNA | Ribonucleic acid |
| ROM | Range of motion |
| RTA | Road traffic accident |
| RUQ | Right upper quadrant |
| SABA | Short-acting beta-antagonist |
| SADQ | Severity of Alcohol Dependence Questionnaire |
| SADS | Sudden arrhythmic death syndrome |
| SAH | Subarachnoid haemorrhage |
| SALT | Speech and language therapy |
| SARC | Sexual assault referral centre |
| SCBU | Special care baby unit |
| SCC | Squamous cell carcinoma |
| SCOFF | Sick, control, one, fat, food |
| SEA | Significant event analysis |
| SENCO | Special educational needs coordinator |
| SGLT-2i | Sodium-glucose co-transporter-2 |
| SHBG | Sex hormone binding globulin |
| SIDS | Sudden infant death syndrome |
| SLE | Systemic lupus erythematosus |
| SLR | Straight leg raise |
| SMART | Self-Management and Recovery Training |
| SNRI | Serotonin and norepinephrine reuptake inhibitor |
| SOB | Shortness of breath |
| SOL | Space-occupying lesion |
| SR | Slow release |

| Acronym/Initialism | Meaning |
| --- | --- |
| SSRI | Selective serotonin reuptake inhibitor |
| STI | Sexually transmitted infection |
| SVT | Supraventricular tachycardia |
| T4 | Thyroxine |
| TCA | Tricyclic antidepressant |
| tds | Three times a day |
| TENS | Transcutaneous electrical nerve stimulation |
| TFT | Thyroid function test |
| TIA | Transient ischaemic attack |
| TM | Tympanic membrane |
| TMJ | Temporomandibular joint disorder |
| TNA | Trigeminal Neuralgia Association |
| TOP | Termination of pregnancy |
| TSH | Thyroid stimulating hormone |
| TSQ | Trauma Screening Questionnaire |
| tTG | Tissue transglutaminase |
| TTGA | Tissue transglutaminase antibody |
| TURP | Transurethral resection of the prostate |
| TV | Transvaginal |
| U&E | Urea and electrolytes |
| UCC | Urgent care centre |
| UI | Urinary incontinence |
| UMN | Upper motor neurone |
| UPSI | Unprotected sexual intercourse |
| URTI | Upper respiratory tract infection |
| USS | Ultrasound scan |
| UTI | Urinary tract infection |
| UV | Ultraviolet |
| VEGF | Vascular endothelial growth factor |
| VF | Ventricular fibrillation |
| VT | Ventricular tachycardia |
| VTE | Venous thromboembolism |
| VZV | Varicella zoster virus |
| WCC | White cell count |
| WHO | World Health Organization |
| WIC | Walk-in centre |
| WPW | Wolfe-Parkinson-White |
| Y-BOCS | Yale Brown Obsessive Compulsive Scale |

Printed in Great Britain
by Amazon

37474012R00368